Medical Spanish

ma

Incredibly Easy!®

3rd edition

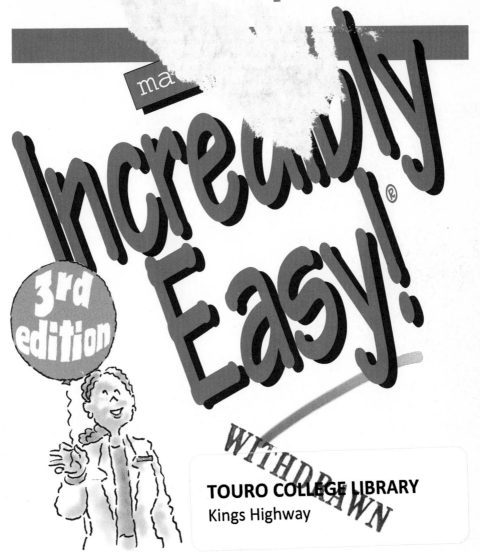

 Wolters Kluwer | Lippincott W
Health

Philadelphia • Baltimore • New York • London
Buenos Aires • Hong Kong • Sydney • Tokyo

D1126812

BP45

Executive Publisher
Judith A. Schilling McCann, RN, MSN

Editorial Director
David Moreau

Clinical Director
Joan M. Robinson, RN, MSN

Art Director
Mary Ludwicki

Editorial Project Manager
Gabrielle Mosquera

Clinical Project Manager
Kate Stout, RN, MSN, CCRN

Translator
Etcetera Language Group, Inc.

Editor
Carol H. Munson

Copy Editors
Kimberly Bilotta (supervisor), Scotti Cohn,
Jeannine Fielding, Amy Furman, Dona Perkins,
Pamela Wingrod

Designer
Georg W. Purvis IV

Illustrator
Bot Roda

Digital Composition Services
Diane Paluba (manager), Joyce Rossi Biletz,
Donald G. Knauss, Donna S. Morris

Associate Manufacturing Manager
Beth J. Welsh

Editorial Assistants
Karen J. Kirk, Linda K. Ruhf, Jeri O'Shea

Indexer
Barbara Hodgson

MSIE3010608

Library of Congress Cataloging-in-Publication Data
Medical Spanish made incredibly easy!. — 3rd ed.
    p. ; cm.
    Includes index.
    Text in English and Spanish.
    1. Spanish language—Conversation and phrase books (for medical personnel) I. Lippincott Williams & Wilkins.
    [DNLM: 1. Medicine—Phrases—English. 2. Medicine—Phrases—Spanish. W 15 M4884 2009]
    PC4120.M3M35 2009
    468.3'42102461—dc22
    ISBN-13: 978-0-7817-8941-7 (alk. paper)
    ISBN-10: 0-7817-8941-9 (alk. paper)   2008010594

7/7/10

Contents

Contributors and consultants

Julie A. Calvery, RN, MS
Instructor
University of Arkansas
Fort Smith

Louise Diehl-Oplinger, RN, MSN, APRN-BC, CCRN, NP-C
Nurse Practitioner–Practice Owner
Lehigh Valley Wellness Center
Phillipsburg, N.J.

Janice D. Hausauer, RN, MS, FNP
Adjunct Assistant Professor
Montana State University College of Nursing
Bozeman

Julia Anne Isen, RN, BS, FNP-C
Family Nurse Practitioner–Primary Care
University of California at San Francisco Medical Center

James F. Murphy, RNC, MS
Educator/Instructor
Rochester (N.Y.) General Hospital, Via Health,
   Department of Education

Rexann G. Pickering, RN, MS, MSN, PhD, CIM, CIP
Administrator, Human Protection
Methodist Healthcare
Memphis

Dana Reeves, RN, MSN
Assistant Professor
University of Arkansas
Fort Smith

Donna Scemons, RN, MSN, MA, CNS, CWOCN, FNP-C
President
Healthcare Systems, Inc.
Castaic, Calif.

Allison J. Terry, RN, MSN, PhD
Director, Center for Nursing
Alabama Board of Nursing
Montgomery

Denise R. York, RNC, MS, MEd, CNS
Professor
Columbus (Ohio) State Community College

Rick Zoucha, APRN,BC, PhD, CTN
Associate Professor
Duquesne University School of Nursing
Pittsburgh

Not another boring foreword

If you're like me, you're too busy to wade through a foreword that uses pretentious terms and umpteen dull paragraphs to get to the point. So let's cut right to the chase! Here's why this book is so terrific:

It will teach you all the important things you need to know about medical Spanish. (And it will leave out all the fluff that wastes your time.)

It will help you remember what you've learned.

It will make you smile as it enhances your knowledge and skills.

Don't believe me? Try these recurring logos on for size:

Pump up your pronunciation—Helps you master difficult words and phrases

Joy's grammar guide—Provides insight into Spanish that helps bring the pieces together

La cultura—Discusses cultural elements that affect health care

La clínica—Offers special phrases relevant to pediatric patients, pregnant patients, and the elderly.

See? I told you! And that's not all. Look for me and my friends in the margins throughout this book. We'll be there to explain key concepts, provide important care reminders, and offer reassurance. Oh, and if you don't mind, we'll be spicing up the pages with a bit of humor along the way, to teach and entertain in a way that no other resource can.

I hope you find this book helpful. Best of luck throughout your career!

Joy

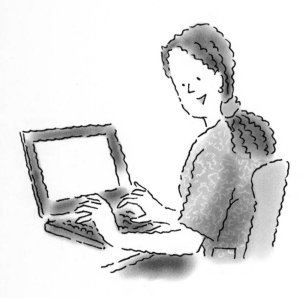

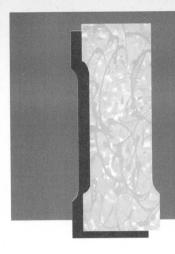

The basics

Pronunciation

Learning basic pronunciation will help you feel more comfortable with the Spanish language. It will also help you communicate more effectively with your Spanish-speaking patients.

You know these

The following letters are common to both Spanish and English. Note that many of the letters (such as B, M, and N) are pronounced similarly in both languages. Others (such as G, H, and R) have a different pronunciation, depending on the situation.

A   Similar to the A in father

B   Similar to the B in abnormal

C   Similar to the English C; it's hard when it precedes A, O, or U (as in escape), soft when it precedes E or I (as in pace)

D   Similar to the D in day when it's at the beginning of a word; similar to the TH in with when in the middle or at the end of a word

E   Similar to the E in sepsis; the Spanish E doesn't end with the glide of the English EY in they

F   Similar to the F in perforate

G   Similar to the G in gout when it precedes A, O, U, or a consonant; similar to the H in hospital when it precedes E or I

H   Always silent

I   Similar to the I in saline and the EE in see

J   Similar to the H in hospital

K   Similar to the K in makeup

L   Similar to the L in sleep

M   Similar to the M in atomic

N   Similar to the N in learning; similar to the M in comma when it precedes B, P, or V; silent when it precedes M

O   Similar to the O in low

P   Similar to the P in spit

Q   Similar to the K in key

R	Similar to the R in ai<u>r</u>y but trilled slightly
S	Similar to the S in ba<u>s</u>ement
T	Similar to the T in s<u>t</u>ent
U	Similar to the U in fl<u>u</u>
V	Same as the Spanish B; similar to the B in sa<u>b</u>le
X	Similar to the X in fle<u>x</u>; similar to the S in me<u>ss</u>age when it precedes a consonant
Y	Similar to the Y in bo<u>y</u>friend; similar to EE in s<u>ee</u> when it's used to denote the word *and*
Z	Similar to the C in <u>c</u>ity or pre<u>c</u>ede

(See *Shorten that vowel.*)

Pump up your pronunciation

Shorten that vowel

Spanish vowels are short and tense, almost clipped. To fine-tune your pronunciation, don't stretch out vowels. For example, *bebé* (baby) is pronounced beh-<u>beh</u>, not bay-bay.

Do you know these?

The following letters are unique to the Spanish alphabet.

CH	Similar to the CH in <u>ch</u>ild
LL	Similar to the YE in <u>y</u>ellow
Ñ	Similar to the NI in on<u>i</u>on
RR	Trilled longer than single R; note that spelling a word with one R or two Rs changes the meaning of the word as in *pero* (but) and *perro* (dog), *caro* (expensive) and *carro* (wagon, cart, car), and *para* (for) and *parra* (grapevine)

Get your accent here

An accent mark indicates that a syllable receives a special stress. For example, *mamá* (mom) is pronounced mah-<u>mah</u>. If no accent mark appears, then the emphasis follows these basic rules of pronunciation.

If a word ends in a vowel, N, or S, emphasis usually falls on the next-to-last syllable—for example:
- <u>fu</u>ma
- nece<u>si</u>ta
- be<u>bi</u>das
- cer<u>ve</u>za.

If a word ends in a consonant other than N or S, stress usually falls on the last syllable—for example:
- us<u>ted</u>
- doc<u>tor</u>
- do<u>lor</u>
- intesti<u>nal</u>.

When one-syllable words have accents, it's to distinguish them from other words that sound alike—for example:
- <u>él</u> (he); <u>el</u> (the)
- <u>sí</u> (yes); <u>si</u> (if)
- <u>tú</u> (you, familiar form); <u>tu</u> (your).

Grammar

Learning grammar basics will help you remember important phrases. It will also help you communicate more effectively with your Spanish-speaking patients.

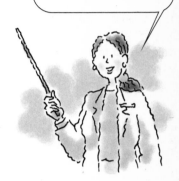

Most nouns ending with A are feminine, but medical words that end in MA, such as *papiloma* and *carcinoma*, are masculine.

Person, place, or thing

Nouns in Spanish are either masculine or feminine. Most nouns ending in O or medical words ending in MA are masculine. Most nouns ending in A are feminine.

Adjectives and nouns ending in E can be either masculine or feminine—their gender is determined by the preceding noun, pronoun, or article—for example:
- *el presidente*
- *la presidente*.

Exceptions to this rule include:
- *mano*, which is always feminine
- *día*, *herbicida*, *insecticida*, *pesticida*, *raticida*, *espermaticida*, and *vermicida*, which are always masculine.

More than one?

A Spanish word is made plural by adding an S or ES to the end:
- Add an S when the word ends in an unaccented vowel: *perro – perros*.
- Add an ES when the word ends in a consonant, Y, or accented vowel: *dolor – dolores*.

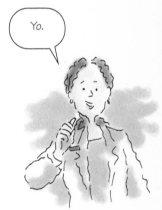

Yo.

Little words

Pronouns in Spanish are either masculine or feminine, singular or plural. The *you* pronoun has two forms: familiar and formal.

Singular forms

I	yo
you	tú (familiar, singular)
	usted (formal, singular); abbreviated Ud. or Vd.
he	él
she	ella

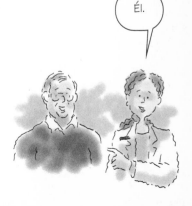

Él.

Plural forms

we	nosotros (masculine)
we	nosotras (feminine)
you	vosotros (masculine familiar)
you	vosotras (feminine familiar)
you	ustedes (formal, plural); abbreviated Uds. or Vds.
they	ellos (masculine, plural)
they	ellas (feminine, plural)

More little words

The articles *the*, *a*, and *an* and the adjectives *this*, *that*, *these*, and *those* can be either masculine or feminine depending on the gender of the noun they modify. *That* and *those* also have different forms to denote distance. (See *Keeping up with contractions*.)

the	el (masculine, singular)
	la (feminine, singular)
	los (masculine, plural)
	las (feminine, plural)
a, an	un (masculine, singular)
	una (feminine, singular)
some	unos (masculine, plural)
	unas (feminine, plural)
this	este (masculine)
	esta (feminine)
that (near)	ese (masculine)
	esa (feminine)
that (far)	aquel (masculine)
	aquella (feminine)
these	estos (masculine)
	estas (feminine)
those (near)	esos (masculine)
	esas (feminine)
those (far)	aquellos (masculine)
	aquellas (feminine)

Mine or yours?

Spanish possessives are masculine or feminine and singular or plural depending on the noun they precede. To make a possessive plural, just add an S to the end of the singular form. *Your* also has two forms: familiar and formal.

Beginnings and endings

Special prefixes and suffixes may be added to Spanish words to denote certain ideas.
• To denote the opposite meaning of the original word, add *des-* to the beginning of the word.
• To denote the diminutive, such as slight or less, use *-ito, -ita, -illo, -illa,* or *-ete.*
• To denote the augmentative, such as very, use *-ísimo* or *-ísima.*
• To make an adverb, add *-mente* to the feminine form of the adjective.
• To indicate the English suffix *-ty* (as in *quantity*), add *-dad* to the end of most Spanish words. (See *T or D?*)
• To denote the location where something is made or sold, add *-ería* to the end of the word.
• To denote the person who makes or sells the object, add *-ero* or *-era* to the end of the word.

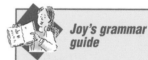

Joy's grammar guide

T or D?

When a Spanish word comes from a verb ending in *-tar, -ter,* or *-tir,* the suffix used is *-tad.* For example, the English word *liberty* comes from the verb *liberate.* The Spanish word for *liberate* is *libertar* (which ends in *-tar*). Hence, to change *liberate* to *liberty* in Spanish, use the suffix *-tad: libertad.*

Joy's grammar guide

Keeping up with contractions

In English, we can choose to form a contraction or not. We can say *I'm happy* or *I am happy*—either way is acceptable. However, in Spanish, when the article *el* (the, masculine singular) is preceded by the prepositions *a* (to, at) or *de* (of, from, about), you must form a contraction.

Al

When you want to say *to the* in Spanish and *the* is *el* (masculine singular), use *al:*

I am going to the doctor this afternoon.   Voy <u>al</u> doctor esta tarde.

Here, *to the doctor* would be *a* (to) *el* (the, masculine singular) *doctor,* so *a* and *el* are contracted together to form *al.*

Del

The same thing happens when you want to use the preposition *de* with *el*—no matter what meaning of *de* you use (of, from, about) use *del:*

The people of the State of New York   El pueblo del Estado de Nueva York

Watch out for him

Be careful not to confuse the article *el* (the) with the pronoun *él* (he, him). *Él* doesn't contract with *a* or *de*—for example:

The book belongs to him.   El libro le pertenece a él.
The book is his.   El libro es de él.

Think you've got a handle on Spanish basics? Try the practice exercises on the next page.

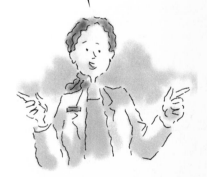

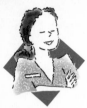

Practice makes perfecto

1. Joy sprained her ankle while skiing and needs crutches for a few days. Help Joy talk about her crutches in Spanish. How would she say "a crutch"? How would she say "the crutches"?

_____ muleta
_____ muletas

_____

_____

_____

_____

2. Joy found a stethoscope in the clinic. Help Joy figure out the stethoscope's owner.

¿_____ estetoscopio?

¿_____ estetoscopio?
¿_____ estetoscopio?

_____

_____

_____

_____

3. Joy is gathering medical supplies. Help Joy express that she has more than one of each item.

El champú
Los _____

La toalla
Las _____

_____

_____

_____

_____

Answer key

1. A crutch
Una muleta
The crutches
Las muletas
2. My stethoscope
¿Mi estetoscopio?
Your stethoscope
¿Su estetoscopio?
Your stethoscope
¿Su estetoscopio?
3. The shampoo; The shampoos
El champú; Los champús
The towel; The towels
La toalla; Las toallas

2 Everyday words and phrases

Fast fact

- To say "Hello, my name is ___" to your patient, say *Hola, me llamo ___.*
- To greet your patient and ask how he's feeling, say *Buenos días. ¿Cómo se siente Ud.?*
- Nurse in Spanish is *enfermera* (feminine) or *enfermero* (masculine). Doctor is *doctora* (feminine) or *doctor* (masculine).

Getting started

If you can greet your patient in his native language when you walk into his room, you'll make him feel more at ease. Here are some phrases that you can use to converse with your patient as well as some phrases to help you learn basic information.

Meet and greet

Hello.	¡Hola!
Good morning.	Buenos días.
Good afternoon.	Buenas tardes.
Good evening.	Buenas noches.
Come in please.	Pase Ud. por favor.
My name is _____. I am your _____. – nurse – doctor (See pages 18 and 19 for more options.)	Me llamo _____. Soy su _____. – enfermera(o) – doctor(a)
Who's the patient?	¿Quién es el (la) paciente?
What's your name?	¿Cómo se llama Ud.?
It's nice to meet you.	Mucho gusto en conocerle.
How are you? (See *First impressions*, page 8.)	¿Cómo está Ud.?

The basics

How are you feeling?	¿Cómo se siente Ud.?
What time is it?	¿Qué hora es?
What day is it?	¿Qué día es hoy?
What's the date?	¿A qué fecha estamos?
Where are you?	¿Dónde está Ud.?

How old are you?	¿Cuántos años tiene Ud.?
Did you come alone?	¿Vino Ud. solo(a)?
Who brought you?	¿Quién lo (la) trajo?
Where were you born?	¿Dónde nació Ud.?
Where do you live?	¿Dónde vive Ud.?
What's your address?	¿Cuál es su dirección?

First impressions

Want to greet your patient in Spanish? Terrific! To help make a good first impression, review your pronunciation. Remember that H is silent and accent marks indicate where to place a stress.

If you want to say "Hello! Good morning," here's how: *¡Hola! Buenos días.*—<u>Oh</u>-lah! <u>Bweh</u>-nohs <u>dee</u>-ahs.

Family matters

Do you live alone?	¿Vive Ud. solo(a)?
Who lives with you?	¿Quién vive con Ud.?
– Your parents?	– ¿Sus padres?
– Your spouse?	– ¿Su esposo(a)?
– Your children?	– ¿Sus hijos?
Your son?	¿Su hijo?
Your daughter?	¿Su hija?
Your grandchildren?	¿Sus nietos?
– Your mother?	– ¿Su madre?
– Your father?	– ¿Su padre?
– Your uncle?	– ¿Su tío?
– Your aunt?	– ¿Su tía?
– Your grandfather?	– ¿Su abuelo?
– Your grandmother?	– ¿Su abuela?
– Your cousin?	– ¿Su primo(a)?
– Your friend?	– ¿Su amigo(a)?
– Your niece?	– ¿Su sobrina?
– Your nephew?	– ¿Su sobrino?
Are you _____?	¿Es Ud. _____?
– single	– soltero(a)
– married	– casado(a)
– divorced	– divorciado(a)
– widowed	– viudo(a)
– separated	– separado(a)
Do you have any children?	¿Tiene Ud. hijos?
– How many?	– ¿Cuántos?

School, work...

Did you go to school?	¿Asistió Ud. a la escuela?
– How many grades did you complete?	– ¿Cuántos años completó Ud.?
– Did you go to college?	– ¿Hizo Ud. estudios universitarios?
Do you work outside the home?	¿Trabaja Ud. fuera de casa?
– What type of work do you do?	– ¿Qué tipo de trabajo hace?
Accountant?	¿Contador(a)?
Architect?	¿Arquitecto(a)?
Banker?	¿Banquero(a)?

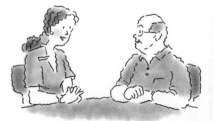

Hello! My name is Joy.

¡Hola! Me llamo Joy.

Bus driver?	¿Conductor(a) de autobuses?
Businessperson?	¿Persona de negocios?
Computer operator?	¿Operador(a) de computadoras?
Designer?	¿Diseñador(a)?
Doctor?	¿Doctor(a)?
Engineer?	¿Ingeniero(a)?
Factory worker?	¿Obrero(a) en una fábrica?
Farmer?	¿Campesino(a)?
Lawyer?	¿Abogado(a)?
Mechanic?	¿Mecánico(a)?
Salesperson?	¿Vendedor(a)? *or* ¿Dependiente?
Secretary?	¿Secretario(a)?
Student?	¿Estudiante?
Taxi driver?	¿Chofer de taxi?
Teacher?	¿Maestro(a)?
Truck driver?	¿Camionero(a)?
Waiter?	¿Camarero?
Waitress?	¿Camarera?
Another type of work?	¿Otro tipo de trabajo?

Where do you work? ¿Dónde trabaja Ud.?

...and play

Do you have any hobbies? ¿Tiene Ud. pasatiempos favoritos?
– Movies? – ¿Cine?
– Music? – ¿Música?
– Painting? – ¿Arte?
– Photography? – ¿Fotografía?
– Reading? – ¿Leer?
– Sewing? – ¿Coser?
– Sports? – ¿Deportes?
  Baseball? ¿Béisbol?
  Basketball? ¿Baloncesto?
  Football? ¿Fútbol americano?
  Golf? ¿Golf?
  Hockey? ¿Hockey?
  Running? ¿Correr?
  Soccer? ¿Fútbol?
  Tennis? ¿Tenis?
– Theater? – ¿Teatro?

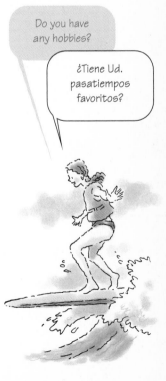

Do you have any hobbies?

¿Tiene Ud. pasatiempos favoritos?

Back to basics

Sometimes it isn't necessary to translate an entire sentence. Instead, you may be able to use one key word or phrase to convey information to your patient.

Yes, no, maybe

please	por favor
thank you	gracias
yes	sí
no	no
maybe	quizás *or* tal vez
sometimes	a veces
never	nunca
always	siempre
date	fecha
signature	firma
good-bye	hasta luego *or* adiós

> Your Spanish is improving!

> ¡Gracias!

Monday, Tuesday, happy days

Monday	lunes
Tuesday	martes
Wednesday	miércoles
Thursday	jueves
Friday	viernes
Saturday	sábado
Sunday	domingo

> Today is Monday, the 5th day of February.

> Hoy es lunes, cinco de febrero.

Turning the calendar

January	enero
February	febrero
March	marzo
April	abril
May	mayo
June	junio

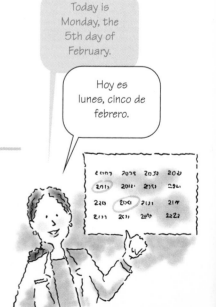

July	julio
August	agosto
September	septiembre
October	octubre
November	noviembre
December	diciembre

Season greetings

spring	la primavera
summer	el verano
fall	el otoño
winter	el invierno

Small numbers

1	uno
2	dos
3	tres
4	cuatro
5	cinco
6	seis
7	siete
8	ocho
9	nueve
10	diez
11	once
12	doce
13	trece
14	catorce
15	quince
16	dieciséis
17	diecisiete
18	dieciocho
19	diecinueve
20	veinte

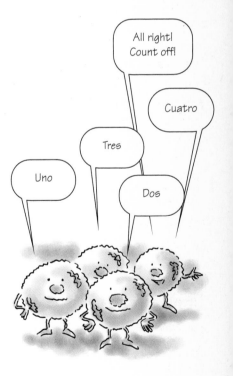

Big numbers

30	treinta
40	cuarenta
50	cincuenta
60	sesenta
70	setenta
80	ochenta
90	noventa
100	cien
1,000	mil
10,000	diez mil
100,000	cien mil
100,000,000	cien millones

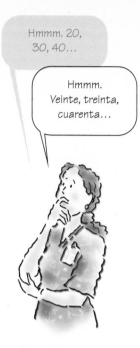

Hmmm. 20, 30, 40…

Hmmm. Veinte, treinta, cuarenta…

Who's on primero?

first	primero(a)
second	segundo(a), dos (in dates)
third	tercero(a), tres (in dates)
fourth	cuarto(a), cuatro (in dates)
fifth	quinto(a), cinco (in dates)
sixth	sexto(a), seis (in dates)
seventh	séptimo(a), siete (in dates)
eighth	octavo(a), ocho (in dates)
ninth	noveno(a), nueve (in dates)
tenth	décimo, diez (in dates)
eleventh	onceavo, once (in dates)
twelfth	doceavo, doce (in dates)
thirteenth	treceavo, trece (in dates)

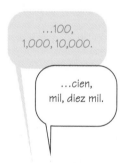

…100, 1,000, 10,000.

…cien, mil, diez mil.

Time is relative

second	segundo
minute	minuto
15 minutes	15 minutos
30 minutes	30 minutos

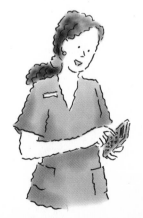

Joy's grammar guide

Morning, afternoon, or night?

Phrases like *por la mañana* (in the morning) or *por la noche* (in the evening) can be very useful. They can help you indicate when medication should be taken or when a patient should return for an appointment.

Preposition preference

Note, however, that some Spanish speakers use the preposition *en* for these phrases, not *por:*

• in the morning—en la mañana
• in the afternoon—en la tarde
• in the evening—en la noche.

hour	hora
in the morning	por la mañana
at noon	al mediodía
in the afternoon	por la tarde
in the evening	por la noche
at bedtime	a la hora de acostarse
at midnight (See *Morning, afternoon, or night?*)	a medianoche

Mealtime

breakfast	el desayuno
lunch	el almuerzo
midafternoon snack	la merienda
dinner	la cena
bedtime snack	el bocadillo a la hora de acostarse

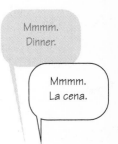

Mmmm.
Dinner.

Mmmm.
La cena.

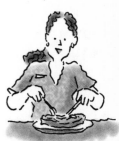

Not just black and white

black	negro
blue	azul
brown	café
gray	gris
green	verde
orange	anaranjado *or* color naranja
pink	rosa *or* rosado

Common regionalisms for "brown" include *marrón, pardo, carmelita,* and *castaño*.

purple	morado *or* violeta
red	rojo
white	blanco
yellow	amarillo

Opposites attract

alive/dead	vivo/muerto
before/after	antes/después
better/worse	mejor/peor
dark/light	oscuro/claro
fat/thin	gordo/delgado
flat/raised	plano/en relieve
healthy/sick	saludable/enfermo
heavy/light	pesado/ligero
high/low	alto/bajo
hot/cold	caliente/frío
large/small	grande/pequeño
long/short	largo/corto
loud/soft	fuerte/suave
many/few	muchos/pocos
on/off	encendido/apagado
open/closed	abierto/cerrado
painful/painless	doloroso/indoloro

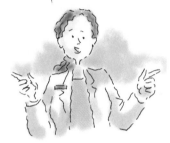

Learn opposites together and then you know two words instead of just one.

When a Spanish-speaking patient says the word *painless,* you may hear the phrase *sin dolor* instead of *indoloro.*

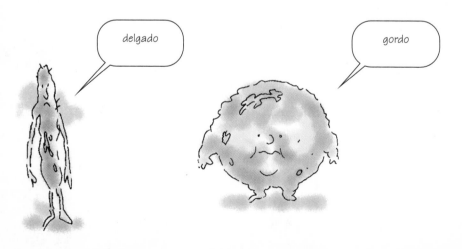

delgado

gordo

regular/irregular	regular/irregular
smooth/rough	liso/áspero
soft/hard	blando/duro
sweet/sour	dulce/agrio
start/stop	arrancar/detener
tall/short	alto/bajo
up/down	arriba/abajo
warm/cool	cálido/fresco
weak/strong	débil/fuerte
wet/dry	mojado/seco

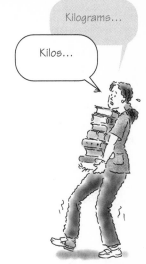

Measuring up

centimeter	centímetro
cup	taza
depth	profundidad
foot	pie
gram	gramo
height	altura
inch	pulgada
kilogram	kilo
length	longitud
liter	litro
meter	metro
milligram	miligramo
ounce	onza
pint	pinta
pound	libra
quart	cuarto de galón
tablespoon	cucharada
teaspoon	cucharadita
volume	volumen
weight	peso
width	ancho or anchura
yard	yarda

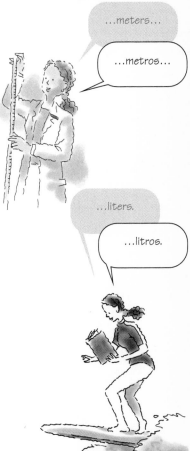

Soup, not soap

Learning cognates (words that sound like their equivalent in another language) can help you develop a vocabulary in Spanish. For example, *litro* sounds very similar to its English equivalent, *liter*. Beware, however, of false cognates—words that sound similar but have very different meanings.

What you hear isn't what you get

Sopa is an example of a false cognate. *Sopa* may sound like *soap,* but it isn't. *Sopa* means *soup,* and *jabón* means *soap.* If your patient asks for *sopa,* he's feeling hungry, not dirty.

Everyday items

blanket	manta or frazada
brush	cepillo
comb	peine
deodorant	desodorante
gown	bata
keys	llaves
lotion	loción
mouthwash	enjuague para la boca
pillow	almohada
pillowcase	funda de almohada
purse	monedero
razor	navaja de afeitar
robe	bata
sanitary napkin	toalla sanitaria
shampoo	champú
shaving cream	crema de afeitar
sheet	sábana
slippers	pantuflas/chanclas
soap (See *Soup, not soap.*)	jabón
tampon	tampón
toothbrush	cepillo de dientes
toothpaste	pasta de dientes
towel	toalla
wallet	monedero
washcloth	paño para lavarse la cara o el cuerpo
water	agua

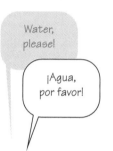

Water, please!

¡Agua, por favor!

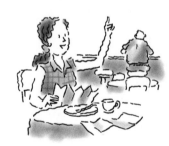

Health care personnel

This list of key health care personnel will help you identify yourself and other caregivers to your patient.

Know your nurses (and others)

admissions clerk	empleado(a) de ingresos
dental hygienist	higienista dental
dentist	dentista
dietitian	nutricionista
doctor	doctor(a)
electrician	electricista
housekeeper	ama de llaves
I.V. nurse	enfermera(o) especialista en procedimientos intravenosos
janitor	empleado(a) de limpieza or conserje
laboratory technician	ayudante de laboratorio
medical assistant	ayudante de medicina
medical student	estudiante de medicina
medical technician	técnico(a) de medicina
medical transcriptionist	persona que transcribe documentos médicos
nurse practitioner	enfermera(o) general
nurse's aid	asistente de enfermera(o)
nursing student	estudiante de enfermería
nutritionist	nutricionista
occupational therapist	terapeuta ocupacional
physical therapist	fisioterapeuta
physician's assistant	asistente del doctor
practical nurse	enfermera(o) auxiliar
radiology technician	radiólogo(a)
registered nurse	enfermera(o) certificada(o)
respiratory therapist	terapeuta de respiración
social worker	trabajador(a) social
volunteer	voluntario(a)

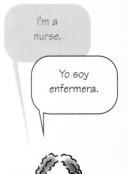

I'm a nurse.

Yo soy enfermera.

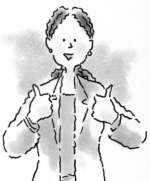

Joy's grammar guide

A doctor by any other name

Knowing the Spanish names for different types of doctors isn't as hard as it may look. Here are some hints to help you.

Sounds similar

The Spanish words for most types of specialists sound very similar to their English counterparts. For example, orthopedist is *ortopedista* (or-toh-peh-<u>dee</u>-sta) and pediatrician is *pediatra* (peh-dee-<u>ah</u>-tra). If you want to mention a specialist to your Spanish-speaking patient, start by thinking of the English word—and you might find the Spanish word very quickly.

Endings, endings

Note also that the English suffix *-ologist* typically corresponds to the Spanish suffix *-ólogo*. Here are some examples:

- cardiologist—cardiólogo
- dermatologist—dermatólogo
- gynecologist—ginecólogo
- neurologist—neurólogo.

Dr. Joe and Dr. Jane

Lastly, remember that a male doctor is *un doctor,* but a female doctor is *una doctora.*

Going down the doctor list

anesthesiologist
  A doctor who puts you to sleep or numbs an area in preparation for surgery or a procedure

anestesista *or* anestesiólogo
  Médico que lo duerme o que adormece el área como preparación para una cirugía o un procedimiento

cardiologist
  A doctor who diagnoses and treats heart disease

cardiólogo
  Médico que efectúa el diagnóstico y tratamiento de enfermedades del corazón

dermatologist
  A doctor who diagnoses and treats skin disorders

dermatólogo
  Médico que efectúa el diagnóstico y tratamiento de trastornos de la piel

endocrinologist
  A doctor who diagnoses and treats problems with the endocrine glands

endocrinólogo
  Médico que efectúa el diagnóstico y tratamiento de problemas en las glándulas endocrinas

gastroenterologist
  A doctor who diagnoses and treats problems with the stomach or intestines

gastroenterólogo
  Médico que efectúa el diagnóstico y tratamiento de problemas en el estómago o intestinos

gynecologist
  A doctor who diagnoses and treats problems with the female genital organs

ginecólogo
  Médico que efectúa el diagnóstico y tratamiento de problemas en los órganos genitales femeninos

hematologist
A doctor who diagnoses and treats problems with the blood

internist
A doctor who diagnoses and treats medical problems

nephrologist
A doctor who diagnoses and treats problems with the kidneys

neurologist
A doctor who diagnoses and treats problems with the brain and nerves

obstetrician
A doctor who delivers babies

oncologist
A doctor who diagnoses and treats cancer

ophthalmologist
A doctor who diagnoses and treats problems with the eyes

orthopedist
A doctor who diagnoses and treats broken bones and joint problems

otolaryngologist
A doctor who diagnoses and treats problems with the ears, nose, and throat

pediatrician
A doctor who takes care of children

pulmonologist
A doctor who diagnoses and treats problems with the lungs

psychiatrist
A doctor who diagnoses and treats problems of mental illness

surgeon
A doctor who performs operations
(See *A doctor by any other name* and *Psst…don't pronounce the P.*)

hematólogo
Médico que efectúa el diagnóstico y tratamiento de problemas en la sangre

internista
Médico que efectúa el diagnóstico y tratamiento de problemas médicos

nefrólogo
Médico que efectúa el diagnóstico y tratamiento de problemas en los riñónes

neurólogo
Médico que efectúa el diagnóstico y tratamiento de problemas en el cerebro y los nervios

obstetra
Médico que efectúa partos

oncólogo
Médico que efectúa el diagnóstico y tratamiento del cáncer

oftalmólogo
Médico que efectúa el diagnóstico y tratamiento de problemas en los ojos

traumatólogo(a)
Médico que efectúa el diagnóstico y tratamiento de huesos fracturados

otorrinonaringólogo
Médico que efectúa el diagnóstico y tratamiento de problemas en la nariz, garganta, y oídos

pediatra
Médico que trata a los niños

neumonólogo
Médico que efectúa el diagnóstico y tratamiento de problemas en los pulmones

psiquiatra
Médico que efectúa el diagnóstico y tratamiento de problemas de enfermedad mental

cirujano
Médico que realiza operaciones

Pump up your pronunciation

Psst…don't pronounce the P

The P in psychologist and psychiatrist is silent in English and in Spanish. Here is a quick guide:
- psicólogo (see-<u>coh</u>-loh-goh)
- psiquiatra (see-kee-<u>ah</u>-trah).

A psychiatrist helps people who have mental illness.

Un psiquiatra ayuda apersonas con enfermedades mentales.

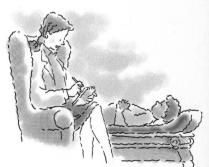

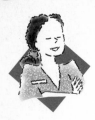

Practice makes perfecto

1. Help Joy greet her patient. Translate what she says into Spanish. Hint: Remember to use *Ud.* (formal you), not *tú* (familiar you).

_____

_____

_____

> How are you feeling?

2. Joy is trying to learn more about her patient. What does Joy want to know? How does her patient respond? Hint: *Cuántos* is used to ask about quantities and age.

_____

_____

_____

> ¿Cuántos años tiene Ud.?

> Cincuenta.

> Cepillo, jabón y pasta de dientes, por favor.

3. A patient is asking Joy for some items for his room. Help Joy understand what the patient wants. Hint: The first item is a brush.

_____

_____

_____

> ¿Quién vive con Ud.?

> Mi madre, mi padre, y mi abuela.

4. Joy is completing a health history for her patient. What's Joy asking? What's the patient's answer? Hint: *Abuela* means grandmother.

_____

_____

_____

Answer key

1. How are you feeling?
¿Cómo se siente Ud.?
2. ¿Cuántos años tiene Ud.?
How old are you?
Cincuenta.
Fifty.
3. Cepillo, jabón, y pasta de dientes, por favor.
Brush, soap, and toothpaste, please.
4. ¿Quién vive con Ud.?
Who lives with you?
Mi madre, mi padre, y mi abuela.
My mother, my father, and my grandmother.

3 Signs and symptoms

Fast fact

- Begin with the phrase *¿Tiene Ud. ___?* (Do you have ___?) or *¿Ha tenido Ud. alguna vez ___?* (Have you ever had ___?).
- To ask your patient about pain in a particular area, use the phrase *dolor de* (pain of), followed by the Spanish word for the body part. (See the illustration on page 22 for a list of major body parts in Spanish.)

Assessing signs and symptoms

Many times during your assessment and history taking, you'll ask your patient about specific signs and symptoms that will alert you to subtle indicators of disease. This easy guide, complete with short phrases in Spanish, will help you understand your patient's concerns and effectively identify his signs and symptoms.

In addition, knowing the names of major body parts in Spanish will help you pinpoint your patient's concerns. (See *The body—El cuerpo*, page 22.)

Rashes, itching, irritation

Do you have or have you ever had _____?	¿Tiene Ud. o ha tenido Ud. alguna vez _____?
– bleeding under the skin	– hemorragia debajo de la piel
– butterfly rash	– erupción en forma de mariposa
– change in skin color	– cambio en color de la piel
– hives	– erupción con pus
– increasing hair loss	– aumento de pérdida de cabello
– itching	– picazón
– papular rash (small, raised bumps)	– erupción papular (ronchas pequeñas)
– rash with filled bubbles	– prurito (comezón)
– red skin or irritation	– enrojecimiento o irritación de la piel
– skin that's:	– piel que está:
scaly	escamosa
oily	aceitosa
dry	seca
– sores	– llagas
– spots on the hands or legs (black, brown, purple, red)	– manchas en las manos o las piernas (negras, cafés, moradas, rojas)
– thin, purple streaks on the skin	– finas líneas púrpuras en la piel

From the neck up

Do you have or have you ever had _____?	¿Tiene Ud. o ha tenido Ud. alguna vez _____?
– difficulty speaking	– dificultad al hablar

The body
El cuerpo

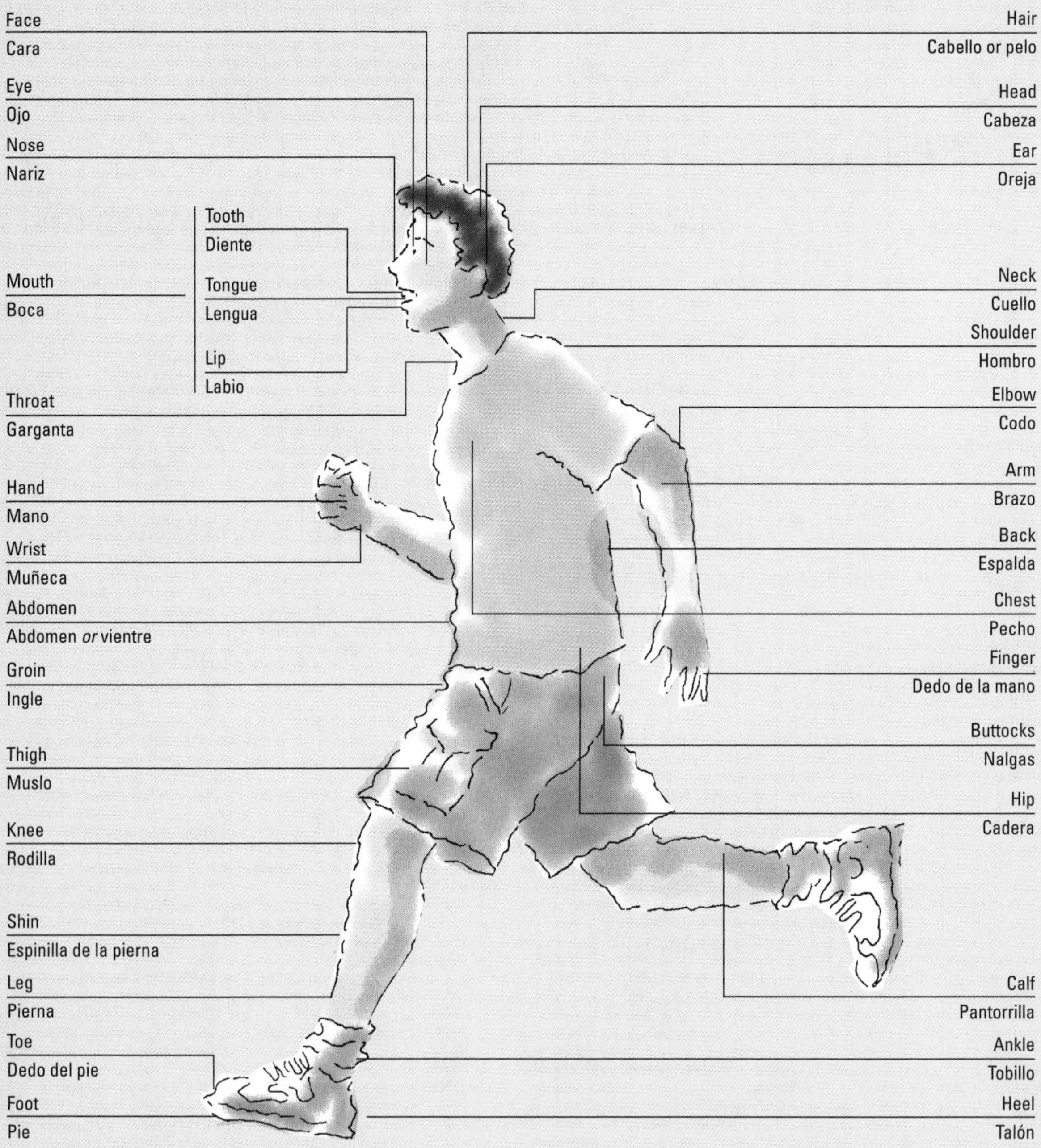

Face
Cara

Eye
Ojo

Nose
Nariz

Tooth
Diente

Mouth
Boca

Tongue
Lengua

Lip
Labio

Throat
Garganta

Hand
Mano

Wrist
Muñeca

Abdomen
Abdomen *or* vientre

Groin
Ingle

Thigh
Muslo

Knee
Rodilla

Shin
Espinilla de la pierna

Leg
Pierna

Toe
Dedo del pie

Foot
Pie

Hair
Cabello or pelo

Head
Cabeza

Ear
Oreja

Neck
Cuello

Shoulder
Hombro

Elbow
Codo

Arm
Brazo

Back
Espalda

Chest
Pecho

Finger
Dedo de la mano

Buttocks
Nalgas

Hip
Cadera

Calf
Pantorrilla

Ankle
Tobillo

Heel
Talón

– decreased salivation

– drooping mouth
– facial numbness
– facial pain
– gum swelling or bleeding
– hoarseness
– increased salivation
– jaw clicking
– jaw locking
– jaw pain
– mouth lesions
– nasal drainage
– nosebleeds
– postnasal drip
– sinus pain
– swelling of:
    the face
    the jaw
    the mouth
    the nose
– throat pain or sore throat
– toothache
(See *Nosing in.*)

– salivación (secreción de saliva) reducida
– caída de la boca
– adormecimiento facial
– dolor facial
– hinchazón o sangrado de las encías
– ronquera
– aumento de salivación
– clic (ruido breve) de la mandíbula
– trismo
– dolor de mandíbula
– lesiones en la boca
– drenaje nasal
– hemorragia por la nariz
– goteo posnasal (detrás de la nariz)
– dolor sinusal
– hinchazón de:
    la cara
    la mandíbula
    la boca
    la nariz
– dolor de garganta
– dolor de muela

Nosing in

If your patient complains of nasal drainage, you may want to know more to determine the exact nature of the patient's symptoms.

The specifics

Here are some phrases to help you:

• Is your nasal discharge___?
  – yellow
  – green
  – bloody
  – white
  – gray
  – clear
• ¿Es su rinorrea_____?
  – amarillo
  – erde
  – con sangre
  – blanco
  – gris
  – sin color/incolora

The eyes (and ears) have it

Do you have or have you ever had _____?

– abnormal eye movements
– area of partial or complete blindness
– blindness in one eye
– bulging of the eyes
– double vision
– drainage from the ear
– earache
– eye drainage
– eye pain
– eye watering or redness
– halo vision
– hearing loss
– involuntary eye movement
– light flashes
– night blindness
– ringing or buzzing in the ears
– sensitivity to light
– sunken eyes
– swelling of the eyes
– tunnel vision
– vision loss
– visual blurring

Tiene Ud. o ha tenido Ud. alguna vez_____?

– movimientos anormales del ojo
– área de ceguera parcial o total
– ceguera en unojo
– protrusión anormal de los ojos
– visión doble
– derrame por el oído
– dolor de oído
– drenaje ocular
– dolor de ojo
– enrojecimento de los ojos
– visión de halo
– sordera
– movimiento ocular involuntario
– destellos de luz
– ceguera nocturna
– zumido en los oídos
– intolerancia visual a la luz
– hundimiento anormal de los ojos
– hinchazón de los ojos
– visión en túnel
– pérdida de visión
– visión borrosa

Joy's grammar guide

Pain locator

When assessing a patient's signs and symptoms, you may want to ask about pain in a particular part of the body. You can do so by using the phrase *dolor de* (+ the body part). For example, if you want to inquire about chest pain, you ask *¿Tiene Ud. dolor de pecho?* If you want to ask a patient if he has a headache, ask *¿Tiene Ud. dolor de cabeza?*

A plethora of pain
Here are some other common examples:

– jaw pain	– dolor de mandíbula
– eye pain	– dolor de ojo
– toothache	– dolor de muela
– earache	– dolor de oído
– abdominal pain	– dolor abdominal
– breast pain	– dolor en los senos
– chest pain	– dolor de pecho
– flank pain	– dolor en el costado
– arm pain	– dolor de brazo
– back pain.	– dolor de espalda.

– visual floaters	– visión con manchas móviles
(See *Pain locator.*)	

Looking at the lungs

Do you have or have you ever had_____?	Tiene Ud. o ha tenido Ud. alguna vez_____?
– blue discoloration of skin	– coloración azulada de la piel
– clubbing of the fingers or toes	– hinchazón en los dedos del pie o de la mano
– cough	– tos
barking	tos fuerte
nonproductive	seca
productive	productive/con secreción
– coughing up blood	– expectoración con sangre
– deep breathing	– respiración rigida
– difficulty breathing	– dificultad respiratoria
– difficulty breathing when lying down	– dificultad al respirar acostado(a)
– fast breathing	– respiración muy rápida
– nasal flaring	– enrojecmiento de la nariz
– wheezing	– respiración jadeante

Hearing about the heart

Do you have or have you ever had _____?
- chest pain
- cramping leg pain
- fast heart rate
- heart attack
- heart flutters
- high blood pressure
- pale skin
- red lesions on the palms of hands and soles of feet
- slow heart rate
- sudden shortness of breath at night

- tender, red or purple lesions on the palms, soles, finger pads, and toes

Tiene Ud. o ha tenido Ud. alguna vez_____?
- dolor de pecho (tórax)
- calambre en la pierna
- ritmo cardiaco acelerado
- ataque cardiaco
- pulsación rápida del corazón
- hipertensión
- palidez
- manchas rojas en la palma de la mano y planta del pie
- lentitud anormal del pulso
- respiración entre cortada repentina por la noche

- lesiones sensibles, rojas, o morades en la palma de la mano, yemas de los dedos de la mano y del pie, y planta del pie

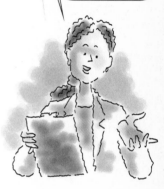

Do you have palpitations? Fast heart rate? Chest pain?

¿Tiene Ud. palpitaciones? ¿Ritmo cardiaco acelerado? ¿Dolor de pecho?

GI info

Do you have or have you ever had _____?
- abdominal distention
- abdominal pain
- abdominal rigidity
- bad breath
- belching
- black, tarry stools
- bloody stools
- breath with fecal odor
- clay-colored stools
- constipation
- diarrhea
- difficulty swallowing
- excessive appetite
- fecal incontinence
- gas
- heartburn
- hiccups
- indigestion
- increased salivation
- loss of appetite
- musty sweet breath odor
- nausea
- rectal bleeding
- rectal pain
- stomach growling

Tiene Ud. o ha tenido Ud. alguna vez_____?
- distensión abdominal
- dolor abdominal
- rigidez abdominal
- mal aliento
- eructo
- heces negras y alquitranadas
- defacación con sangre
- aliento con olor a defacación
- defacación con color de arcilla
- estreñimiento
- diarrea
- dificultad para tragar
- apetito excesivo
- incontinencia fecal
- flatulencia
- indigestión
- hipo
- indigestión
- aumento de saliva
- pérdida del apetito
- olor dulzón rancio del aliento
- náuseas
- sangrado rectal
- dolor rectal
- gruñido del estómago

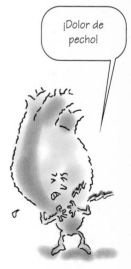

¡Dolor de pecho!

– vomiting	– vómitos
– vomiting of blood	– vómitos con sangre
– yellow skin	– piel amarilla

Checking the breast and genitourinary system

Do you have or have you ever had
_____?

Tiene Ud. o ha tenido Ud. alguna
vez_____?

– abnormally light or infrequent menstruation	– menstruación insualmente liviana o poco frecuente
– bladder distention	– distensión de la vejiga
– blood in the urine	– sangre en la orina
– breast dimpling	– pequeoños hoyuelos en los senos
– breast enlargement	– desarrollo excessivo de los senos
– breast nodules	– nódulos en los senos
– breast pain	– dolor en los senos
– breast ulcers	– úlcera en los senos
– decreased urine	– disminició de orina
– genital lesions	– lesiones genitales
– impotence (no erection)	– impotencia
– increased urination	– aumento de orina
– long or heavy menstruation	– menstruación larga o abundante
– nightime urination	– micción noctura
– nipple changes	– cambios en los pezones
– nipple discharge (excretion)	– supuración (excreción) del pezón
– orange peel skin on the breast	– celulitis en los pechos
– painful intercourse	– dolor al tener relaciones sexuales
– painful menstrual periods	– períodos menstruales dolorosos
– painful urination	– dolar al orinar
– prolonged erection	– erección prolongada
– scrotal swelling	– hinchazón escrotal
– side pain	– dolor de costado
– urethral discharge (excretion)	– supuración (excreción) de la uretra
– urinary frequency	– orinar con frecuencia
– urinary hesitancy	– vacilación urinaria
– urinary incontinence	– incontinencia urinaria
– urinary urgency	– urgencia urinaria
– urine cloudiness	– orina turbia
– uterine bleeding	– hemorragia uterina
– vaginal bleeding, postmenopausal	– sangramiento vaginal posmenopáusico
– vaginal discharge (excretion)	– supuración (excreción) vaginal

Brain matters, part one

Do you have or have you ever had
_____?

Tiene Ud. o ha tenido Ud. alguna
vez_____?

– amnesia (loss of memory)	– amnesia (pérdida de memoria)
– aura	– aura
– confusion	– confusión
– decreased level of consciousness	– disminución del nivel de conciencia

– difficulty talking	– dificultad para hablar
– difficult walking	– dificultad al caminar
– dizziness	– vertigo (máreos)
– drooling	– babeo (continuo)
– footdrop	– pie cáido
– headache	– dolor de cabeza
– insomnia	– insomnio
– loss of consciousnses	– desmayo
– muscle spasms	– espasmo muscular
– muscle twitching	– torsión de los muscúlos
– sleepiness	– adormecimiento
– swallowing problems	– dificultad al tragar

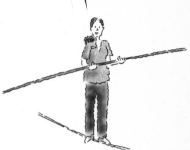

Have you ever had dizziness?

¿Ha tenido Ud. alguna vez vértigo?

Brain matters, part two

Do you have or have you ever had _____?	Tiene Ud. o ha tenido Ud. alguna vez_____?
– eyelid droop	– cáida de los párpados
– neck pain	– dolor de cuello
– neck stiffness	– el cuello rígido o tieso
– numbness or tingling	– adormecimiento o hormigueo
– paralysis	– parálisis
– racoon eyes	– ojos de "mapache" o equimosis
– seizure	– convulsiones
– taste abnormalities	– anormalidades del paladar
– tics (twitching)	– movimientos involuntarios
– tremors	– temblores
– vertigo (spinning or dizzy feeling)	– vértigo

Arms and legs

Do you have or have you ever had _____?	¿Tiene Ud. o ha tenido Ud. alguna vez _____?
– arm pain	– dolor de brazo
– back pain	– dolor de espalda
– bruises	– contusiones
– bumps	– chichones
– enlarged finger joint	– coyunturas agrandadas de los dedos
– leg pain	– dolor de pierna
– muscle spasms	– músculos espasmódicos
– muscle weakness	– debilidad en los músculos
– swelling, generalized	– edema generalizada
of the arm	del brazo
of the fingers	de los dedos
of the leg	de la pierna

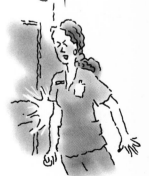

Have you ever had bumps or bruises?

¿Ha tenido Ud. alguna vez chichones o contusiones?

Immune system issues

Do you have or have you ever had
_____?

– breath with ammonia odor
– breath with fruity odor
– cold intolerance
– craving or eating nonfoods
– enlarged lymph nodes

– excessive thirst
– fatigue
– fever
– heat intolerance
– moon face
– salt craving
– skin, bronze
– skin, clammy
– skin, mottled
– sweating
– weight gain
– weight loss

¿Tiene Ud. o ha tenido Ud. alguna vez
_____?

– aliento con olor a amoníaco
– aliento con olor a fruta
– intolerancia al frío
– ingestión de sustancias extrañas
– agrandamiento de los nódulos
  linfáticos

– sed excesiva
– fatiga
– fiebre
– intolerancia al calor
– cara redonda
– gran deseo de sal
– piel bronce
– piel fría y húmeda
– piel abigarrada
– diaforesis
– aumento de peso
– disminución de peso

All the rest

Do you have or have you ever had
_____?

– anger
– agitation
– anxiety
– chills
– depression

¿Tiene Ud. o ha tenido Ud. alguna vez
_____?

– enojo
– agitación
– ansiedad
– escalofríos
– depresión

Positioning the patient

During your examination, you may want your patient to assume different positions. Use the following phrases to help you communicate the different positions to your patient.

Bending, leaning, lying, speaking

Bend backward.	Inclínese Ud. hacia atrás.
Bend forward.	Inclínese Ud. hacia adelante.
Don't talk.	No hable Ud.
Lean backward.	Recuéstese Ud.
Lean forward.	Inclínese Ud. hacia adelante.
Lie down.	Acuéstese Ud.
Lie on your:	Acuéstese Ud.:
– back.	– boca arriba.
– left side.	– del lado izquierdo.
– right side.	– del lado derecho.
– stomach.	– boca abajo.
Put your arms over your head.	Colóquese los brazos sobre la cabeza.
Roll over.	Dé Ud. una vuelta.
Say "Ahhh."	Diga Ud. "Ahhh."
Sit down.	Siéntese Ud.
Sit up.	Enderécese Ud.
Stand up.	Póngase Ud. de pie.
Turn to the side.	Voltéese Ud. hacia un lado.
Whisper.	Murmure Ud.

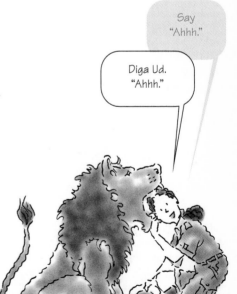

Say "Ahhh."

Diga Ud. "Ahhh."

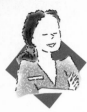

Practice makes perfecto

1. Help Joy assess her patient's signs and symptoms by filling in her questions. First, Joy wants to know if her patient has or has ever had headaches.

_____

_____

_____

_____

> ¿Tiene Ud. o
> _____
> dolores de cabeza?

2. Now Joy wants to know if her patient has ever had nosebleeds.

_____

_____

_____

_____

> ¿Ha tenido Ud.
> alguna vez
> _____?

3. Now Joy wants to assess GI symptoms. She begins by asking if her patient has ever had yellowing of the skin.

_____

_____

_____

_____

> ¿Ha tenido
> Ud. alguna vez
> _____?

4. Now Joy is helping a patient move around the room. You can help Joy by translating her request into Spanish.

_____

_____

_____

_____

> Sit down,
> please.

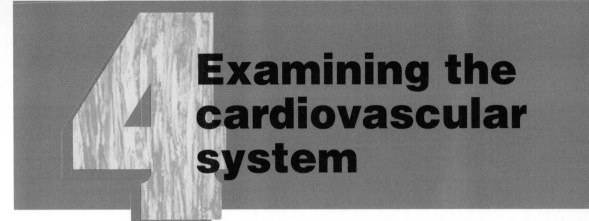

Examining the cardiovascular system

Fast fact

Key words for examining the cardiovascular system include:
- *dolor de pecho* (chest pain)
- *fatiga* (fatigue).

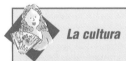

La cultura

The health care delay

Even though Latinos are the fastest growing ethnic group in the United States, many members of the Latino population face difficulties in accessing the health care system. Latino patients may delay seeking health care due to cultural differences, income, language barriers, and lack of health insurance benefits. As a result, some patients may seek health care only when symptoms have become advanced.

Health problems

Health problems that may be discussed during the cardiovascular examination include chest pain, dizziness, fluid retention, and fatigue. (See *The health care delay*.) To learn anatomical terms that may be relevant to your patient's condition, see *Heart—El corazón*, page 32, and *Coronary circulation—La circulación coronaria*, page 33.

Does it hurt?

Do you have chest pain or discomfort?	¿Tiene Ud. alguna vez dolor de pecho o molestia?
–How would you describe it? Constant? Intermittent?	– ¿Cómo lo describiría? ¿Constante? ¿Intermitente?
Does it hurt when you take a deep breath? (See *Dolor de pecho*, page 33.)	¿Duele cuando respira profundo?
Have you ever had this pain before? – When? – How was it treated? – How often have you had the pain?	¿Ha sentido este dolor anteriormente? – ¿Cuándo? – ¿Cómo fue tratado? – ¿Con cuánta frecuencia ha sentido el dolor?

Where does it hurt?

Where in your chest do you feel the pain? – Point to where you feel the pain.	¿En qué parte del pecho siente Ud. el dolor? – Indica Ud. dónde siente el dolor.
Does it radiate to any other area?	¿Se irradia este dolor a otra parte del cuerpo?
(See *Point and speak*, page 34.)	

Heart
El corazón

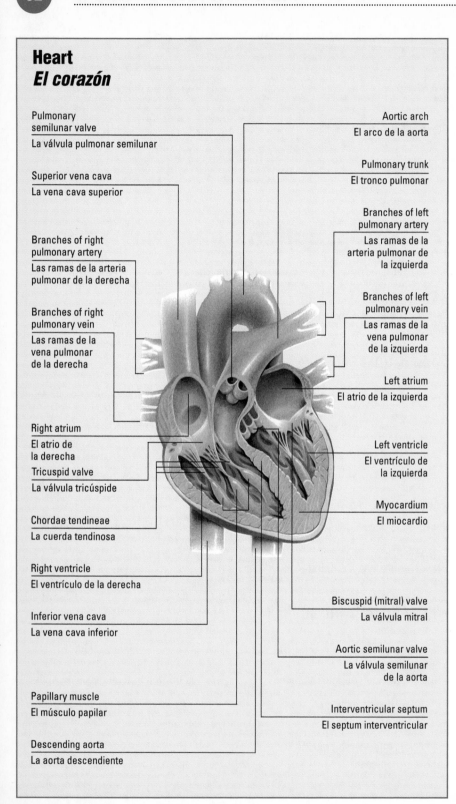

Pulmonary
semilunar valve
La válvula pulmonar semilunar

Superior vena cava
La vena cava superior

Branches of right
pulmonary artery
Las ramas de la arteria
pulmonar de la derecha

Branches of right
pulmonary vein
Las ramas de la
vena pulmonar
de la derecha

Right atrium
El atrio de
la derecha

Tricuspid valve
La válvula tricúspide

Chordae tendineae
La cuerda tendinosa

Right ventricle
El ventrículo de la derecha

Inferior vena cava
La vena cava inferior

Papillary muscle
El músculo papilar

Descending aorta
La aorta descendiente

Aortic arch
El arco de la aorta

Pulmonary trunk
El tronco pulmonar

Branches of left
pulmonary artery
Las ramas de la
arteria pulmonar de
la izquierda

Branches of left
pulmonary vein
Las ramas de la
vena pulmonar
de la izquierda

Left atrium
El atrio de la izquierda

Left ventricle
El ventrículo de
la izquierda

Myocardium
El miocardio

Biscuspid (mitral) valve
La válvula mitral

Aortic semilunar valve
La válvula semilunar
de la aorta

Interventricular septum
El septum interventricular

Remember
these words at
the heart of the
cardiovascular
system.

Coronary circulation
La circulación coronaria

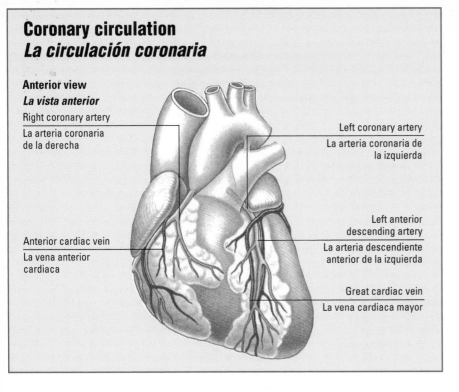

Anterior view
La vista anterior

Right coronary artery
La arteria coronaria de la derecha

Left coronary artery
La arteria coronaria de la izquierda

Left anterior descending artery
La arteria descendiente anterior de la izquierda

Anterior cardiac vein
La vena anterior cardiaca

Great cardiac vein
La vena cardiaca mayor

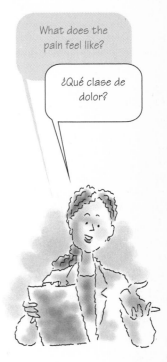

What does the pain feel like?

¿Qué clase de dolor?

What does it feel like?

What does the pain feel like?	¿Qué clase de dolor?
– Crushing or squeezing?	– ¿Siente que lo aplasta o oprime?
– Someone or something heavy pressing on your chest?	– ¿Como si algo pesado estuviera oprimiendo su pecho?
– Pressure or tightness?	– ¿Siente presión o tensión?
– Dull ache?	– ¿Es un dolor agudo?
– Burning sensation?	– ¿Sensación de ardor?
– Sharp or stabbing like a knife?	– ¿Agudo o punzante como un cuchillo?
– Ripping or tearing sensation?	– ¿Siente que es un dolor desgarrante?
– Heartburn-type pain?	– ¿Siente como si le quemara el pecto?
Do you have any other symptoms with the pain?	¿Tiene otros sintomas con el dolor?
– Anxiety?	– ¿Ansiedad?
– Arm pain?	– ¿Dolor en los brazos?
– Back pain?	– ¿Dolor en la espalda?
– Dizziness	– ¿Mareos?
– Fainting?	– ¿Desmayos?
– Fatigue?	– ¿Fatiga?
– Feeling of doom?	– ¿Sensación de muerte?
– Jaw pain?	– ¿Dolor de mandíbula?
– Nausea?	– ¿Náuseas?
– Restlessness?	– ¿Inquietud?

Pump up your pronunciation

Dolor de pecho

When assessing the cardio-vascular system, remember how to pronounce *dolor de pecho* (chest pain):
dolor de pecho—do-<u>lohr</u> deh <u>peh</u>-cho.

Point and speak

When you're facing a language barrier, nonverbal communication is especially important. For example, you can point to an area of your chest when asking where pain is occurring. However, don't let hand gestures take the place of verbal communication. Be sure to ask the necessary question in Spanish at the same time you use a hand gesture. This serves two purposes:

 It can prevent confusion because knowing the right word is more specific than relying on hand gestures.

It shows the patient that you're really trying to communicate, despite a language difference.

– Shortness of breath?	– ¿Respiración entrecortada?
– Sweating?	– ¿Sudor?
– Vomiting?	– ¿Vómitos?
– Weakness?	– ¿Debilidad?
Does anything make it worse?	¿Hay algo que empeora el dolor?
– Standing?	– ¿Pararse?
– Walking?	– ¿Caminar?
– Climbing stairs?	– ¿Subir escaleras?
Does anything make it better?	¿Hay algo que alivia el dolor?
– Lying down?	– ¿Acostarse?
– Resting?	– ¿Descansar?
– Taking medication?	– ¿Tomar medicamentos?

How long have you felt it?

How long have you been having this chest pain?	¿Hace cuánto tiempo que Ud. tiene este dolor de pecho?
– Did it start recently?	– ¿Comenzó hace poco?
– Over the last few hours, days, or weeks?	– ¿Hace unas horas, días, o semanas?

How long does an attack last?

How long does an attack last?	¿Cuánto tiempo dura el ataque?
– Seconds?	– ¿Segundos?
– Minutes?	– ¿Minutos?
– Hours?	– ¿Horas?
– Days?	– ¿Días?

(See *Morning, afternoon, or night?*)

Feeling fatigue?

Do you tire more easily than you used to?	¿Se cansa Ud. con más facilidad que antes?

Joy's grammar guide

Morning, afternoon, or night?

When assessing chest pain, it may be helpful to ask when the patient feels pain. For example, you can ask the patient:

Do you feel chest pain:
 – in the morning?
 – in the afternoon?
 – in the evening?

¿Siente este dolor de pecho:
 – en la mañana?
 – en la tarde?
 – en la noche?

Since when?

If you want to ask in a more general way when the pain started, you can ask *¿desde cuándo?* (since when?).

Get ready for the answer

Here's how the patient might respond:
 – One hour ago.
 – Two hours ago.
 – Since this morning.
 – Since last night.

 – Hace una hora.
 – Hace dos horas.
 – Desde la mañana.
 – Desde anoche.

What type of activity causes you to feel fatigued?
– How long can you perform this activity before you feel fatigued?

– Does rest relieve the fatigue?

¿Qué tipo de actividad le hace sentirse fatigado(a)?
– ¿Por cuánto tiempo puede Ud. hacer esa actividad antes de sentirse fatigado(a)?

– ¿El reposo le mitiga la fatiga?

Tight fit

Do your shoes or rings feel tight?

Do your ankles or feet feel swollen?

How long have you felt this way?

Have you gained or lost weight recently?

¿Le aprietan los zapatos o los anillos?

¿Siente Ud. que se le hinchan los tobillos o los pies?

¿Hace cuánto tiempo que se siente así?

¿Aumentó o perdió peso recientemente?

Pounding, racing, and skipping

Does your heart ever feel like it's:
– pounding?
– racing?
– skipping beats?

When does this feeling occur?
– While resting?
– During an activity?

¿Siente Ud. alguna vez que el corazón:
– le late violentamente?
– le late aceleradamente?
– se saltea latidos?

¿Cuándo ocurre esta sensación?
– ¿Mientras descansa?
– ¿Mientras hace alguna actividad?

What type of activity causes you to feel fatigued?

¿Qué tipo de actividad le hace sentirse fatigado(a)?

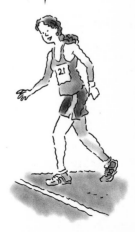

– After an activity?	– ¿Después de desempeñar una actividad?
– After exercising?	– ¿Después de hacer ejercicio?
– After walking up steps?	– ¿Después de subir escalones?
– After eating?	– ¿Después de comer?

Rating respirations

Have you ever experienced shortness of breath?	¿Alguna vez ha sentido Ud. que le falta la respiración?
– When did it occur?	– ¿Cuándo ocurrió?
– What makes it better?	– ¿Qué lo mejora?
– What makes it worse?	– ¿Qué lo empeora?
Is shortness of breath related to any activity?	¿Está relacionado con alguna actividad?
– Which activity?	– ¿Con qué actividad?
Is shortness of breath accompanied by coughing?	¿Va acompañado de tos?
How many pillows do you use when you sleep?	¿Cuántas almohadas usa para dormir?

Looking at the legs

Do you have any ulcers or sores on your legs?	¿Tiene Ud. úlceras o llagas en las piernas?
– Are they getting better?	– ¿Se están mejorando?
– Are they getting worse?	– ¿Se están empeorando?
– How long have you had them?	– ¿Hace cuánto tiempo que las tiene?
– Have you ever been treated for them?	– ¿Alguna vez ha recibido Ud. tratamiento para ellas?
– How were they treated?	– ¿Qué tratamiento se les dió?
Do you notice any change in the feeling in your legs?	¿Ha notado Ud. algún cambio en la sensación de las piernas?
Do you have pain in your legs?	¿Siente dolor en las piernas?
– When?	– ¿Cuándo?
Do your legs ever look red, blue, or purple?	¿Alguna vez nota que sus piernas están rojas, azules, o violáceas?
– When?	– ¿Cuándo?

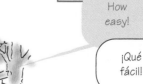

How easy!

¡Qué fácil!

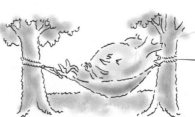

Medical history

In the medical history, investigate if the patient was born with a heart problem as well as if he has a history of high blood pressure, high cholesterol, or diabetes.

A long-time problem?

Were you born with a heart problem?

– What was it?
– When was it treated?
– How was it treated?

¿Nació Ud. con algún problema cardiaco?

– ¿Qué pasó?
– ¿Cuándo recibió tratamiento?
– ¿Cómo se le trató?

Not just any fever

Have you had rheumatic fever?
– When?
– Have any heart problems resulted from the rheumatic fever?

¿Ha tenido Ud. fiebre reumática?
– ¿Cuándo?
– ¿Le han resultado enfermedades del corazón a causa de la fiebre reumática?

Should I be hearing things?

Have you ever been told you had a heart murmur?
– Who told you about it?
– When did you find out about it?
– How was it treated?

¿Alguna vez se le ha dicho que tenía un soplo cardiaco?
– ¿Quién se lo dijo?
– ¿Cuándo se enteró Ud. de esto?
– ¿Cómo fue tratado?

What else have you got?

Do you have any of the following conditions?
– High blood pressure? (See *Asking the pregnant patient about high blood pressure.*)

– High cholesterol?
– Diabetes mellitus?
– Heart failure?

¿Tiene Ud. alguna de las siguientes enfermedades?
– ¿Presión sanguínea alta?

– ¿Colesterol alto?
– ¿Diabetes melitus?
– ¿Problemas cardiacos?

Have you ever had _____?
– a heart attack
– a cardiac catheterization
– a stent placed
– an angioplasty
– any type of heart surgery
– a pacemaker inserted
– a defibrillator inserted

¿Se le hizo alguna vez_____?
– un ataque cardiaco
– una cateterización cardiaca
– insertó alguna vez una cínula
– una angioplastía
– un tipo de cirugía cardiaca
– insertó alguna vez un marca pasos
– insertó alguna vez un desfribilador

When was the disorder first diagnosed?

¿Cuándo se le diagnosticó por primera vez este trastorno?

How is it treated?	¿Cómo se trata?
How has it affected your lifestyle? (See *Alto o alta?*)	¿Cómo ha afectado su modo de vida?

Medications

What prescription medications do you take?	¿Qué medicamentos bajo receta toma?
– What are they for?	– ¿Para qué son?
What over-the counter medications do you take?	¿Qué medicamentos de venta libre toma?
– How often do you take them?	– ¿Con cuánta frecuencia los toma?
What herbal remedies do you take?	¿Qué remedios a base de hierbas toma?
– How often do you take them?	– ¿Con cuánta frecuencia los toma?
What illicit drugs do you use?	¿Qué drogas ilícitas usa?
– How often do you use them?	– ¿Con cuánta frecuencia las usa?
Are you allergic to any medications?	¿Es alérgico(a) a algún medicamento?

Joy's grammar guide

Alto o alta?

Remember that adjectives in Spanish may change, depending on the gender of the noun they're modifying. A masculine noun gets a masculine adjective, which may end in *-o*. Likewise, a feminine noun gets a feminine adjective, which may end in *-a*. So if you're asking about high cholesterol, it's *colesterol alto,* but high blood pressure is *presión sanguínea alta.*

Family history

Be sure to ask about a family history of heart disease, high blood pressure, high cholesterol, or diabetes mellitus. (See *All in the family.*)

Family heartache

Has anyone in your family been treated for heart disease?	¿Algún miembro de su familia ha recibido tratamiento para alguna enfermedad cardiaca?
– How was the person related to you?	– ¿Cómo estába Ud. emparentado a esa persona?
– What was the disorder?	– ¿Qué desorden tuvo?
– At what age did it occur?	– ¿A qué edad le ocurrió?
Has anyone in your family died suddenly of an unknown cause?	¿Algún miembro de su familia ha muerto repentinamente por causa desconocida?

Blood pressure, cholesterol, and diabetes

Does anyone in your family have medical problems?	¿Hay alguien en su familia que tenga problemas médicos?
– High blood pressure?	– ¿La presión sanguínea alta?
– High cholesterol?	– ¿Colesterol alto?
– Diabetes mellitus?	– ¿Diabetes melitus?
At what age did the disorder develop?	¿A qué edad se le desarrolló la enfermedad?
How is it treated?	¿Qué tratamiento recibe?

Has anyone in your family been treated for heart disease?

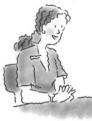

¿Algún miembro de su familia ha recibido tratamiento por alguna enfermedad cardiaca?

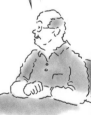

Yes, my father.

Sí, mi padre.

Joy's grammar guide

All in the family

Use this family tree to help you ask about your patient's family medical history.

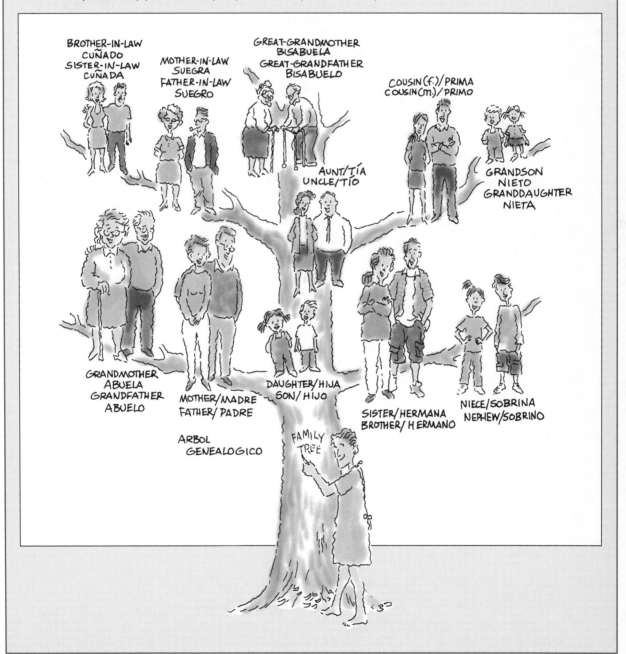

BROTHER-IN-LAW
CUÑADO
SISTER-IN-LAW
CUÑADA

MOTHER-IN-LAW
SUEGRA
FATHER-IN-LAW
SUEGRO

GREAT-GRANDMOTHER
BISABUELA
GREAT-GRANDFATHER
BISABUELO

COUSIN (f.) / PRIMA
COUSIN (m.) / PRIMO

AUNT/TÍA
UNCLE/TÍO

GRANDSON
NIETO
GRANDDAUGHTER
NIETA

GRANDMOTHER
ABUELA
GRANDFATHER
ABUELO

MOTHER/MADRE
FATHER/PADRE

DAUGHTER/HIJA
SON/HIJO

SISTER/HERMANA
BROTHER/HERMANO

NIECE/SOBRINA
NEPHEW/SOBRINO

ARBOL
GENEALOGICO

FAMILY
TREE

Lifestyle

Questions about lifestyle factors are central to any cardiovascular assessment. These questions discuss tobacco use, alcohol use, sleep patterns, exercise habits, and more.

Tobacco talk

Do you smoke or chew tobacco?
– What do you smoke?
   Cigarettes?
   Cigars?
   Pipes?
– How long have you smoked or chewed tobacco?
– How many cigarettes, cigars, or pipes of tobacco do you smoke per day?
– How much tobacco do you chew per day?
– Did you ever stop smoking or chewing tobacco?
   For how long?
   What method did you use to stop?

   Did you ever start again?

¿Ud. fuma o masca tabaco?
– ¿Qué fuma?
   ¿Cigarrillos?
   ¿Cigarros (puros)?
   ¿Pipas?
– ¿Hace cuánto tiempo que fuma o masca tabaco?
– ¿Cuántos cigarrillos, cigarros (puros), o pipas de tabaco fuma Ud. al día?
– ¿Cuánto tabaco masca al día?
– ¿Dejó Ud. el hábito alguna vez?

   ¿Cuánto tiempo duró sin fumar?
   ¿Qué método usó Ud. para dejar de fumar?
   ¿Volvió Ud. a fumar o mascar tabaco?

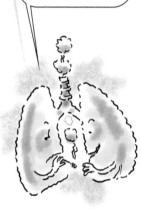

How long have you smoked or chewed tobacco?

¿Hace cuánto tiempo que fuma o masca tabaco?

Cheers!

Do you drink alcoholic beverages?
– What type?
   Beer?
   Wine?
   Hard liquor?

How often do you drink?

How many drinks per day?

Did you drink more frequently in the past?

Did you stop drinking?

When did you stop?

¿Toma Ud. bebidas alcohólicas?
– ¿Qué clase?
   ¿Cerveza?
   ¿Vino?
   ¿Aguardiente?

¿Con qué frecuencia bebe Ud.?

¿Cuántos tragos bebe al día?

¿Bebía Ud. más frecuentemente en el pasado?

¿Dejó de beber?

¿Cuándo dejó de beber?

Sweet dreams

How long do you sleep each night?

Do you feel rested each morning?

Do you feel tired later in the day?

¿Cuántas horas duerme Ud. cada noche?

¿Se siente Ud. descansado a la mañana siguiente?

¿Se siente Ud. cansado más tarde en el día?

Do you take naps?	¿Toma Ud. siestas?
– When do you take them?	– ¿Cuándo las toma?
– How long do you nap?	– ¿Por cuánto tiempo duerme la siesta?

It happens at night

Have you been told that you snore during sleep?	¿Se le ha dicho que ronca?
Do you awaken during the night to urinate?	¿Se despierta Ud. durante la noche para orinar?
Do you ever have shortness of breath or coughing spells during the night?	¿Alguna vez tiene la respiración entrecortada o accesos de tos por la noche?
– When do they occur?	– ¿Cuándo los tiene?
– How frequently do they occur?	– ¿Con qué frecuencia ocurren?
Every night?	¿Todas las noches?
A few times a week?	¿Unas cuantas veces a la semana?
A few times a month?	¿Unas cuantas veces al mes?
Do you become short of breath when you lie flat?	¿Le falta a Ud. la respiración cuando se acuesta de espaldas?
How many pillows do you use at night?	¿Cuántas almohadas usa Ud. en la noche?
– Has this number changed recently?	– ¿Ha cambiado últimamente este número?

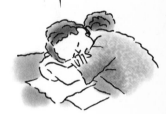

Have you been told that you snore during sleep?

¿Se le ha dicho que ronca?

Day in, day out

Describe your typical day.	Describa un día típico en su vida.
What are your daily activities during the week?	¿Cuáles son sus actividades diarias durante la semana?
What are your daily activities on weekends?	¿Cuáles son sus actividades diarias durante los fines de semana?

Ready, 10 jumping jacks

Do you exercise routinely?	¿Hace Ud. ejercicio rutinariamente?
– Which exercises do you perform?	– ¿Qué tipo de ejercicio hace?
– How often do you exercise?	– ¿Con qué frecuencia hace ejercicio?
– How intensely do you exercise?	– ¿Con qué intensidad hace el ejercicio?
– Do you ever have trouble breathing or chest pain while exercising?	– ¿Alguna vez le cuesta respirar o siente dolor en el pecho al ejercitarse?
– How long do you spend exercising?	– ¿Por cuánto tiempo hace Ud. ejercicio?
Did a health care professional prescribe your exercise plan?	¿Le recetó el ejercicio una persona especialista en el cuidado de la salud?
– Who?	– ¿Quién fue?

It's too darn hot

Do environmental factors, such as temperature extremes, humidity, and pollution, affect your ability to exercise?

– Do any of these factors affect the way you feel after exercise?

Has your exercise level changed from that of 6 months, 1 year, or 5 years ago?

– What caused this change?

Have you noticed any change in your ability to perform your usual activities of daily living (such as dressing, grooming, walking, and eating)?

¿Las condiciones ambientales tales como temperaturas extremas, la humedad, y la contaminación, afectan su habilidad de hacer ejercicio?
– ¿Alguno de esos factores afectan la manera en que se siente después de hacer ejercicio?

¿Ha cambiado su nivel de hacer ejercicio en relación al de hace 6 meses, 1 año o 5 años?
– ¿Qué fue lo que causó el cambio?

¿Ha notado Ud. algún cambio en su habilidad de realizar las actividades normales de su vida cotidiana (tal como vestirse, asearse, caminar, y comer)?

Just for fun

Do you participate in any recreational activities, such as hobbies and sports?
– How frequently do you engage in them?
– How do you feel after these activities?

– Has your level of involvement in these activities changed recently?
– What caused this change?

¿Participa Ud. en actividades de recreo, tales como pasatiempos y deportes?
– ¿Con qué frecuencia participa?

– ¿Cómo se siente Ud. después de participar en estas actividades?

– ¿Ha cambiado recientemente su nivel de participación en estas actividades?
– ¿Qué fue lo que causó este cambio?

Home sweet home

Do you live in a house or an apartment?

– How many floors does it have?
– Must you climb steps to get inside?

– Must you climb steps to get from room to room?
     How many?
– On which levels are the bathroom, bedroom, and kitchen?

¿Vive Ud. en una casa o en un apartamento?
– ¿Cuántos pisos tiene?
– ¿Tiene Ud. que subir escalones para entrar?
– ¿Tiene que subir escalones para ir de un cuarto a otro?
     ¿Cuántos?
– ¿En qué pisos están el baño, el dormitorio, y la cocina?

Stormy weather

Do certain weather conditions affect your symptoms?
– What are the conditions?
– How do they affect your symptoms?

¿Le afectan sus síntomas las condiciones atmosféricas?
– ¿Cuáles son las condiciones?
– ¿Qué efecto tienen en sus síntomas?

Do certain weather conditions affect your symptoms?

¿Le afectan sus síntomas las condiciones atmosféricas?

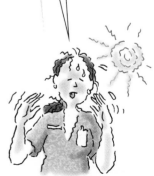

The stress factor

How often do you experience stress?	¿Con qué frecuencia siente Ud. estrés?
– Rarely	– Raramente
– Once in awhile	– De vez en cuando
– Very often	– Con frecuencia
Are you ever overwhelmed by stress?	¿Se siente Ud. alguna vez abrumado(a) por el estrés?
What causes you to feel stress?	¿Cuáles son las causas del estrés?
– Work	– El trabajo
– School	– La escuela
– Family	– La familia
– Marriage	– El matrimonio
– Finances	– Las finanzas
What physical feelings do you have when you're stressed?	¿Qué síntomas físicos siente Ud. cuando está estresado(a)?

Do the dishes, take out the trash

What are your responsibilities at home?	¿Cuáles son sus responsabilidades típicas en casa?
What are the responsibilities of your spouse and children?	¿Cuáles son las responsabilidades típicas de su cónyuge y de sus hijos?
Have your responsibilities at home changed since you developed a health problem?	¿Han cambiado sus responsabilidades en casa desde que se tuvo un problema de salud?
– How do you feel about these changes?	– ¿Cuál es su impresión acerca de estos cambios?

It's a working life

Are you currently employed?	¿Tiene Ud. empleo actualmente?
What's your occupation?	¿Cuál es su profesión o trabajo?
How many hours a day do you work?	¿Cuántas horas al día trabaja Ud.?
How many days a week do you work?	¿Cuántos días por semana trabaja Ud.?
What are your responsibilities?	¿Cuáles son sus responsabilidades?
What are the physical demands of your job?	¿Cuáles son las exigencias físicas de su trabajo?
– How much lifting do you do?	– ¿Tiene que levantar cosas pesadas?
– How much walking?	– ¿Cuánto tiene Ud. que caminar?
– Do you work in a hot, cold, humid, dusty, smoky, noisy, or outdoor environment?	– ¿Trabaja Ud. en un sitio caluroso, frío, húmedo, con mucho polvo, humo o ruido, o a la intemperie?
Do your financial resources and insurance cover your medical needs?	¿Cubren sus recursos financieros y seguro sus necesidades médicas?

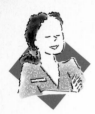

Practice makes perfecto

1. Joy wants to ask her patient if she ever has chest pain. Help her finish her question.

_____
_____
_____
_____

> ¿Ha tenido Ud. alguna vez _____?

2. Joy wants to know how long this patient has been experiencing chest pain. Help her finish her question.

_____
_____
_____
_____

> ¿_____ ha tenido este dolor de pecho?

> ¿Que_____?

3. Joy is asking a patient about his medical history. Help Joy ask her patient what medication he takes.

_____
_____
_____
_____

4. To complete her examination, Joy asks a patient about family history. Help Joy ask the patient if anyone in his family has heart problems or diabetes.

_____
_____
_____
_____

> ¿Algún miembro de su familia sufre de problemas _____?

Answer key

1. Do you ever have chest pain?
¿Ha tenido Ud. alguna vez <u>dolor de pecho</u>?

2. How long have you been having this chest pain?
<u>¿Hace cuánto tiempo que</u> ha tenido este dolor de pecho?

3. What medication do you take?
¿Qué <u>medicamentos toma</u>?

4. Does anyone in your family have a heart problem or diabetes?
¿Algún miembro de su familia sufre de problemas <u>cardiacos o de diabetes</u>?

5 Examining the respiratory system

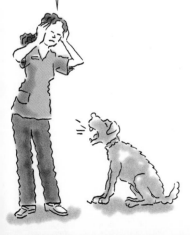

Do you have a cough? What does it sound like? Barking?

¿Tiene Ud. tos? ¿Qué sonido tiene? ¿Tos perruna?

Health problems

When examining the respiratory system, be sure to ask about chest pain, coughing, weight gain, shortness of breath, swelling in the ankles, and medication use. To learn the Spanish words for anatomical terms, see *Respiratory system—El sistema respiratorio*, page 46.

Aches and pains

Do you have chest pain?	¿Tiene Ud. dolor de pecho?
– Is it intermittent?	– ¿Es intermitente?
– Is it constant?	– ¿Es constante?
– Where's it located?	– ¿Dónde se localiza el dolor?
– Do any activities produce the pain?	– ¿Qué actividad o actividades producen el dolor?
What relieves the pain?	¿Qué alivia el dolor?
Does it hurt when you breathe normally or when you breathe deeply?	¿Tiene Ud. el dolor cuando respira normalmente o cuando respira profundamente?
Does it hurt when you cough?	¿Le duele cuando tose?

Who's confused?

Do you ever feel confused, restless, or faint?	¿Alguna vez siente Ud. confusión, desasosiego o desmayo?
– When does the feeling occur?	– ¿Cuándo ocurre esto?
– How long does it last?	– ¿Cuánto tiempo dura?

Cataloging a cough

Do you have a cough?	¿Tiene Ud. tos?
– What does it sound like?	– ¿Qué sonido tiene?
Hacking?	¿Tos seca?
Barking?	¿Tos perruna?
Congested?	¿Congestionada?

Respiratory system
El sistema respiratorio

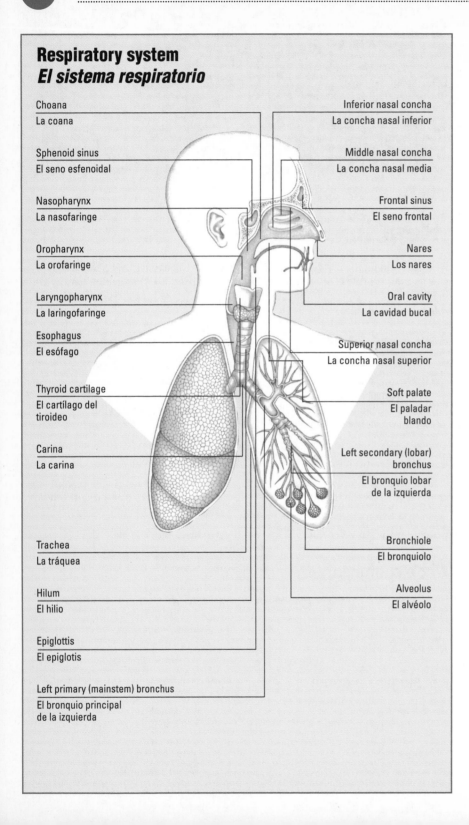

Choana
La coana

Sphenoid sinus
El seno esfenoidal

Nasopharynx
La nasofaringe

Oropharynx
La orofaringe

Laryngopharynx
La laringofaringe

Esophagus
El esófago

Thyroid cartilage
El cartílago del tiroideo

Carina
La carina

Trachea
La tráquea

Hilum
El hilio

Epiglottis
El epiglotis

Left primary (mainstem) bronchus
El bronquio principal de la izquierda

Inferior nasal concha
La concha nasal inferior

Middle nasal concha
La concha nasal media

Frontal sinus
El seno frontal

Nares
Los nares

Oral cavity
La cavidad bucal

Superior nasal concha
La concha nasal superior

Soft palate
El paladar blando

Left secondary (lobar) bronchus
El bronquio lobar de la izquierda

Bronchiole
El bronquiolo

Alveolus
El alvéolo

Do you cough up sputum? | ¿Expectora Ud.?
– How much do you cough up each day? | – ¿Cuánto expectora Ud. al día?
– What color is it? | – ¿De qué color es?
    Red? | ¿Rojo?
    Pink? | ¿Rosado?
    With streaks of blood? | ¿Sanguino lento?
    Yellow? | ¿Amarillo?
    Green? | ¿Verde?
    White? | ¿Blanco?
    Clear? | ¿Transparente o claro?
– Does it smell? | – ¿Tiene dos?
– Is it thick? | – ¿Es el esputo denso?
– Is it thin? | – ¿Es el esputo claro?
– What time of day do you cough up the most sputum? | – ¿A qué hora del día expectora Ud. más?
    Morning? | ¿Por la mañana?
    Night? | ¿Por la noche?
    After meals? | ¿Después de las comidas?

> Note that the Spanish word *expectora* (cough up) looks like *expectorate*.

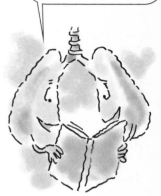

Gaining weight?

Do you suffer from foot or ankle swelling? | ¿Sufre Ud. de inflamación (hinchazón) del tobillo?

Have you noticed any weight gain recently? | ¿Ha notado Ud. algún aumento de peso recientemente?
– How much weight have you gained? | – ¿Cuánto peso ha aumentado?
– In what time frame? | – ¿En qué tiempo?

Losing breath

Do you have shortness of breath? | ¿Sufre Ud. de falta de respiración?
– Is it constant? | – ¿Es constante?
– Is it intermittent? | – ¿Es intermitente?

What makes it better? | ¿Qué disminuye el dolor?

What makes it worse? | ¿Qué aumenta el dolor?

Do your lips or nail beds ever turn blue? | ¿Alguna vez se le ponen azules los labios o el lecho de la uña?

Does body position affect your breathing? | ¿Le afecta la respiración la postura del cuerpo?
– How? | – ¿Cómo?

Does time of day affect your breathing? | ¿Le afecta la respiración la hora del día?
– What time of day? | – ¿A qué hora del día se siente peor?
(See *Respiration transformation*.)

How many pillows do you use to sleep? | ¿Cuántas almohadas usa para dormir?

Do you snore? | ¿Ronca?

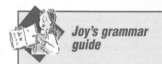

Joy's grammar guide

Respiration transformation

Note that the English suffix -tion typically corresponds to the Spanish suffix -*ción,* which is pronounced "see-yohn." Therefore, the English word respiration becomes the Spanish word *respiración* (res-pee-rah-see-y<u>ohn</u>). Other common examples include:

- constitution   constitución
- dilation   dilatación
- extraction   extracción
- limitation   limitación
- regulation   regulación
- rehabilitation   rehabilitación
- retention.   retención.

Walk, run, or climb

Does a particular activity affect your breathing?
– Which activity?
    Bathing?
    Walking?
    Running?
    Climbing stairs?
    Other?

How many stairs can you climb before you feel short of breath?

How many blocks can you walk before you feel short of breath?

¿Alguna actividad en particular afecta su respiración?
– ¿Qué actividad?
    ¿Bañarse?
    ¿Caminar?
    ¿Correr?
    ¿Subir escaleras?
    ¿Otra?

¿Cuántos escalones puede Ud. subir antes de sentir falta de respiración?

¿Cuántas calles puede caminar antes de sentir falta de respiración?

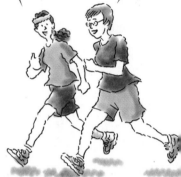

> Does a particular activity affect your breathing?

> ¿Alguna actividad en particular afecta su respiración?

> Yes, running.

> Sí, correr.

Inquiring about inhalers

Do you ever use over-the-counter nasal sprays or inhalers?
– What kind do you use?
– How frequently do you use them?
– When did you last take these drugs?

– Do they help you?

Do you use a nebulizer or other breathing treatment?
– What condition does it treat?

– What dose do you use?
– How often do you have a treatment?

– Do you ever experience any adverse effects from the treatment?
– Do you follow special instructions for using the treatment?
– When did you last do a treatment?
(See *Over-the-counter opportunity.*)

¿Usa Ud. alguna vez rociadores nasales o inhaladores?
– ¿Qué clase usa Ud.?
– ¿Con qué frecuencia lo usa Ud.?
– ¿Cuándo fue la última vez que tomó estos medicamentos?

– ¿Lo ayudan?

¿Usa Ud. un nebulizador u otro tratamiento para respirar?
– ¿Para qué enfermedad usa Ud. el tratamiento?
– ¿Qué dosis se le dió?
– ¿Con qué frecuencia sigue Ud. un tratamiento?

– ¿Alguna vez tiene Ud. efectos adversos a causa del tratamiento?
– ¿Sigue Ud. instrucciones especiales para el uso del tratamiento?
– ¿Cuándo recibió el último tratamiento?

Oxygen at home?

Do you use oxygen at home?
– Do you use a cannula or a mask?
– How much do you use?
– How often do you use it?
    Continuously?
    Intermittently?

¿Usa Ud. oxígeno en casa?
– ¿Usa Ud. una cánula o máscara?
– ¿Cuánto lo usa?
– ¿Con qué frecuencia la usa?
    ¿Continuamente?
    ¿Intermitentemente?

Pump up your pronunciation

Over-the-counter opportunity

Practicing the following pronunciations will help you find out what medications your patient may be taking for respiratory symptoms:
• nasal spray – *rociador nasal* (ross-i-a-<u>dor</u> nah-<u>zahl</u>)
• inhaler – *inhalador* (en-al-a-<u>dor</u>)
• medication – *medicamento* (me-dee-ka-<u>men</u>-to)
• prescription – *de receta* (de re-<u>se</u>-ta)
• over-the-counter – *sin necesidad de receta* (seen ne-seh-see-<u>dath</u> de reh-<u>se</u>-ta).

– How long have you been using oxygen at home?
(See *Get it right with oxygen*.)

– ¿Hace cuánto tiempo que Ud. usa oxígeno en casa?

Pump up your pronunciation

Medical history

In the medical history, determine if the patient has a history of respiratory problems or has had tuberculosis, a chest X-ray, a flu or pneumonia vaccination, or a sinus infection.

Past problems

Have you had any lung problems?

¿Ha tenido Ud. problemas de los pulmones?

– Bronchitis?
– Asthma?
– Tuberculosis?
– Pneumonia?
– Influenza?
– Sinus problems?
– Emphysema?
– Heart failure?
– Allergies?
– Other?

– ¿Bronquitis?
– ¿Asma?
– ¿Tuberculosis?
– ¿Pulmonía?
– ¿Gripe?
– ¿Sinusitis?
– ¿Enfisema?
– ¿Insuficiencia cardiaca?
– ¿Alergias?
– ¿Otros?

How long did the problem last?

¿Cuánto tiempo le duró el problema?

How was the problem treated?

¿Qué tratamiento recibió?

Medications

What prescription medications do you take?
– What are they for?

¿Qué medicamentos bajo receta toma?
– ¿Para qué son?

What over-the-counter medications do you take?
– How often do you take them?

¿Qué medicamentos de venta libre toma?
– Con cuánta frecuencia los toma?

What herbal remedies do you take?
– How often do you take them?

¿Qué remedios a base de hierbas toma?
– ¿Con cuánta frecuencia los toma?

What illicit drugs do you use?
– How often do you use them?

¿Qué drogas ilícitas usa?
– ¿Con cuánta frecuencia las usa?

Are you allergic to any medications?

¿Es alérgico/a a algún medicamento?

Exposing exposure

Have you been exposed to anyone with a respiratory disease?

¿Ha estado Ud. expuesto(a) a alguna persona que tenga una enfermedad respiratoria?

Get it right with oxygen

Although the Spanish word *oxígeno* may look like its English equivalent, oxygen, it's pronounced a bit differently. Remember that the Spanish letter G sounds like the English letter H. In addition, *oxígeno* has a stress mark on the second syllable. Therefore, *oxígeno* is pronounced ox-<u>ee</u>-heh-no.

– What type of disease? – ¿Qué clase de enfermedad?
– When were you exposed? – ¿Cuándo estuvo Ud. expuesto(a)?

Did you get sick from being exposed? ¿Se enfermó a raíz de la exposición?

Do you get a flu or pneumonia vaccine? ¿Se vacuna contra la gripe o la neumonía?

– When was your last one? – ¿Cuándo se vacunó por última vez?

Talking about tests

Have you had chest surgery? ¿Lo han operado del pecho?

Have you had surgery on your___? ¿Fue operado___?
– lungs – de los pulmones
– sinuses – de los senos nasales
– mouth, nose, or throat – de la boca, nariz o garganta

Have you had a diagnostic study of the lungs? ¿Le han hecho una revisión de los pulmones?
– What type? – ¿De qué tipo?
– Why did you have it? – ¿Por qué tuvo la cirugía o por qué se le hizo el estudio?

When was your last chest X-ray? ¿Cuándo se le tomó a Ud. la última radiografía de los pulmones?

– What was the result? – ¿Cuál fue el resultado?

When was your last tuberculosis test? ¿Cuándo se le hizo el último análisis para la tuberculosis?

– What was the result? – ¿Cuál fue el resultado?

Do you use home remedies for respiratory problems? ¿Usa Ud. remedios caseros para sus problemas respiratorios?
– What do you use? – ¿Qué usa Ud.?

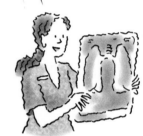

When was your last chest X-ray?

¿Cuándo se le tomó a Ud. la última radiografía de los pulmones?

Asking about allergies

Do you have allergies? ¿Tiene Ud. alergias?
– What are they? – ¿Qué son?
– Do they cause any of these symptoms: – ¿Le causan alguno de los siguientes síntomas:

    trouble breathing? dificultad para respirar?
    runny nose? le gotea la nariz?
    itching eyes? picazón en los ojos?
    congestion? congestión?
    other symptoms? otros síntomas?
– What do you do to relieve the symptoms? – ¿Qué hace Ud. para aliviar síntomas?

Recent reactions

In the last 2 months, have you had:
– fever?
– chills?
– fatigue?
– night sweats?

Have you ever had a blood test that showed you had anemia?
– When?

Do you ever have sinus pain?

Do you ever have nasal discharge or postnasal drip?

Do you ever have a bad taste in your mouth or bad breath?

¿En los últimos dos meses ha tenido:
– fiebre?
– escalofríos?
– fatiga?
– sudores nocturnos?

¿Alguno de sus análisis de sangre ha indicado que tenía anemia?
– ¿Cuándo?

¿Le han dolido alguna vez los senos nasales?

¿Ha tenido alguna vez secreción nasal o goteo posnasal?

¿Tiene alguna vez mal sabor en la boca o mal aliento?

Family history

Ask the patient about a family history of emphysema, asthma, respiratory allergies, and tuberculosis.

Checking the family tree

Has any member of your family had:

– emphysema?
– asthma?
– respiratory allergies?
– tuberculosis?
– sarcoidosis?

Did you have contact with the family member who had tuberculosis?
– When?
– Does the family member live with you?

Was the family member treated?
– How?

¿Algún miembro de su familia tuvo alguna de las siguientes enfermedades:
– enfisema?
– asma?
– alergias del sistema respiratorio?
– tuberculosis?
– sarcoidosis?

¿Estuvo Ud. en contacto con el miembro de la familia que tuvo tuberculosis?
– ¿Cuándo?
– ¿Vive con Ud.?

Su familiar, ¿fue tratado?
– ¿Cómo?

Lifestyle

Ask the patient about lifestyle issues, such as smoking and sleep patterns. Also ask about factors at home or work that might cause respiratory problems, such as pets, excessive stress, and workplace irritants.

Smoke or chew?

Do you smoke or chew tobacco?
– What do you smoke?
    Cigarettes?
    Cigars?
    Pipes?
– How long have you smoked or chewed tobacco?
– How many cigarettes, cigars, or pipes of tobacco do you smoke each day?
– How much tobacco do you chew each day?
– Did you ever stop?

    For how long did you stop?
    What method did you use to stop?

    Did you start again?
– Have you smoked or chewed tobacco in the past?
    What influenced you to stop?

¿Fuma Ud. o masca tabaco?
– ¿Qué fuma Ud.?
    ¿Cigarrillos?
    ¿Cigarros (puros)?
    ¿Pipas?
– ¿Hace cuánto tiempo que Ud. fuma o masca tabaco?
– ¿Cuántos cigarrillos, cigarros (puros), o pipas de tabaco fuma Ud. al día?
– ¿Cuánto tabaco masca Ud. diariamente?
– ¿Dejó Ud. alguna vez de fumar o mascar tabaco?
    ¿Por cuánto tiempo lo dejó?
    ¿Qué método usó Ud. para dejar de fumar o mascar?
    ¿Volvió a empezar?
– ¿Ha Ud. fumado o mascado tabaco en el pasado?
    ¿Qué influenció sobre Ud. para parar?

Sleep easy?

How many pillows do you use when you sleep?
– Are you using more or fewer pillows than you used to?

Have your sleep patterns changed because of breathing problems?

How many hours of sleep do you get each night?

Do you snore?

Do you wake up during the night?

Do you feel rested in the morning?

¿Cuántas almohadas usa Ud. para dormir?
– ¿Usa Ud. más o menos almohadas de las que usaba antes?

¿Han cambiado sus hábitos de dormir a causa de sus problemas respiratorios?

¿Cuántas horas duerme por noche?

¿Ronca?

¿Se despierta durante la noche?

¿Se siente descansado al levantarse a la mañana?

Who's at home?

How many people live with you?	¿Cuántas personas viven con Ud.?
Do you have pets? (See *The animal family*.)	¿Tiene Ud. animales en la casa?
– How many?	– ¿Cuántas?
– What type of pets do you have?	– ¿Qué tipo de mascotas tiene Ud.?
– Does the animal's fur or feathers bother you?	– ¿Le molestan a Ud. el pelaje o las plumas del animal?
– How does it bother you?	– ¿Cómo le molestan?
Runny nose?	¿Le gotea a Ud. la nariz?
Cough?	¿Tose?
Wheezing?	¿Respira con dificultad?
Other?	¿Otro síntoma?
What type of home heating do you have?	¿Qué tipo de calefacción tiene Ud. en casa?
Are there any respiratory irritants in your home, such as fresh paint, cleaning sprays, or heavy cigarette smoke?	¿Hay en su casa agentes irritantes que le afectan la respiración, tales como pintura fresca, nebulización de productos de limpieza, o humo de cigarrillos?
Do you have steps leading to or in your home?	¿Tiene escalones para entror en su casa o escaleras en su casa?
Do you have to walk up and down them often?	¿Tiene que subirlos o bajarlos con frecuencia?

Stressed out

Does stress at home or work affect your breathing?	¿Le afecta la respiración el estrés en casa o en el trabajo?
Do you have any special measures for stress management?	¿Toma Ud. algunas medidas especiales para controlar el estrés?
– What are they?	– ¿Cuáles son?

Occupational obstacles

What's your current occupation?	¿Cuál es su ocupación o empleo actual?
What were your previous occupations?	¿Qué otros empleos ha tenido anteriormente?
Are you exposed to any known respiratory irritants at work?	¿Sabe Ud. si está expuesto en su trabajo a agentes irritantes que afecten su respiración?
– Do you use safety measures during exposure?	– ¿Usa Ud. medidas de seguridad mientras está expuesto(a)?

The animal family

Because pets can cause or aggravate respiratory problems, it's important to ask your patient if he has pets at home. Note that, in Spanish, the word for pets is *animales* (think "animals") or *mascota* (think "mascot"). To understand your patient's response, consult this list of common pets:

• bird	pájaro
• cat	gato
• dog	perro
• ferret	hurón
• hamster	hámster
• snake.	culebra.

Do you have pets?

¿Tiene Ud. animales en la casa?

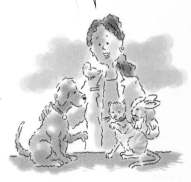

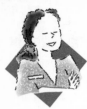

Practice makes perfecto

1. Joy wants to ask her patient if she suffers shortness of breath. Can you finish her question?

_____

_____

_____

_____

¿Sufre Ud. _____?

¿_____ rociadores nasales o inhaladores?

2. Joy is asking a patient about medications. Can you help her ask the patient if she uses over-the-counter nasal sprays or inhalers?

_____

_____

_____

_____

¿En los últimos dos meses ha tenido _____?

3. Joy is asking a patient about recent medical history. Can you help her ask the patient if he has had fever or chills in the last 2 months?

_____

_____

_____

_____

4. Joy wants to ask a patient if he smokes. Can you supply the correct verb?

_____

_____

_____

_____

¿_____ Ud.?

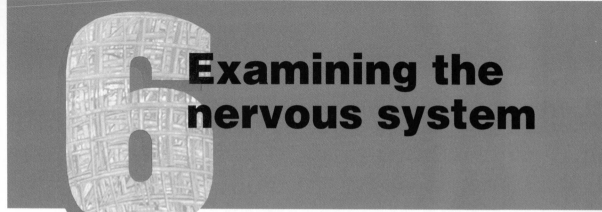

Examining the nervous system

Fast fact

Key terms for examining the nervous system include:
- *dolor de cabeza* (headache)
- *ataque epiléptico* (seizure)
- *derrame cerebral* (stroke).

Health problems

This chapter provides words and phrases to use during an examination of the patient's nervous system. Using the anatomical illustrations of the brain, spinal cord, and spinal nerves may facilitate more in-depth communication with your patient. (See *Brain—El cerebro*, page 56, and *Spinal cord and spinal nerves—La columna vertebral y los nervios espinales*, page 57.)

Topics you might discuss during an examination of the nervous system include auditory changes, difficulty speaking and swallowing, fainting, dizziness, headaches, seizures, memory changes, muscle spasms and incoordination, numbness, and visual changes.

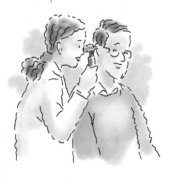

How is your hearing?

¿Cómo está su audición?

Hearing things

How is your hearing?	¿Cómo está su audición?
Have you had any changes in your hearing?	¿Ha notado Ud. algún cambio en su audición, es decir en su percepción de los sonidos?
– Describe the change.	– Describa el cambio.
– Does it affect one ear? Which one?	– ¿Le afecta a Ud. un oído? ¿Cuál?
When did the change start?	¿Cuándo empezó el cambio?
Do you wear a hearing aid?	¿Usa Ud. un audífono?
– In which ear?	– ¿En cuál oído?
– Does it help?	– ¿Le ayuda?
– Do you wear it all the time?	– ¿Lo usa Ud. todo el tiempo?

Say what?

Do you have difficulty speaking?	¿Tiene Ud. dificultad al hablar?
– What happens when you try to speak?	– ¿Qué ocurre cuando Ud. trata de hablar?
– When did you first notice this?	– ¿Cuándo notó Ud. esto por primera vez?
How often does it happen?	¿Con cuánta frecuencia ocurre?

Brain
El cerebro

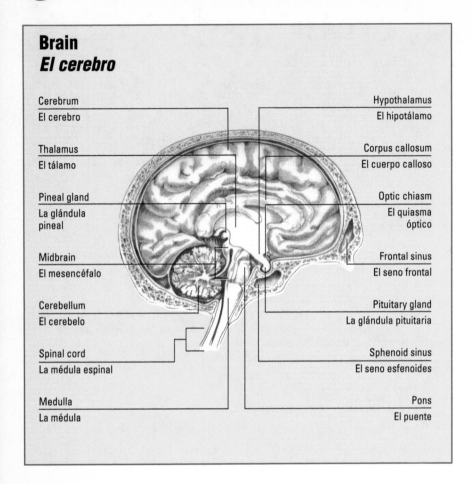

Cerebrum	Hypothalamus
El cerebro	El hipotálamo
Thalamus	Corpus callosum
El tálamo	El cuerpo calloso
Pineal gland	Optic chiasm
La glándula pineal	El quiasma óptico
Midbrain	Frontal sinus
El mesencéfalo	El seno frontal
Cerebellum	Pituitary gland
El cerebelo	La glándula pituitaria
Spinal cord	Sphenoid sinus
La médula espinal	El seno esfenoides
Medulla	Pons
La médula	El puente

Do you have difficulty expressing the words you're thinking?	¿Tiene Ud. dificultad en expresar las palabras que piensa?
– What happens?	– ¿Qué ocurre?
– When did you first notice this?	– ¿Cuándo notó Ud. esto por primera vez?
Do you have difficulty understanding what people are saying?	¿Tiene Ud. dificultad para comprender lo que dice la gente?
Do you have difficulty swallowing?	¿Tiene Ud. dificultad al tragar?
Do you choke on food or liquids?	¿Se atraganta Ud. a menudo al comer o bebes?
Do you feel like there's a lump in your throat?	¿Siente Ud. que tiene un nudo en la garganta?

Up, down, and all around

Do you have problems with your balance?	¿Tiene Ud. problemas de equilibrio?
Do you have dizzy spells?	¿Tiene Ud. accesos de vértigo?

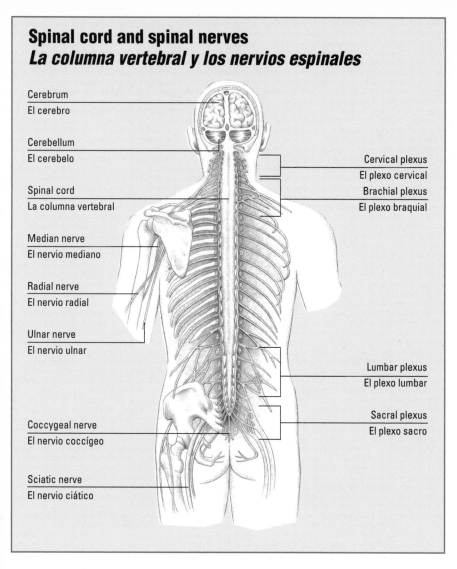

Spinal cord and spinal nerves
La columna vertebral y los nervios espinales

Cerebrum
El cerebro

Cerebellum
El cerebelo

Spinal cord
La columna vertebral

Median nerve
El nervio mediano

Radial nerve
El nervio radial

Ulnar nerve
El nervio ulnar

Coccygeal nerve
El nervio coccígeo

Sciatic nerve
El nervio ciático

Cervical plexus
El plexo cervical

Brachial plexus
El plexo braquial

Lumbar plexus
El plexo lumbar

Sacral plexus
El plexo sacro

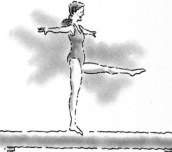

Do you have problems with your balance?

¿Tiene Ud. problemas de equilibrio?

– How often do they occur?
– Are they associated with any activity?

– How long do they last?

When did you first notice the dizzy spells?

What relieves them?

What makes them worse?

Have they gotten worse since they first started?

– ¿Con qué frecuencia ocurren?
– ¿Están relacionados con alguna actividad?

– ¿Cuánto tiempo duran?

¿Cuándo notó Ud. estos accesos por primera vez?

¿Qué es lo que los mitiga?

¿Qué es lo que los agrava?

¿Se han empeorado desde la primera vez que aparecieron?

Lights out

Have you ever fainted or blacked out, even if only for a few moments?

¿Alguna vez se ha desmayado Ud. o perdido el conocimiento, aunque sólo haya sido por unos momentos?

– When did this happen?
– Has it happened more than once?
– How long did the episode last?

– ¿Cuándo ocurrió esto?
– ¿Le ha ocurrido más de una vez?
– ¿Cuánto tiempo duró el incidente?

What happened before you fainted?

¿Qué ocurrió antes de que se desmayara?

Do you have difficulty recalling blocks of time?

¿Tiene Ud. dificultad en recordar espacios de tiempo?

All about (head)aches

How often do you get headaches?

¿Con qué frecuencia le dan dolores de cabeza?

– Frequently?
– Rarely?

– ¿Con frecuencia?
– ¿Raramente?

How long do the headaches last?

¿Cuánto duran los dolores de cabeza?

Do the headaches seem to follow a pattern?
– What kind of pattern?
(See *All kinds of time*.)

¿Siguen los dolores de cabeza un patrón específico?
– ¿Qué clase de patrón?

When does it hurt?

When do you usually get a headache?

¿Por lo general, a qué hora le dan los dolores de cabeza?

– In the early morning?
– During the day?
– At night?
– At certain times of the month?
– With certain types of weather?
    Rain?
    Cold?
    Heat?
    Humidity?
    Summer?
    Fall?
    Winter?
    Spring?

– ¿Temprano por la mañana?
– ¿Durante el día?
– ¿Por la noche?
– ¿En cierta parte del mes?
– ¿Con ciertos cambios del tiempo?
    ¿La lluvia?
    ¿El frío?
    ¿El calor?
    ¿El tiempo húmedo?
    ¿En el verano?
    ¿En el otoño?
    ¿En el invierno?
    ¿En la primavera?

Where does it hurt?

Where do you feel the pain?
– Across your forehead?
– Behind your eyes?

¿Dónde siente Ud. el dolor?
– ¿En la frente?
– ¿Detrás de los ojos?

Joy's grammar guide

All kinds of time

When assessing your patient's symptoms, it's helpful to know phrases related to time, duration, and frequency. Use this guide as a quick reference to help you remember:
• when?—*¿cuándo?*
• how long?—*¿cuánto tiempo?*
• at what time?—*¿a qué hora?*

– Along your temples?   – ¿En las sienes?
– In the back of your head?   – ¿En la parte de atrás de la cabeza?

What does it feel like?

What kind of pain do you feel?   ¿Qué tipo de dolor siente?
– Sharp?   – ¿Agudo?
– Stabbing?   – ¿Punzante?
– Dull ache?   – ¿Sordo?
– Throbbing?   – ¿Palpitante?
– Pressure?   – ¿Presión?
– Other?   – ¿Otro?

What else happens?

Do you have any other signs or symptoms along with the headaches?   ¿Tiene Ud. otros síntomas junto con los dolores de cabeza?
– What are they?   – ¿Cuáles son?
    Nausea?   ¿Náuseas?
    Vomiting?   ¿Vómitos?
    Stiff neck?   ¿Tortícolis?
    Blurred vision?   ¿Visión borrosa?
    Sensitivity to light?   ¿Sensibilidad a la luz?

What do you use to relieve the headaches?   ¿Qué hace Ud. para mitigar el dolor de cabeza?

You must remember this

Have you noticed a change in your ability to remember things?   ¿Ha notado Ud. algún cambio en su habilidad de recordar cosas?
– How would you describe this change?   – ¿Cómo describiría Ud. este cambio?
    A loss of recent memory?   ¿Pérdida de la memoria reciente?
    A loss of past events?   ¿Pérdida de memoria de eventos en tiempos pasados?

Have you noticed any change in your mental alertness or ability to concentrate?   ¿Ha notado Ud. algún cambio en su agudeza mental o en su habilidad de concentrarse?
– What kind of change?   – ¿Qué tipo de cambio?

Do you have difficulty following conversations or television programs?   ¿Tiene Ud. dificultad en seguir el hilo de una conversación o de un programa de la televisión?

Do you have difficulty concentrating on activities that you once enjoyed, such as reading and watching movies?   ¿Tiene Ud. dificultad en concentrarse en actividades que anteriormente disfrutaba, tal como leer o mirar películas?

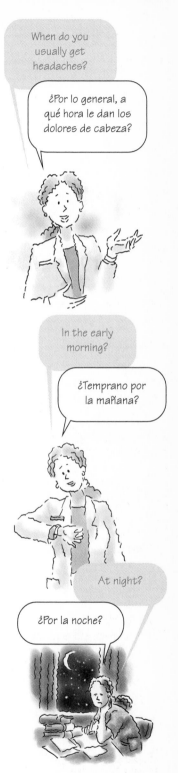

When do you usually get headaches?

¿Por lo general, a qué hora le dan los dolores de cabeza?

In the early morning?

¿Temprano por la mañana?

At night?

¿Por la noche?

Muscle beach

How would you rate your muscle strength?
– Very strong?
– Strong?
– Moderate?
– Weak?
– Very weak?

¿Cómo clasificaría Ud. su fortaleza muscular?
– ¿Muy fuerte?
– ¿Fuerte?
– ¿Moderada?
– ¿Débil?
– ¿Muy débil?

Have you recently noticed any change in strength?
– When did the change start?
– Is it constant or intermittent?
– Is one side stronger than the other?

¿Ha notado Ud. últimamente algún cambio en su fortaleza?
– ¿Cuándo comenzó el cambio?
– ¿Es constante o intermitente?
– ¿Tiene más fuerza de un lado que del otro?

How would you descibe your muscle co-ordination?

¿Cómo describiría su coordinación muscular?

Do you often drop things?

¿Se le caen con frecuencia objetos de la mano?

– How often?
– How recently have you noticed this?

– ¿Con qué frecuencia?
– ¿Hace cuánto tiempo ha notado Ud. esto?

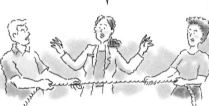

How would you rate your muscle strength?

¿Cómo clasificaría Ud. su fortaleza muscular?

Getting somewhere

Do you have difficulty walking?
– What kind of difficulty?
   Loss of balance?
   Staggering gait?
   Shuffling gait?
   Weakness?
   Loss of sensation?

¿Tiene Ud. dificultad al andar?
– ¿Qué tipo de dificultad?
   ¿Pierde el equilibrio?
   ¿Anda tambaleándose?
   ¿Arrastra los pies al caminar?
   ¿Siente debilidad?
   ¿Ha perdido sensación?

Do you use any assistive devices?
– What do you use?
   Cane?
   Walker?
   Wheelchair?

¿Usa Ud. algún aparato de asistencia?
– ¿Qué usa Ud.?
   ¿Bastón?
   ¿Andador?
   ¿Silla de ruedas?

Do you need to hold on to chairs and tables when you walk?

¿Necesita Ud. apoyarse en las sillas y las mesas cuando camina?

Do you have tremors or muscle spasms in your hands?

¿Tiene Ud. temblores o espasmos musculares en las manos?

Pins and needles

Do you have tremors or muscle spasms in your hands?
– Arms?
– Legs?
– When did you first notice it?
– Has it gotten worse or better?

¿Tiene Ud. temblores o espasmos musculares en las manos?
– ¿Los brazos?
– ¿Las piernas?
– ¿Cuándo los notó Ud. por primera vez?
– ¿Se han empeorado o mejorado?

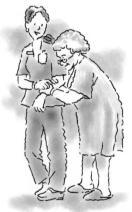

Do you have any of the following with the spasms?
– Numbness?
– Tingling?
– Feeling of cold?

What do you do to relieve the spasms? (See *For better or worse*.)

¿Tiene Ud. alguno de los siguientes síntomas junto con los espasmos?
– ¿Adormecimiento?
– ¿Hormigueo?
– ¿Sensación de frío?

¿Qué hace para aliviar los espasmos?

Pump up your pronunciation

For better or worse

When assessing a patient's symptoms, it's helpful to ask whether a symptom is improving *(mejorado)* or becoming worse *(empeorado)*. Use this quick pronunciation guide to help you ask these questions:

• Is it improving?—*¿Se ha mejorado?* (se ah meh-ho-<u>ra</u>-do)

• Is it becoming worse?—*¿Se ha empeorado?* (se ah em-pe-o-<u>ra</u>-do)

This won't hurt a bit

Have you noticed any change in your ability to feel textures?
– What type of change?

¿Ha notado Ud. algún cambio en su habilidad de palpar texturas?
– ¿Qué tipo de cambio?

Do you have any numbness?
– Tingling?
– Other unusual sensations?
– When did you first notice them?

¿Siente Ud. adormecimiento?
– ¿Hormigeo?
– ¿Otras sensaciones raras?
– ¿Cuándo notó Ud. esto por primera vez?

– Where are they located?
    Arms?
    Fingers?
    Legs?
    Feet?
    Toes?
– What, if anything, relieves them?

– What makes them worse?

– ¿Dónde las siente Ud.?
    ¿En los brazos?
    ¿En los dedos?
    ¿En las piernas?
    ¿En los pies?
    ¿En los dedos del pie?
– ¿Qué es lo que las mitiga, si hay algo que las mitigue?
– ¿Qué hace que empeoren?

Eye spy an eye problem

How would you describe your eyesight?
– Excellent?
– Good?
– Fair?
– Poor?

¿Cómo describiría Ud. su vista?
– ¿Excelente?
– ¿Buena?
– ¿Regular?
– ¿Mala?

Do you wear eyeglasses?
– Why do you need them?
    Near-sightedness?
    Far-sightedness?

    Other problem?

¿Usa Ud. lentes?
– ¿Por qué los necesita Ud.?
    ¿Miopía (ser corto de vista)?
    ¿Hipermetropía (mala vista de cerca)?
    ¿Otro problema?

Do you have:
– blurred vision?
– double vision?
– other vision disturbances such as blind spots?

¿Tiene Ud.:
– visión borrosa?
– visión doble?
– otros problemas de la vista tal como puntos ciegos de la retina?

Do you have blurred vision?

¿Tiene Ud. visión borrosa?

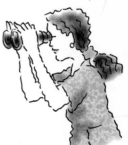

Medical history

In the medical history, ask if your Spanish-speaking patient has a history of seizures, headaches, or strokes or has ever had a head injury. For elderly patients, be sure to ask about memory loss and falls. (See *Asking elderly patients about memory loss and falls.*)

Medications

Here's how to ask the patient about his medication regimen.

What prescription medications do you take?	¿Qué medicamentos bajo receta toma?
– What are they for?	– ¿Para qué son?
What over-the-counter medications do you take?	¿Qué medicamentos de venta libre toma?
– How often do you take them?	– ¿Con cuánta frecuencia los toma?
What herbal remedies do you take?	¿Qué remedios a base de hierbas toma?
– How often do you take them?	– ¿Con cuánta frecuencia los toma?
What illicit drugs do you use?	¿Qué drogas ilícitas usa?
– How often do you use them?	– ¿Con cuánta frecuencia las usa?
Are you allergic to any medications?	¿Es alérgico(a) a algún medicamento?

Knock on the head

Have you ever had a head injury?	¿Ha tenido Ud. alguna vez una herida en la cabeza?
– When?	– ¿Cuándo?
– How would you describe what happened?	– ¿Cómo describiría Ud. lo que ocurrió?
– Do you have any lasting effects?	– ¿Le quedan a Ud. efectos perdurables?
Have you ever been treated by a neurologist or neurosurgeon?	¿Ha estado Ud. alguna vez bajo el cuidado de un neurólogo o de un neurocirujano?
– Why were you treated?	– ¿Por qué recibió tratamiento?
– What treatment was used?	– ¿Qué tratamiento se usó?

Seizure stats

Have you ever had a seizure?	¿Alguna vez ha tenido Ud. un ataque epiléptico?
– When?	– ¿Cuándo?
– What happened before the seizure?	– ¿Qué pasó antes del ataque epiléptico?
– What happened to you during the seizure?	– ¿Qué le pasó durante el ataque?

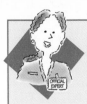

La clinica

Asking elderly patients about memory loss and falls

Elderly patients are at particular risk for memory loss and for injury caused by falls. Here are some questions to help assess symptoms related to these situations:

Have you developed tremors?	¿Se le han desarrollado temblores?
Have you noticed any change in your memory or thinking abilities, vision, hearing, or sense of smell or taste?	¿Ha notado Ud. algún cambio en su memoria o en su habilidad de pensar, en la visión, el oído o el sentido del olfato o del gusto?

Talk about the walk

Are you less agile than you used to be?	¿Es Ud. menos ágil de lo que lo era antes?
Do you trip or fall more frequently?	¿Se tropieza o se cae Ud. con más frecuencia?
How would you describe your walking pattern?	¿Cómo describiría Ud. su manera de andar?
Has your walking pattern changed?	¿Ha cambiado?

– Did you get hurt during the seizure?	– ¿Se lastimó durante el ataque?
– How long did the seizure last?	– ¿Cuánto tiempo duró el ataque?
– Can you remember anything about the seizure?	– ¿Recuerda Ud. lo que ocurrió durante el ataque epiléptico?
When was your first seizure?	¿Cuándo fue su primer ataque epiléptico?
How often do you have seizures?	¿Con cuánta frecuencia sufre los ataques?
– How are they treated?	– ¿Cómo son tratados?

Stroke effects

Have you ever had a stroke?	¿Ha tenido Ud. alguna vez un derrame cerebral?
– When did it occur?	– ¿Cuándo lo tuvo?
– What happened to you when you had the stroke?	– ¿Qué le pasó cuando tuvo el derrame cerebral?
– Could you speak?	– ¿Podía Ud. hablar?
– Could you move your arms and legs?	– ¿Podía mover los brazos y las piernas?
– Which side of your body could you not move?	– ¿Qué lado del cuerpo no podía Ud. mover?
Right side?	¿El lado derecho?
Left side?	¿El lado izquierdo?
– Was this the first time you had a stroke?	– ¿Fue ésta la primera vez que Ud. tuvo un derrame cerebral?
– What treatment did you receive for the stroke?	– ¿Qué tratamiento recibió Ud. para el derrame cerebral?
– Do you have any lasting effects from the stroke?	– ¿Tiene Ud. aún algún efecto perdurable del derrame cerebral?

Do you have high blood pressure?

How is it treated?
– Were you ever told you have an irregular heartbeat?
– Is it being treated?
– How?

¿Tiene hipertensión?

¿Cómo es tratada?
– ¿Alguna vez le dijeron que tiene el ritmo cardiaco irregular?
– ¿Está siendo tratado?
– ¿Cómo?

Family history

Ask the patient about a family history of neurologic disease as well as high blood pressure, stroke, diabetes mellitus, heart disease, epilepsy, cerebral palsy, and Down syndrome.

Family brainworks

Has any member of your family had a neurologic disease, such as a brain tumor, a degenerative disease, or senility?

– Which relative?
– How was it treated?

¿Hay algún miembro de su familia que haya tenido una enfermedad neurológica, tal como un tumor cerebral, una enfermedad degenerativa, o senilidad?

– ¿Qué pariente?
– ¿Qué tratamiento se le dió?

Going down the list

Have any of your immediate family members (mother, father, or siblings) had the following?

– High cholesterol?
– High blood pressure?
– Stroke?
– Diabetes mellitus?
– Heart disease?
– Epilepsy?
– Cerebral palsy?
– Down syndrome?
– Multiple sclerosis?

¿Hay algún miembro de su familia inmediata (madre, padre o hermano[a]) que haya tenido alguna de las siguientes?

– ¿Colesterol alto?
– ¿Alta presión sanguínea?
– ¿Derrame cerebral?
– ¿Diabetes melitus?
– ¿Enfermedad del corazón?
– ¿Epilepsia?
– ¿Parálisis cerebral?
– ¿Síndrome de Down?
– ¿Esclerosis múltiple?

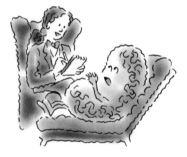

Has any family member had a neurologic disease?

¿Hay algún miembro de su familia que haya tenido una enfermedad neurológica?

Lifestyle

Ask the patient if he's exposed to toxins or chemicals at home or at work and ask about activities that might impair the neurologic system. If the patient is disabled, ask how the disability has affected his daily life.

Chemical contacts

Are you exposed to toxins or chemicals in your home or on the job, such as:

– insecticides?
– petroleum distillates?
– lead?

¿Está Ud. expuesto a algún producto tóxico o químico en su casa o en su trabajo, tales como:

– insecticidas?
– destilados de petróleo?
– plomo?

Do it again

On the job, do you perform strenuous or repetitive activities?
– What type of activities?
    Do you sit?
    Stand?
    Walk?

En su trabajo, ¿realiza Ud. actividades extenuantes o repetitivas?
– ¿Qué tipo de actividades?
    ¿Se sienta?
    ¿Se para?
    ¿Anda Ud.?

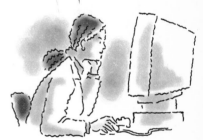

On the job, do you perform any repetitive activities?

En su trabajo, ¿realiza Ud. actividades repetitivas?

Role reversal

How has your disability affected you?

¿Cómo le ha afectado su incapacidad?

Has it made you feel differently about yourself?

¿Le ha hecho sentirse diferente?

Can you do the things for yourself that you would like to do?

¿Puede valerse por sí mismo(a)?

Can you fulfill your usual family responsibilities?
– If not, who has assumed them?

¿Puede atender sus responsabilidades normales con su familia?
– Si Ud. no puede con ellas, entonces ¿quién las ha asumido?

Does anyone help you at home?

¿Tiene a alguien que lo ayude en su casa?

Does your problem affect your ability to perform your daily activities?
– How?

Su problema, ¿afecta su capacidad de realizar las actividades cotidianas?
– ¿Cómo?

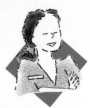

Practice makes perfecto

1. Joy is asking her patient if she has difficulty speaking. Can you finish her question?

_____

_____

_____

_____

> ¿Tiene Ud. _____?

2. Now Joy wants to ask if her patient has difficulty swallowing. Can you help?

_____

_____

_____

_____

> ¿Tiene Ud. _____?

3. Joy wants to ask a patient if he has had a head injury. Finish the question for Joy.

_____

_____

_____

_____

> ¿Ha tenido Ud. alguna vez _____?

4. Because the patient responded "yes," Joy wants to know when the head injury occurred. Can you help her ask the question?

_____

_____

_____

_____

> ¿_____?

Examining the GI system

Health problems

This chapter provides words and phrases you may use when examining the GI system. For a listing of anatomical terms, see *Gastrointestinal system—El sistema gastrointestinal*, page 68.

Common topics discussed during examination of the GI system include problems with changes in bowel habits, loss of appetite, difficulty swallowing, nausea and vomiting, indigestion, pain, and changes in weight.

Change in habits?

When did you last have a bowel movement or pass gas?	¿Cuándo fue la última vez que Ud. tuvo una evacuación intestinal o flato?
How often do you have regular bowel movements? – Once daily? – More than once daily? – Every other day? – Other?	¿Con qué frecuencia tiene Ud. evacuaciones intestinales regulares? – ¿Una vez al día? – ¿Más de una vez al día? – ¿Un día sí y un día no? – ¿Otra?

Color and consistency

What color are your bowel movements? – Brown? – Black? – Clay-colored? – Green? – Other?	¿De qué color es su material fecal? – ¿Parda? – ¿Negra? – ¿Color de arcilla? – ¿Verde? – ¿Otro?
Do you ever see blood in your bowel movements?	¿Ha notado sangre en su material fecal?
Have you noticed any change in your normal pattern of bowel movements? – Describe the change. 　More frequent? 　Less frequent?	¿Ha notado Ud. algún cambio en el patrón regular de sus evacuaciones intestinales? – Describa el cambio. 　¿Más frecuente? 　¿Menos frecuente?

Gastrointestinal system
El sistema gastrointestinal

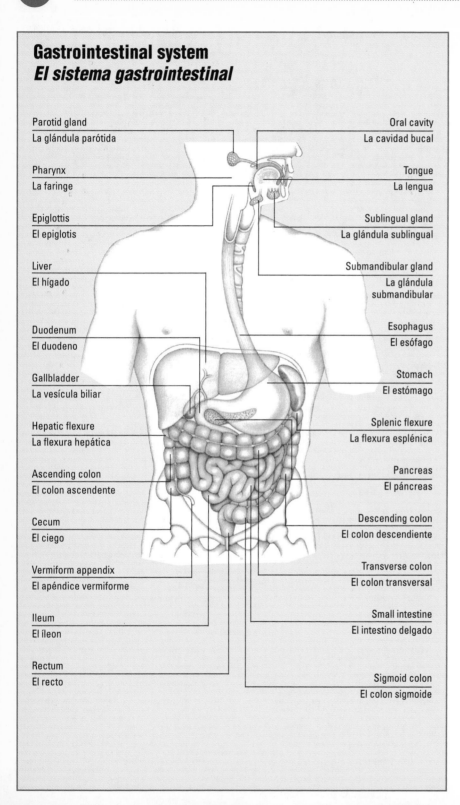

Parotid gland
La glándula parótida

Pharynx
La faringe

Epiglottis
El epiglotis

Liver
El hígado

Duodenum
El duodeno

Gallbladder
La vesícula biliar

Hepatic flexure
La flexura hepática

Ascending colon
El colon ascendente

Cecum
El ciego

Vermiform appendix
El apéndice vermiforme

Ileum
El íleon

Rectum
El recto

Oral cavity
La cavidad bucal

Tongue
La lengua

Sublingual gland
La glándula sublingual

Submandibular gland
La glándula submandibular

Esophagus
El esófago

Stomach
El estómago

Splenic flexure
La flexura esplénica

Pancreas
El páncreas

Descending colon
El colon descendiente

Transverse colon
El colon transversal

Small intestine
El intestino delgado

Sigmoid colon
El colon sigmoide

A possibly painful discussion

Do you have diarrhea?
– How often does it occur?
– How do you treat it?

¿Tiene diarrea?
– ¿Con qué frecuencia?
– ¿Cómo la trata?

Do you suffer from constipation?

¿Sufre Ud. de estreñimiento?

How often does it occur?
– When did it start?

¿Con qué frecuencia?
– ¿Cuándo comenzó a sufrir de esto?

Do you have abdominal pain?
– Where's the pain?

¿Tiene dolor abdominal?
– ¿Dónde se localiza el dolor?

How do you treat the pain?

¿Cómo trata el dolor?

Have you noticed swelling in your abdomen?

¿Ha notado Ud. algo de inflamación del abdomen?

Do you have other symptoms such as abdominal cramping?

¿Tiene otros síntomas, tales como retorcijones abdominales?

Hard to swallow

Do you have difficulty swallowing?
– When does it occur?
    With all foods?
    With liquids?

¿Tiene Ud. dificultad al tragar?
– ¿Cuándo ocurre esto?
    ¿Con todo lo que come?
    ¿Con líquidos?

Do you have heartburn or indigestion?
– When does it occur?
    In the morning?
    In the afternoon?
    In the evening?
    During sleep?

¿Sufre Ud. de acidez o indigestión?
– ¿Cuándo la tiene?
    ¿Por la mañana?
    ¿Por la tarde?
    ¿Por la noche?
    ¿Mientras Ud. duerme?

Is this heartburn or indigestion associated with eating or drinking?
– When?
– What did you eat? Drink?

¿La acidez o indigestión está asociada a la comida o la bebida?
– ¿Cuándo?
– ¿Qué comió Ud.? ¿Bebió?

How do you treat the heartburn or indigestion?

¿Cómo trata la acidez o indigestión?

> Do any specific foods or liquids bother you?
>
> ¿Hay algunos alimentos o líquidos en particular que le molestan?

Just not hungry

Have you had a recent change in appetite?
– Are you more hungry or thirsty?
– Are you less hungry or thirsty?

¿Ha tenido Ud. recientemente un cambio en su apetito?
– ¿Siente más hambre o sed?
– ¿Siente menos hambre o sed?

Have you had a recent change in diet?

¿Ha tenido Ud. recientemente un cambio de dieta?

Do any specific foods or liquids bother you?
– Which foods or liquids?

¿Hay algunos alimentos o líquidos en particular que le molestan?
– ¿Qué alimentos o líquidos?

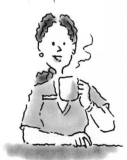

Unpleasant recurrence

Have you had any nausea?	¿Ha tenido Ud. náuseas?
– When did it occur?	– ¿Cuándo la tuvo?
Did you vomit?	¿Vomitó Ud.?
– How much did you vomit?	– ¿Cuánto vomitó?
A cup?	¿Una taza?
A quart?	¿Un litro?
More?	¿Más?
– What color was the vomitus?	– ¿De qué color fue el vómito?
Clear?	¿Transparente?
Green?	¿Verde?
Red?	¿Roja?
Black?	¿Negro?
How long did the vomiting last?	¿Durante cuánto tiempo vomitó?

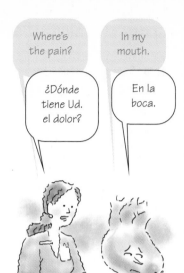

Where's the pain?

In my mouth.

¿Dónde tiene Ud. el dolor?

En la boca.

Does it hurt?

Do you have pain?	¿Tiene Ud. algún dolor?
Point to the area of the pain.	Señale el lugar del dolor.
Describe the pain.	Describa el dolor.
Does the pain interfere with any activity?	¿Interfiere el dolor en alguna actividad?
– Can you walk upright?	– ¿Puede Ud. caminar derecho(a)?
Were you drinking coffee or alcohol before the stomach pain began?	¿Estaba Ud. tomando café o bebidas alcohólicas antes que le comenzara el dolor de estómago?

When doesn't it hurt?

What relieves the pain?	¿Qué es lo que le mitiga el dolor?
– Food?	– ¿Comida?
– Drink?	– ¿Algo de beber?
– Medication?	– ¿Medicamento?
What makes the pain worse?	¿Qué empeora el dolor?
Does the pain affect other parts of the abdomen?	¿El dolor le afecta otras partes del abdomen (vientre)?
– Please point to the area.	– Por favor señale el lugar del dolos.
When does the pain occur in relation to eating?	¿Cuándo siente Ud. el dolor en relación con las comidas?
– Before meals?	– ¿Antes de las comidas?
– Immediately after meals?	– ¿Inmediatamente después de comer?
– Two to 3 hours after meals?	– ¿Dos o 3 horas después de comer?

What else happens?

Do you have other signs or symptoms with this pain?	¿Tiene Ud. otros síntomas junto con el dolor?
– Fever?	– ¿Fiebre?
– General discomfort?	– ¿Malestar?
– Nausea?	– ¿Náuseas?
– Vomiting?	– ¿Vómito?
– Redness?	– ¿Enrojecimiento?
– Swelling such as in the mouth?	– ¿Hinchazón, como por ejemplo en la boca?

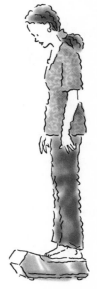

Have you recently had an unintentional weight change?

¿Recientemente ha cambiado de peso sin proponérselo?

On the scale

How much do you weigh?	¿Cuánto pesa Ud. actualmente?
Have you recently had an unintentional weight change?	¿Recientemente ha cambiado de peso sin proponérselo?
– How much weight did you lose or gain?	– ¿Cuánto peso perdió o aumentó?
– Over how long a time?	– ¿Cuánto tiempo le tomó bajar ese peso?

Medications

What prescription medications do you take?	¿Qué medicamentos bajo receta toma?
– What are they for?	– ¿Para qué son?
What over-the-counter medications do you take?	¿Qué medicamentos de venta libre toma?
– How often do you take them?	– ¿Con qué frecuencia los toma?
What herbal remedies do you take?	¿Qué medicamentos herbales toma?
– How often do you take them?	– ¿Con qué frecuencia los toma?
What illicit drugs do you use?	¿Qué drogas ilícitas usa?
– How often do you use them?	– ¿Con qué frecuencia las usa?
Are you allergic to any medications?	¿Es alérgico(a) a algún medicamento?

Taking anything?

Do you take medications for heartburn or indigestion?	¿Toma medicamentos para la acidez o la indigestión?
Do you take antacids?	¿Toma Ud. antiácidos?
– How often do you take them?	– ¿Con qué frecuencia los toma?
Once daily?	¿Una vez al día?
Twice daily?	¿Dos veces al día?
Three times daily?	¿Tres veces al día?
Four times daily?	¿Cuatro veces al día?
More often?	¿Con más frecuencia?

Do you use laxatives?   ¿Usa Ud. laxantes?
– Which laxatives?   – ¿Qué laxantes?
– How often?   – ¿Con qué frecuencia?

Do you use enemas?   ¿Usa Ud. enemas?
– Which enemas?   – ¿Qué enemas?
– How often?   – ¿Con qué frecuencia?

Medical history

When taking your patient's medical history, ask about any major or chronic illnesses as well as eating disorders, allergies, and recent swelling.

Major trouble

Have you had any major illnesses or do you have any chronic illnesses?   ¿Ha tenido alguna enfermedad significativa o tiene alguna enfermedad crónica?
– Cancer?   – ¿Cáncer?
– Trauma?   – ¿Trauma?
– Extensive dental work?   – ¿Trabajo dental extenso?
– Peptic ulcer disease?   – ¿Úlcera péptica?
– Gastroesophageal reflux disease?   – ¿Reflujo gastroesofágico?
– Diabetes mellitus?   – ¿Diabetes mellitus?
– Chronic lung disease?   – ¿Enfermedad pulmonar crónica?

Have you ever had an eating disorder, such as anorexia nervosa or bulimia?   ¿Ha sufrido Ud. de algún trastorno relacionado con las comidas, tal como anorexia nerviosa o bulimia?

Have you had problems with alcohol?   ¿Tiene problemas de alcoholismo?

Have you ever had hepatitis?   ¿Ha tenido hepatitis alguna vez?
– Diverticulitis?   – ¿Diverticulitis?
– What type of hepatitis?   – ¿Quetipo dehepatitis?
– Cirrhosis?   – ¿Cirrosis?

Long, long time

Have you had any problems with your mouth that have lasted for a long time?   ¿Ha tenido Ud. algún problema con la boca que haya durado por mucho tiempo?

– Throat?   – ¿Con la garganta?
– Abdomen?   – ¿Con el abdomen?
– Rectum?   – ¿Con el recto?

Have you ever had surgery on your: ¿Ha tenido Ud. alguna vez cirugía:
– mouth?   – de la boca?
– throat?   – de la garganta?
– abdomen?   – del abdomen?
– rectum?   – del recto?

Assessing allergies

Do you have any food allergies such as to milk products?

¿Tiene Ud. alguna alergia a alimentos, como por ejemplo a los productos lácteos?

– What happens when you have an allergic reaction?

– ¿Qué pasa cuando Ud. tiene una reacción alérgica?

Have you noticed a change in the size of your abdomen?

¿Ha notado Ud. algún cambio en el tamaño de su abdomen?

Do you have any difficulty breathing?

¿Tiene Ud. dificultad al respirar?

Here and there

Have you lived in or traveled to a foreign country?
– When?
– Where?

¿Ha vivido Ud. o viajado por algún país extranjero?
– ¿Cuándo?
– ¿Dónde?

Swelling, weakness, and numbness

Have you noticed any swelling in your neck?
– Underarms?
– Groin?

¿Ha notado Ud. alguna hinchazón en el cuello?
– ¿En las axilas?
– ¿En la ingle?

Have you had any nerve problems such as weakness in your hands or fingers?

¿Ha tenido Ud. algún problema con los nervios, tal como debilidad en las manos o los dedos?

– Numbness or tingling in your hands or fingers?

– ¿Adormecimiento u hormigueo en las manos o dedos?

Do you have eye pain, tearing, redness, or intolerance of light?

¿Tiene Ud. dolor en el ojo, lagrimeo, enrojecimiento, o intolerancia a la luz?

> Have you lived in or traveled to a foreign country?
>
> ¿Ha vivido Ud. o viajado por algún país extranjero?

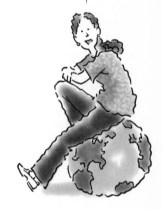

Family history

Ask your patient about a family history of cardiovascular disease, GI disorders, diabetes mellitus, food intolerance, and obesity.

Serious situations

Does anyone in your family have a history of:

– cardiovascular disease?
– Crohn's disease?
– diabetes mellitus?

¿Hay algún miembro de su familia que tenga un historial de alguna de las siguientes:

– enfermedad cardiovascular?
– enfermedad de Crohn?
– diabetes melitus?

– GI tract disorders?	– desarreglos en la región gastrointesti-nal?
– sickle cell anemia?	– anemia drepanocita?
– food intolerance?	– intolerancia a ciertos alimentos?
– obesity?	– obesidad?
– cancer?	– cáncer?

Has anyone in your family had colon or rectal cancer or polyps?	¿Hay algún miembro de su familia que haya tenido cáncer del recto o del colon o pólipos?
– Who?	– ¿Quién?
– When was it diagnosed?	– ¿Cuándo se le diagnosticó?
– How was it treated?	– ¿Qué tratamiento recibió?
– Did they have surgery?	– ¿Tuvieron que operarlo(a)?
– Do they have a colostomy bag?	– ¿Tiene un saco de colostomía?

Has anyone in your family had colitis?	¿Hay algún miembro de su familia que haya tenido colitis?
– Who?	– ¿Quién?
– When was it diagnosed?	– ¿Cuándo se le diagnosticó?
– How was it treated?	– ¿Qué tratamiento recibió?
– Did they have surgery?	– ¿Tuvieron que operarlo(a)?
– Do they have a colostomy bag?	– ¿Tiene un saco de colostomía?
– Do they take medication?	– ¿Toma medicamentos?

Lifestyle

Ask your patient about lifestyle factors, such as sleep patterns, nutrition, coping skills, and self-image.

Up all night

Do any GI symptoms ever cause you to awaken at night?	¿Algún síntoma gastrointestinal lo(a) despierta por la noche?
– What happens?	– ¿Qué pasa?
– How long do the symptoms last?	– ¿Cuánto duran los síntomas?
– What relieves the symptoms?	– ¿Qué es lo que le mitiga los síntomas?
– What do you do to get back to sleep?	– ¿Qué hace Ud. para volver a dormirse?

Food findings

How many times a day do you eat?	¿Cuántas veces por día come?
Which foods do you eat during the day?	¿Qué come Ud. durante el curso de un día?
Are there foods you can't eat?	¿Hay alimentos que Ud. no puede comer?
– What are these foods?	– ¿Cuáles son?
– Why can't you eat these foods?	– ¿Por qué no puede comer estos alimentos?

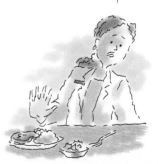

Are there foods that you can't eat?

¿Hay alimentos que Ud. no puede comer?

– How do these foods affect you?

– ¿Cómo le afectan estos alimentos si Ud. los come?

Fluid facts

How many servings do you drink of the following each day?
– Coffee? Decaf?
– Tea? Decaf?
– Soda?
– Cocoa?
– Water?
– Energy drink?
– Alcohol?

¿Cuántas porciones de las siguientes bebidas toma Ud. al día?
– ¿Café? ¿Descafeinado?
– ¿Té? ¿Descafeinado?
– ¿Gaseosa?
– ¿Cocoa?
– ¿Aqua?
– ¿Bebida energizante?
– ¿Alcohol?

How much fluid do you drink during the day?

¿Cuánto líquido bebe Ud. al día?

Brushing up

How do you care for your teeth and gums?

¿Qué cuidado da Ud. a sus dientes y encías?

Do you have any problems with your teeth or gums that interfere with your ability to eat?

¿Tiene algún problema con sus dientes o encías que interfieran con su habilidad de comer?

When was your last dental visit?
– Do you wear dentures?
– Do the dentures fit well?

¿Cuándo fue su última visita dental?
– ¿Tiene dentadura postiza?
– ¿Calza bien su dentadura postiza?

Mealtime

Who does the food shopping?

¿Quién hace sus compras de comestibles?

Do you have adequate storage and refrigeration?

¿Tiene Ud. una despensa y refrigerador adecuados?

Who prepares the meals?

¿Quién prepara las comidas?

Where's your food prepared?

¿Dónde se preparan los alimentos?

Do you eat alone or with others?

¿Come Ud. solo(a) o con otras personas?

Who prepares the meals?

¿Quién prepara las comidas?

La clinica

Talking to the parent or caregiver of a child with GI problems

Use these questions to ask a parent or caregiver about the child's GI problems:

Characteristics

What's the color of the child's bowel movements?	¿De qué color es la defecación del (de la) niño(a)?
How many bowel movements a day does the child have?	¿Cuántas veces por día defeca el niño/la niña?
Describe the consistency of the child's bowel movements.	Describa la consistencia de la evacuatión intestinal de la criatura.
Do the child's bowel movements ever appear large, bulky, and frothy and float in the toilet bowl?	¿Hay veces que la evacuación del (de la) niño(a) parece ser grande, abultada, y espumosa y flota en el retrete?
Is the odor especially strong?	¿Es el olor especialmente fuerte?

Behavior

Does the child want to eat despite forceful vomiting?	¿Quiere la criatura comer a pesar de que vomita violentamente?
What special words does the child use for having a bowel movement?	¿Cuáles son las palabras especiales que el (la) niño(a) usa para decir que quiere evacuar?
At what age was the child toilet trained?	¿A qué edad se entrenó al (a la) niño(a) a usar el retrete?
–Did any problems occur?	–¿Tuvo problemas con esto?
Does the child seem to have more "accidents" when ill?	¿Tiene la criatura más "accidentes" cuando está enferma?
Do you suspect that the child sometimes deliberately holds back bowel movements?	¿Sospecha Ud. que a veces el (la) niño(a) retiene intencionalmente la defecación?
Is the child under any unusual stress?	¿Está la criatura bajo un estrés inusual?

House plans

Do you live in a house or apartment?	¿Vive Ud. en una casa o en un apartamento?
– How many floors does it have?	– ¿Cuántos pisos tiene?
– Where's the bathroom?	– ¿Dónde está el baño?
Can you make it to the bathroom to move your bowels?	¿Puede llegar hasta el baño sin dificultad para evacuar?
– If not, what do you do?	– Si no puede Ud. llegar a tiempo, ¿qué hace Ud. para compensar el problema?

Mood and food

Have you been depressed or felt anxious recently?

¿Se ha sentido Ud. deprimido(a) o preocupado(a) últimamente?

Does the stress of your job, daily schedule, or other factors influence your eating or bowel patterns?

¿Su estrés en el trabajo, su horario diario u otros factores le influyen en sus patrones de comida o en su evacuación intestinal?

– How?

– ¿Cómo?

Do you use food or drink to help you get through a stressful event?

¿Toma Ud. alimentos o bebidas para ayudarle a llevar a cabo eventos estresantes?

Do you like yourself physically?

¿Se siente Ud. satisfecho(a) con su físico?

Do you think you need to lose weight?
– Gain weight?

¿Piensa que debe bajar de peso?
– ¿Subir de peso?

Are you content with your present weight?
(See *Talking to the parent or caregiver of a child with GI problems* and *End with the right gender.*)

¿Está Ud. satisfecho(a) con su peso actual?

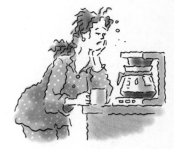

Do you use food or drink to help you through a stressful event?

¿Toma Ud. alimentos o bebidas para ayudarle a llevar a cabo eventos estresantes?

Joy's grammar guide

End with the right gender

Because Spanish is a gender-specific language, certain words get either an *-o* or an *-a* at the end, depending on whether you're speaking to a man or a woman. In the text, this is indicated by the ending *-o(a)*. For example, to ask a male patient if he's content with his present weight, you say *¿Está Ud. satisfecho con su peso actual?* To ask a female patient the same question, say *¿Está Ud. satisfecha con su peso actual?*

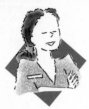

Practice makes perfecto

1. Joy wants to ask her patient if she has heartburn, but she can't remember the right word. Can you help her?

_____

_____

_____

_____

> ¿Sufre Ud. de _____?

2. Joy wants to ask a patient if he uses enemas. Can you supply the correct verb?

_____

_____

_____

_____

> ¿_____ Ud. enemas?

3. Joy wants to ask this patient about his recent medical history. Can you help her ask him if he has noticed any swelling in his neck?

_____

_____

_____

_____

> ¿Ha notado Ud. alguna hinchazón _____?

4. Joy is asking a patient about lifestyle changes and wants to know if she has been depressed lately. Can you finish her question?

_____

_____

_____

_____

> ¿Se ha sentido Ud. _____ últimamente?

Answer key

1. Do you have heartburn?
   ¿Sufre Ud. de <u>acidez</u>?
2. Do you use enemas?
   ¿<u>Usa</u> Ud. enemas?
3. Have you noticed any swelling in your neck?
   ¿Ha notado Ud. alguna hinchazón <u>en el cuello</u>?
4. Have you been depressed recently?
   ¿Se ha sentido Ud. <u>deprimida</u> últimamente?

8 Examining the genitourinary and reproductive systems

Female reproductive health

Topics that may be discussed during an examination of the female reproductive system include menstrual bleeding and irregularities, breast changes, vaginal discharge, and menstrual cycle changes. (See *Say it right*, page 80.)

For anatomical illustrations that may help build your vocabulary and facilitate communication, see *Female genitalia—Los órganos genitales femeninos*, page 80, and *Female breast—El seno de la mujer*, page 81.

Checking changes

Have you noticed any changes in your breasts?	¿Qué cambios ha notado Ud. en los senos?
How would you describe the change? – Lump? – Thickening? – Swelling? – Skin dimpling? – Nipple dimpling?	¿Cómo describiría Ud. este cambio? – ¿Bulto? – ¿Endurecimiento? – ¿Hinchazón? – ¿Hoyuelos en la piel? – ¿Hoyuelos en los pezones?
When did you first notice the change? – Has it improved? – Has it worsened?	¿Cuándo notó Ud. el cambio por primera vez? – ¿Se ha mejorado? – ¿Se ha empeorado?
Have you noticed any changes to your underarms?	¿Ha notado Ud. algún cambio en las axilas?
Describe the change. – How long ago did you notice it? – Has the condition improved? – Has the condition worsened?	Describa el cambio. – ¿Hace cuánto tiempo lo notó? – ¿Ha mejorado la afección? – ¿Ha empeorado la afección?

Female genitalia
Los órganos genitales femeninos

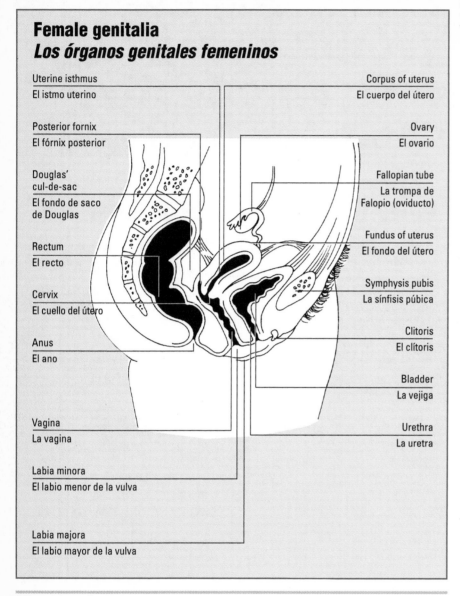

Uterine isthmus
El istmo uterino

Posterior fornix
El fórnix posterior

Douglas'
cul-de-sac
El fondo de saco
de Douglas

Rectum
El recto

Cervix
El cuello del útero

Anus
El ano

Vagina
La vagina

Labia minora
El labio menor de la vulva

Labia majora
El labio mayor de la vulva

Corpus of uterus
El cuerpo del útero

Ovary
El ovario

Fallopian tube
La trompa de
Falopio (oviducto)

Fundus of uterus
El fondo del útero

Symphysis pubis
La sínfisis púbica

Clitoris
El clítoris

Bladder
La vejiga

Urethra
La uretra

Say it right

Use this quick guide to help you pronounce key terms for examining the female reproductive system:
- blood—*sangre* (<u>sahn</u>-greh)
- menstruation—*menstruación* (men-stroo-ah-see-<u>on</u>)
- menopause—*menopausia* (mehn-oh-<u>paw</u>-see-ah)
- breast—*seno* (<u>seh</u>-noh).

Have you noticed any nipple discharge?

¿Ha notado Ud. alguna descarga del pezón?

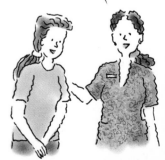

Unwanted excess

Have you noticed any nipple discharge?

– How long ago did you notice it?
– Has it become more pronounced lately?

Does this discharge occur with only one nipple?
– Which nipple?

What color is the discharge?

¿Ha notado Ud. alguna descarga del pezón?
– ¿Hace cuánto tiempo que Ud. la notó?
– ¿Ha aumentado ultimamente?

¿Viene esta descarga sólo de un pezón?

– ¿De cuál?

¿De qué color es la descarga?

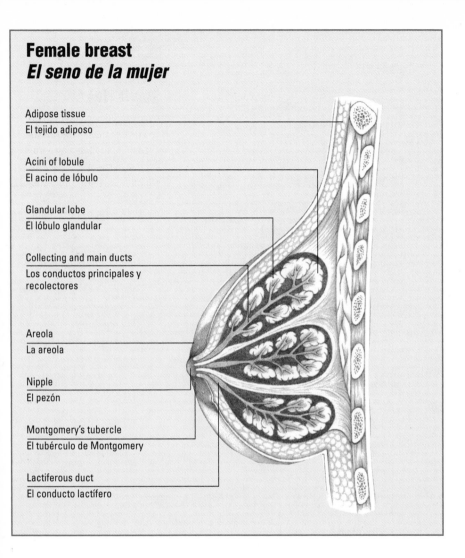

Female breast
El seno de la mujer

Adipose tissue
El tejido adiposo

Acini of lobule
El acino de lóbulo

Glandular lobe
El lóbulo glandular

Collecting and main ducts
Los conductos principales y recolectores

Areola
La areola

Nipple
El pezón

Montgomery's tubercle
El tubérculo de Montgomery

Lactiferous duct
El conducto lactífero

– Red?
– Clear?
– Pink?
– Green?
– Brown?

Does the discharge occur:
– spontaneously?
– with manual pressure?

Does the discharge have an odor?

Do you have any rash, redness, or irritation on either nipple?

Do you have any breast pain?
– Where?

– ¿Roja?
– ¿Transparente?
– ¿Rosada?
– ¿Verde?
– ¿Parda (color café)?

¿Ocurre la descarga:
– espontáneamente?
– bajo presión manual?

¿Tiene olor la secreción?

¿Tiene Ud. algo de erupción o eczema en uno u otro de los pezones?

¿Tiene dolor en el pecho?
– ¿Dónde?

– Describe the pain.   – Describa el dolor.
– Has it improved?   – ¿Ha mejorado?
– Has it worsened?   – ¿Ha empeorado?

Medications

What prescription medications do you take?

¿Qué medicamentos bajo receta toma?

– What are they for?

– ¿Para qué son?

What over-the counter medications do you take?

¿Qué medicamentos de venta libre toma?

– How often do you take them?

– ¿Con qué frecuencia los toma?

What herbal remedies do you take?

¿Qué medicamentos herbales toma?

– How often do you take them?

– ¿Con qué frecuencia los toma?

What illicit drugs do you use?

¿Qué drogas ilícitas usa?

– How often do you use them?

– ¿Con qué frecuencia las usa?

Are you allergic to any medications?

¿Es alérgico(a) a algún medicamento?

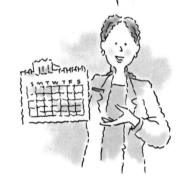

When was the first day of your last menstrual period?

¿Cuándo fue el primer día de su último periodo menstrual?

That time again

When was the first day of your last menstrual period?

¿Cuándo fue el primer día de su último periodo menstrual?

Was that period normal compared with your previous periods?

¿Fue ese periodo normal en comparación con los periodos anteriores?

How often do your periods occur?

¿Con qué frecuencia tiene Ud. sus periodos menstruales?

– Are they regular?

– ¿Con regularidad?

How long do your periods normally last?

¿Normalmente cuántos días duran sus periodos menstruales?

Is your period over?

¿Terminó su periodo?

– When did it end?

– ¿Cuándo terminó?

It's all in the activity

Do you ever have vaginal bleeding during or after intercourse?

¿Tiene Ud. alguna vez sangrado vaginal después de tener relaciones?

– When?

– ¿Cuándo?

– How much?

– ¿Cuánto?

– For how long?

– ¿Por cuánto tiempo?

Do you have pain during intercourse?

¿Tiene Ud. dolor al tener relaciones sexuales?

– After?

– ¿Después?

Much ado about menstrual flow

How would you describe your menstrual flow?	¿Cómo describiría Ud. su flujo menstrual?
– Heavy?	– ¿Fuerte?
– Moderate?	– ¿Moderado?
– Light?	– ¿Ligero?
Do you ever bleed between periods?	¿Ha tenido Ud. alguna vez sangrado entre sus periodos menstruales?
– How much do you bleed?	– ¿Cuánto sangra?
– For how long do you bleed?	– ¿Durante cuánto tiempo sangra?
What color is your menstrual flow?	¿De qué color es su flujo menstrual?
– Red?	– ¿Rojo?
– Bright red?	– ¿Rojo vivo?
– Dark brown-red?	– ¿Rojo café oscuro?
– Pink?	– ¿Rosado?
Are there any blood clots?	¿Contiene coágulos de sangre?
– Few?	– ¿Pocos?
– Moderate number?	– ¿Un número moderado?
– Many?	– ¿Muchos?
How many sanitary napkins or tampons do you use on each day of your period?	¿Cuántas almohadillas sanitarias o tampones usa Ud. cada uno de los días de su periodo?
– Has the number changed recently?	– ¿Ha cambiado esto últimamente?
Has it increased?	¿Ha aumentado?
Has it decreased?	¿Ha aminorado?

This hurts

Do you have cramping pain?	¿Tiene retorcijones?
– When does the pain occur?	– ¿Cuándo tiene Ud. el dolor?
Before your periods?	¿Antes de sus periodos?
During your periods?	¿Durante sus periodos?
After your periods?	¿Después de sus periodos?
Another time?	¿En otro momento?
Please point to where you feel the pain.	Por favor, señale dónde siente dolar.
Does it radiate to other areas?	¿Se extiende a otra región?
– Please point to where it radiates.	– Por favor, señale hacia donde le extiende.

Putting your finger on pain

What does the pain feel like?	¿Cómo siente Ud. el dolor?
– Dull and cramping?	– ¿Sordo y con retortijones?
– Sharp and stabbing, like a knife?	– ¿Agudo y punzante, como una cuchillada?

– Pressure or tightness?	– ¿Presión o tensión?
– Burning sensation?	– ¿Sensación de ardor?
How long does the pain last?	¿Cuánto tiempo dura el dolor?
– Is it constant?	– ¿Es constante?
– Is it intermittent?	– ¿Es intermitente?
How long have you had the pain?	¿Hace cuánto tiempo que Ud. tiene el dolor?
– Did it start recently? When?	– ¿Comenzó hace poco? ¿Cuándo?
What relieves it?	¿Qué le da alivio?
What makes it worse?	¿Qué lo empeora?

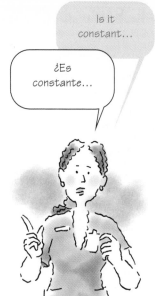

Is it constant...

¿Es constante...

Thin or thick

Do you have any vaginal discharge?	¿Tiene Ud. alguna descarga vaginal?
– When did it start?	– ¿Cuándo comenzó?
– How long have you had it?	– ¿Hace cuánto tiempo que Ud. la tiene?
– How much discharge have you noticed?	– ¿Cuánta descarga ha notado Ud.?
What color is the vaginal discharge?	¿De qué color es la descarga vaginal?
– Red?	– ¿Roja?
– Yellow?	– ¿Amarilla?
– White?	– ¿Blanca?
– Clear?	– ¿Transparente?
What's the consistency of the discharge?	¿Qué consistencia tiene la descarga vaginal?
– Cheesy?	– ¿Ni fluida ni espesa?
– Thin?	– ¿Fluida?
– Thick?	– ¿Espesa?
Does the discharge have any odor?	¿La descarga vaginal tiene algún olor?
– Can you describe the odor? Foul? Sweet?	– ¿Puede Ud. describir el olor? ¿Tiene muy mal olor? ¿Dulzón?

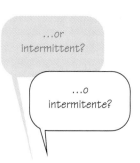

...or intermittent?

...o intermitente?

What else?

Have you experienced any other signs or symptoms, such as:	¿Ha tenido Ud. otros síntomas, tales como:
– vaginal itching?	– picazón vaginal?
– burning on urination?	– ardor al orinar?
– fever?	– fiebre?
– chills?	– escalofríos?
– swelling?	– hinchazón?
– lower back pain?	– dolor en la región lumbar?
Have you noticed any genital sores or ulcers?	¿Ha notado Ud. algunas llagas genitales o úlceras?

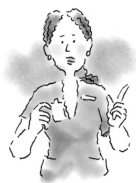

Does your sexual partner have any signs or symptoms of an infection, such as:
– genital sores?
– penile discharge?

¿Tiene su compañero sexual algunos indicios o sítomas de una infección como:
– llagas genitales?
– descarga del pene?

Do you have sex with multiple partners?

¿Tiene sexo con múltiples compañeros(as)?

Do you have anal sex?

¿Tiene relaciones sexuales anales?

What type of birth control do you use?
– Condoms?
– Hormones?
     What type?
– Other?

¿Qué tipo de contraceptivo usa?
– ¿Condones?
– ¿Hormonas?
     ¿Qué tipo?
– ¿Otra?

Have you ever had a sexually transmitted disease or other genital or reproductive system infection?

¿Ha tenido Ud. alguna vez una enfermedad transmitida sexualmente u otra infección genital o del sistema reproductivo?

– What was the infection?
     Human immunodeficiency virus (HIV) or acquired immunodeficiency syndrome (AIDS)?
     Chlamydia?
     Gonorrhea?
     Syphilis?
     Herpes?
     Other?
– How was it treated?
– Did any complications develop?
– What were the complications?

– ¿Cuál fue el problema?
     ¿Virus de inmunodeficiencia humana (VIH) o síndrome de inmunodeficiencia adquirida (SIDA)?
     ¿Clamidiosis?
     ¿Gonorrea?
     ¿Sífilis?
     ¿Herpes genitales?
     ¿Otra?
– ¿Qué tratamiento se le dió?
– ¿Se le desarrolló alguna complicación?
– ¿Cuál fue la complicación?

Life cycle change

At what age did you begin to menstruate?

¿A qué edad comenzó Ud. la menstruación?

Have you gone through menopause?
– At what age?

¿Ha tenido Ud. la menopausia?
– ¿A qué edad?

Did you experience any problems during menopause, such as:
– hot flashes?
– night sweats?
– excessive weight gain?
– mood swings?
– other?

¿Durante la menopausia tuvo Ud. algún problema, tal como:
– accesos repentinos de calor?
– sudores nocturnos?
– aumento de peso excesivo?
– cambios de humor?
– otro?

What did you do to relieve your problems?
– Did you take hormone replacement therapy?
– Did you take herbs?

¿Qué hizo Ud. para mitigarlos?
– ¿Hizo una terapia de reemplezo de hormonas?
– ¿Tomó hierbas?

During menopause, did you experience hot flashes?

¿Durante la menopausia, sintió Ud. accesos repentinos de calor?

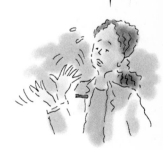

A cutting question

Have you had surgery for a reproductive system problem?
– When?
– What type of surgery?
– Was your uterus removed?
– Were your ovaries removed?

¿Ha tenido Ud. cirugía a causa de un problema en el sistema reproductivo?
– ¿Cuándo?
– ¿Qué tipo de cirugía?
– ¿Se le ha extirpado el útero?
– ¿Se le han extirpado los ovarios?

Have you ever been told you have:
– endometriosis?
– cysts on your ovaries?
– fibroids on your uterus?
– pelvic inflammatory disease?
– cancer of your ovaries, uterus, or vagina?

¿Le han dicho alguna vez que Ud. tiene:
– endometriosis?
– quistes ováricos?
– fibromas en su útero?
– enfermedad inflamatoria pélvica?
– cáncer de ovario, útero, o vagina?

Have you ever received radiation therapy to your reproductive organs?
– When?

¿Se hizo terapia de radiación en sus órganos reproductivos?
– ¿Cuándo?

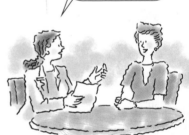

Have you ever been pregnant?

¿Ha estado Ud. embarazada alguna vez?

Motherhood and more

Have you ever been pregnant?
– How many times?
– How many living children do you have?

¿Ha estado Ud. embarazada alguna vez?
– ¿Cuántas veces?
– ¿Cuántos hijos que aún viven tiene Ud.?

Have you ever had a miscarriage or abortion?
– How many times?

¿Alguna vez ha tenido Ud. un aborto espontáneo o inducido?
– ¿Cuántas veces?

At what age did you bear your children?

¿A qué edad tuvo Ud. a sus hijos?

Have you ever had problems during pregnancy?
– What was the problem?
    Bleeding?
    Nausea or vomiting?
    High blood pressure?
    Diabetes?
    Heart disease?
    Physical injury or trauma?
    Infection?
    Another medical condition?
– When in the pregnancy did the problem occur?
    During the first 3 months?
    During the second 3 months?
    During the third 3 months?
    During labor?
    After delivery?
– What treatment did you receive?

¿Ha tenido Ud. alguna vez problemas durante el embarazo?
– ¿Cuál fue el problema?
    ¿Sangrado?
    ¿Náuseas o vómitos?
    ¿Presión sanguíne a alta?
    ¿Diabetes?
    ¿Enfermedad cardiaca?
    ¿Lesión física o trauma?
    ¿Infección
    ¿Otra enfermedad médica?
– ¿Cuándo ocurrió esto?

    ¿Durante el primero trimestre?
    ¿Durante el segundo trimestre?
    ¿Durante el tercer trimestre?
    ¿Durante el parto?
    ¿Después del parto?
– ¿Qué tratamiento se le dió?

¿Ha estado Ud. embarazada alguna vez?

Bed rest?	¿Descanso en cama?
Medications?	¿Medicamentos?
Surgery?	¿Cirugía?
Did these problems continue after you delivered your baby?	¿Siguió Ud. teniendo esos problemas después del parto?
– Which ones?	– ¿Cuáles?
Did you have a vaginal or cesearean delivery?	¿Tuvo un parto vaginal o una cesaria?
Did any of your infants have a medical problem?	¿Tuvo alguno de sus bebés un problema?
– What type of problem?	– ¿Qué tipo de problema?
Breathing problem?	¿Respiratorio?
Blood sugar problems?	¿Problemas de azúcar en sangre?
Infection?	¿Infección?
Weight — too low? Too high?	¿Peso muy bajo o excesivo?
Genetic disease?	¿Enfermedad genetica?
Did you breast-feed your infants?	¿Les dió Ud. de mamar a sus hijos?

History

Have you ever had problems conceiving?	¿Ha tenido Ud. problemas para concebir?
– Were you treated for this?	– ¿Qué tratamiento se le dió, si es que se le dió algún tratamiento?
– Were your treated with:	– ¿Se la trató con:
medication?	medicamentos?
surgery?	cirugía?
artificial insemination?	inseminación artificial?
in vitro fertilization?	fertilización in vitro?
Have you ever had breast surgery?	¿Ha tenido Ud. cirugía de los senos?
– When?	– ¿Cuándo?
– For what reason?	– ¿Por qué razón?
When was your last Pap smear?	¿Cuándo fue el último Papanicolau?
– Was it normal?	– ¿Fue normal?
– Did you follow up with your doctor?	– ¿Hizo un seguimiento con su médico?
Have you ever had a mammogram?	¿Se le ha tomado una mamografía?
– When?	– ¿Cuándo?
– Was it normal?	– ¿Fue normal?
Do you have any medical problems?	¿Tiene algún problema médico?
– Diabetes mellitus?	– ¿Diabetes mellitus?
– Heart disease?	– ¿Enfermedad cardiaca?
– High blood pressure?	– ¿Presión sanguínea alta?
– Other?	– ¿Otro?

Medications

What prescription medications do you take?
– What are they for?

¿Qué medicamentos bajo receta toma?
– ¿Para qué son?

What over-the-counter medications do you take?
– How often do you take them?

¿Qué medicamentos de venta libre toma?
– ¿Con qué frecuencia los toma?

What herbal remedies do you take?
– How often do you take them?

¿Qué medicamentos herbales toma?
– ¿Con qué frecuencia los toma?

What illicit drugs do you use?
– How often do you use them?

¿Qué drogas ilícitas usa?
– ¿Con qué frecuencia las usa?

Are you allergic to any medications?

¿Es alérgico(a) a algún medicamento?

Family facts

Has anyone in your family ever had reproductive problems, such as:

¿Algún miembro de su familia ha tenido alguna vez problemas del sistema reproductivo, tales como:

– difficulty conceiving?
– spontaneous abortion?
– menstrual difficulties?
– multiple births?
– congenital anomalies?
– difficult pregnancies?

– dificultad para concebir?
– aborto espontáneo?
– dificultades con la menstruación?
– nacimiento múltiple?
– anomalías congénitas?
– embarazos difíciles?

Has anyone in your family had:
– high blood pressure?
– diabetes mellitus?
– gestational diabetes?
– obesity?
– heart disease?
– cancer?
    Who?
    Where was the cancer?
    How was it treated?

¿Algún miembro de su familia ha tenido:
– presión sanguínea alta?
– diabetes melitus?
– diabetes gestacional?
– obesidad?
– enfermedad del corazón?
– ¿cáncer?
    ¿Quién?
    ¿Dónde tuvo el cáncer?
    ¿Qué tratamiento se le dió?

Has any member of your immediate family had gynecologic surgery?

– Who?
– What type of surgery?
    Ovaries removed?
    Uterus removed?
    Biopsy of the uterus?
    Breast surgery?
    Laparoscopic surgery?
    Endometriosis treatment?

¿Hay algún miembro de su familia inmediata que haya tenido cirugía ginecológica?
– ¿Quién?
– ¿Qué tipo de cirugía?
    ¿Se extirparon los ovarios?
    ¿Se extirpó el útero?
    ¿Se hizo biopsia del útero?
    ¿Cirugía de mamas?
    ¿Laparoscopía?
    ¿Tratamiento por endometriosis?

Did your mother, grandmother, aunt, or siblings have breast cancer?	¿Ha tenido su madre o cualquiera de sus hermanas cáncer del seno?
– Was the cancer in one or both breasts?	– ¿Tuvo o tuvieron el cáncer en uno o en los dos senos?
– How was it treated?	– ¿Qué tratamiento se les dió?
Chemotherapy?	¿Quimioterapia?
Radiation?	¿Radiación?
Surgery?	¿Cirugía?

Male reproductive health

Topics that may be discussed during an examination of the male reproductive system include penile discharge, sexual difficulties, and scrotal swelling. (See *Say it correctly*.)

To facilitate more detailed communication, see the anatomic terms in *Male genitalia—Los órganos genitales masculinos*, page 90.

A different look?

Have you noticed any changes in the skin color on your penis or scrotum?	¿Ha notado Ud. algún cambio en el color de la piel del pene o del escroto?
– What is the color?	– ¿De qué color es?
Are you circumcised?	¿Se le hizo a Ud. la circuncisión?
– Can you retract and replace the foreskin easily?	– ¿Puede Ud. contraer y reponer el prepucio con facilidad?
Have you noticed any of the following in your genital area?	¿Ha notado alguno de los siguientes en su área genital?
– Sore?	– ¿Llagas?
– Lump?	– ¿Bultos?
– Ulcer?	– ¿Úlceras?
When did you first notice it?	¿Cuándo fue la primera vez le notó?
How was it treated?	¿Córro fue tratado?

Personal problems

Do you have difficulty with erection or ejaculation?	¿Tiene Ud. alguna dificultad con la erección o la eyaculación?
– What type of difficulty?	– ¿Qué clase de dificultad?
Premature ejaculation?	¿Eyaculación precoz?
Delayed ejaculation?	¿Eyaculación regresiva?
Retrograde (backward) ejaculation?	¿Eyaculación retrógrada (cuando el semen entra en la vejiga en vez de salir por la uretra)?
Difficulty achieving an erection?	¿Dificultad para lograr una erección?
Difficulty maintaining an erection?	¿Dificultad para mantener una erección?

Pump up your pronunciation

Say it correctly

Use this quick guide to help you pronounce key terms for examining the male reproductive system:

• penis—*pene* (<u>peh</u>-neh)
• scrotum—*escroto* (eh-<u>scrow</u>-toh)
• ejaculation—*eyaculación* (eh-yak-oo-lah-see-<u>ohn</u>)
• groin—*ingle* (<u>een</u>-gleh).

Male genitalia
Los órganos genitales masculinos

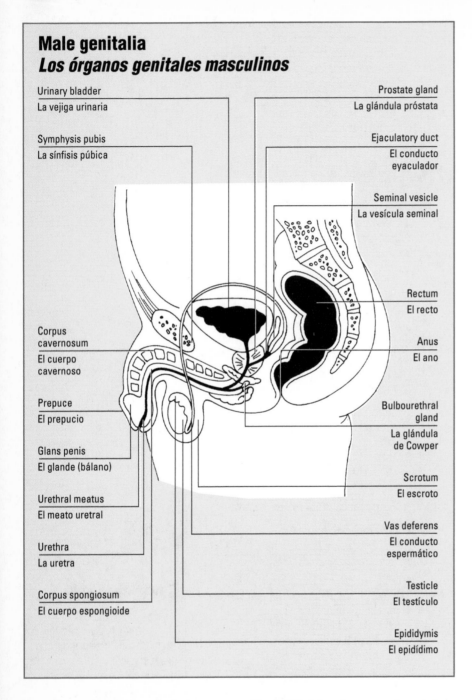

Urinary bladder
La vejiga urinaria

Symphysis pubis
La sínfisis púbica

Corpus cavernosum
El cuerpo cavernoso

Prepuce
El prepucio

Glans penis
El glande (bálano)

Urethral meatus
El meato uretral

Urethra
La uretra

Corpus spongiosum
El cuerpo espongioide

Prostate gland
La glándula próstata

Ejaculatory duct
El conducto eyaculador

Seminal vesicle
La vesícula seminal

Rectum
El recto

Anus
El ano

Bulbourethral gland
La glándula de Cowper

Scrotum
El escroto

Vas deferens
El conducto espermático

Testicle
El testículo

Epididymis
El epidídimo

> Knowing these terms in Spanish will help you talk with your patient about his problems.

Do you ever experience pain during erection or ejaculation?

¿Siente Ud. dolor alguna vez durante la erección o la eyaculación?

Do you ever have erections even when you aren't aroused?

¿Ha tenido erecciones alguna vez aun cuando no estaba excitado?

Do you have erections at other times such as upon awakening?	¿Tiene Ud. erecciones en otras ocasiones, por ejemplo, al despertar?
Do you take any medication to achieve an erection?	¿Toma algún medicamento para lograr una erección?
– Which medication?	– ¿Qué medicamento?
– How often do you take it?	– ¿Con qué frecuencia lo toma?

Pinpointing pain

Do you have pain in your penis, testes, or scrotum?	¿Tiene Ud. dolor en el pene, los testículos o el escroto?
– Where?	– ¿Dónde?
– When did it start?	– ¿Cuándo le empezó el dolor?
When does the pain occur?	¿Cuándo tiene el dolor?
Does the pain radiate?	¿Se extiende el dolor?
– Where?	– ¿Dónde?
What does the pain feel like?	¿Qué tipo de dolor siente Ud.?
– Dull ache?	– ¿Dolor sordo?
– Burning sensation?	– ¿Sensación de ardor?
– Pressure?	– ¿Presión?
– Pulling sensation?	– ¿Tirantez?
– Sharp and stabbing, like a knife?	– ¿Agudo y punzante, como una cuchillada?
What aggravates the pain?	¿Qué es lo que agrava el dolor?
What relieves the pain?	¿Qué es lo que lo mitiga?

Does the pain radiate?

¿Se extiende el dolor?

¡Sí!

Color and consistency

Have you noticed any discharge from your penis?	¿Ha notado Ud. alguna descarga del pene?
– What color is it?	– ¿De qué color es?
Yellow?	¿Amarilla?
Clear?	¿Transparente?
Bloody?	¿Ensangrentada?
Other?	¿Otra?
– What's the discharge's consistency?	– ¿Cuál es la consistencia de la descarga?
Thin?	¿Fluida?
Thick?	¿Espesa?
When did the discharge start?	¿Cuándo comenzó la secreción?
How long have you had it?	¿Por cuánto tiempo la tuvo?
Does the discharge have an odor?	¿Tiene olor la secreción?

Swell guide

Have you noticed any swelling in your scrotum?
– When did it start?
– How long have you had it?

¿Ha notado Ud. alguna hinchazón del escroto?
– ¿Cuándo le comenzó?
– ¿Hace cuánto tiempo que la ha tenido?

How would you describe the swelling?
– Constant?
– Intermittent?

¿Cómo describiría Ud. la hinchazón?
– ¿Constante?
– ¿Intermitente?

What relieves the swelling?

¿Qué es lo que le hace bajar la hinchazón?

What aggravates the swelling?

¿Qué es lo que agrava la hinchazón?

Has the swelling improved or worsened since it started?

¿Ha mejorado o empeorado la hinchazón desde que comenzó?

Do you have children?

¿Tiene Ud. hijos?

Pictures in your wallet?

Do you have children?
– How many?
– What are their ages?

¿Tiene Ud. hijos?
– ¿Cuántos?
– ¿Qué edad tienen?

Have you ever had a problem with infertility?
– Is it a current concern?

¿Ha tenido Ud. alguna vez algún problema de esterilidad?
– ¿Es esto una preocupación actual?

Surgery, hernia, and injury

Have you ever had surgery on the genitourinary tract or for a hernia?
– Where?
– When?
– Why?

¿Se le ha hecho alguna vez una cirugía en el sistema genitourinario o de hernia?
– ¿Dónde?
– ¿Cuándo?
– ¿Por qué?

Did you experience any complications after surgery?
– What were the complications?

¿Tuvo Ud. alguna complicación después de la cirugía?
– ¿Cuáles fueron las complicaciones?

How were they treated?

¿Qué tratamiento se le dió?

Have you ever had an injury to the genitourinary tract?
– What happened?
– When did it occur?
– What symptoms have developed as a result?

¿Ha tenido Ud. alguna vez una lesión en el sistema genitourinario?
– ¿Qué ocurrió?
– ¿Cuándo ocurrió?
– ¿Qué síntomas ha tenido a causa de esto?

STD tales

Have you ever been diagnosed as having a sexually transmitted disease (STD) or any other infection in the genitourinary tract?
– What was the problem?
      HIV or AIDS?
      Chlamydia?
      Gonorrhea?
      Syphilis?
      Herpes?
      Other?
– How long did it last?
– How was it treated?
– Did any complications develop?
      What were the complications?

¿Se le ha diagnosticado alguna vez una enfermedad transmitida sexualmente o cualquier otra infección del sistema genitourinario?
– ¿Cuál fue el problema?
      ¿VIH o SIDA?
      ¿Clamidiosis?
      ¿Gonorrea?
      ¿Sífilis?
      ¿Herpes genitales?
      ¿Otra?
– ¿Cuánto tiempo le duró?
– ¿Qué tratamiento se le dió?
– ¿Tuvo alguna complicación?
      ¿Cuáles fueron las complicaciones?

History issues

Do you have a history of:
– diabetes mellitus?
– heart disease, such as arteriosclerosis?

– high blood pressure?
– neurologic disease, such as multiple sclerosis or amyotrophic lateral sclerosis?
– cancer of the genitourinary tract?

Do you have a history of an endocrine disorder, such as hypogonadism?

– When was it diagnosed?
– How was it treated?

Do you have a history of undescended testes?
– How was it diagnosed?
– How was it treated?

Has anyone in your family had infertility problems?
– Who?
– How was it treated?

Has anyone in your family had an inguinal hernia?
– Who?
– How was it treated?

¿Ha tenido Ud.:
– diabetes melitus?
– enfermedad del corazón, tal como arteriosclerosis?

– presión sanguínea alta?
– enfermedades neurológicas, como esclerosis múltiple o esclerosis amiotrófica lateral?
– cáncer del sistema genitourinario?

¿Tiene Ud. un historial de algún trastorno endocrino, tal como hipogonadismo?
– ¿Cuándo se le diagnosticó?
– ¿Qué tratamiento se le dió?

¿Tiene Ud. un historial de testículos no descendidos (criptorquidia)?
– ¿Cómo se le diagnosticó?
– ¿Qué tratamiento se le dió?

¿Hay algún miembro de su familia que haya tenido problemas de esterilidad?
– ¿Quién?
– ¿Qué tratamiento se le dió?

¿Hay algún miembro de su familia que haya tenido una hernia?
– ¿Quién?
– ¿Qué tratamiento se le dió?

More than friends

Are you sexually active?

¿Tiene Ud. relaciones sexuales actualmente?

– When was the last time you had intercourse?

– ¿Cuándo fue la última vez que tuvo relaciones sexuales?

– Do you have more than one partner?

– ¿Tiene Ud. más de un(a) compañero(a)?

– Do you have anal sex?

– ¿Tiene relaciones sexuales anales?

Do you take any precautions to prevent contracting an STD or AIDS?

¿Toma Ud. precauciones para no contagiarse de una enfermedad sexual o SIDA?

– What precautions do you take?
   Use a condom?
   Limit the number of sexual partners?
   Avoid I.V. drug use?

   Make sure your partner was tested for any STD at the time you were treated?

– ¿Qué precauciones toma Ud.?
   ¿Usa un condón o preservativo?
   ¿Limita la cantidad de compañeros sexuales?
   ¿Evita inyectarse drogas por viá introvenosa?
   ¿Se aseguró de que su compañero(a) sexual fuera examinado(a) de una enfermedad sexual cuando lo trataron a Ud.?

Do any cultural or religious factors affect your beliefs or practices regarding sexuality and reproduction?

¿Hay algún factor cultural o religioso que afecte sus creencias o hábitos con respecto a su sexualidad y su procreación?

Meeting needs

Is your sexual preference heterosexual, homosexual, or bisexual?

¿Es su preferencia sexual heterosexual, homosexual, o bisexual?

Have you noticed any changes in your sexual interest, frequency of intercourse, or sexual functioning?

¿Ha notado Ud. algún cambio en su interés sexual, frecuencia de coito o en su desempeño sexual?

Are you experiencing any sexual difficulty?

¿Tiene Ud. actualmente alguna dificultad sexual?

– Does it affect your emotional and social relationships?

– ¿Le afecta esta dificultad en sus relaciones emocionales y sociales?

– Are you satisfied with the communication between you and your partner about your sexual needs?

– ¿Está Ud. satisfecha(o) de la comunicación entre Ud. y su compañero(a) con respecto a sus necesidades sexuales?

Urinary function

During examination of the male or female urinary system, you may ask questions about burning, hesitancy, and pain on urination as well as changes in urinary elimination patterns and the presence of urethral discharge. (See *Say it bien*.)

To learn Spanish words for anatomical structures of the kidney, see *Kidney—El riñón*, page 96.

Sound the fire alarm

Do you ever feel a burning sensation when you urinate?	¿Hay veces que Ud. siente una sensación de ardor cuando orina?
– How often?	– ¿Con qué frecuencia?
Every time?	¿Cada vez que Ud. orina?
Frequently?	¿Con frecuencia?
Occasionally?	¿De vez en cuando?
Where do you feel the burning sensation?	¿Dónde siente Ud. el ardor?
– At the urethral opening?	– ¿En la abertura de la uretra?
– Around the urethral opening?	– ¿Alrededor de la uretra?
– Inside the urethra?	– ¿Dentro de la uretra?

Pump up your pronunciation

Say it *bien*

Use this quick guide to help you pronounce key terms for examining the urinary system:

- urine—*orina* (oh-<u>ree</u>-na)
- burning—*ardor* (ar-<u>dor</u>)
- hesitancy—*vacilacion* (va-see-la-see-<u>on</u>)
- leakage—*pérdida* (<u>per</u>-dee-da).

How many trips?

How often do you urinate each day?	¿Con qué frecuencia orina Ud. al día?
– Once per day?	– ¿Una vez?
– Twice per day?	– ¿Dos veces?
– Three times per day?	– ¿Tres veces?
– Four times per day?	– ¿Cuatro veces?
– More often?	– ¿Con más frecuencia?
How does your bladder feel after you urinate?	¿Cómo se siente su vejiga después de orinar?
– Full?	– ¿Llena?
– Empty?	– ¿Vacía?

How often do you urinate each day?

¿Con qué frecuencia orina Ud. al día?

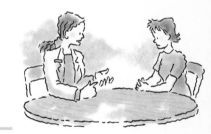

Consulting the color chart

What color is your urine?	¿De qué color es su orina?
– Colorless?	– ¿Incolor(a)?
– Light yellow?	– ¿Amarilla pálida?
– Dark yellow?	– ¿Amarilla oscura?
– Red?	– ¿Roja?
– Brown?	– ¿Parda?
– Black?	– ¿Negra?
Does your urine ever appear cloudy?	¿Hay veces que la orina parece estar turbia?
– How often does this occur?	– ¿Con qué frecuencia ocurre esto?
Every time?	¿Cada vez que orina?

Kidney
El riñón

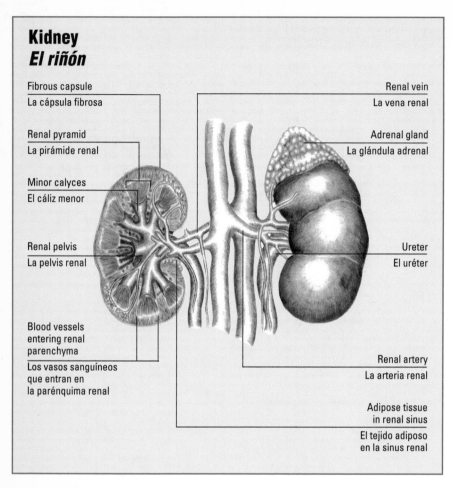

Fibrous capsule
La cápsula fibrosa

Renal pyramid
La pirámide renal

Minor calyces
El cáliz menor

Renal pelvis
La pelvis renal

Blood vessels
entering renal
parenchyma
Los vasos sanguíneos
que entran en
la parénquima renal

Renal vein
La vena renal

Adrenal gland
La glándula adrenal

Ureter
El uréter

Renal artery
La arteria renal

Adipose tissue
in renal sinus
El tejido adiposo
en la sinus renal

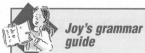

Joy's grammar guide

What's the frequency?

When examining your patient, it's helpful to pinpoint how often a particular symptom occurs. Use this quick phrase guide to ask your Spanish-speaking patient about the frequency of a symptom:
• every time—*cada vez*
• frequently—*con frecuencia*
• occasionally—*de vez en cuando.*

Frequently?
Occasionally?

Do you ever pass gas in your urine?
– How often does this occur?
    Every time?
    Frequently?
    Occasionally?
(See *What's the frequency?*)

¿Con frecuencia?
¿De vez en cuando?

¿Hay veces que Ud. pasa gas en la orina?
– ¿Con qué frecuencia ocurre esto?
    ¿Cada vez que orina?
    ¿Con frecuencia?
    ¿De vez en cuando?

Reluctant to start

Do you ever have difficulty starting or maintaining a urine stream?
– How often does this occur?
    Every time?
    Frequently?
    Occasionally?

¿Hay veces que Ud. tiene dificultad en comenzar o mantener un flujo de orina?
– ¿Con qué frecuencia ocurre esto?
    ¿Cada vez que orina?
    ¿Con frecuencia?
    ¿De vez en cuando?

Have you noticed a change in the size or force of your urine stream?	¿Ha notado Ud. algún cambio en el tamaño o la fuerza del flujo de su orina?
– Is it a trickle?	– ¿Es un flugo muy pequeño?
– Is it prolonged?	– ¿Es prolongado?
– Is it fast and strong?	– ¿Es rápido y fuerte?

Ouch! That hurts!

Do you have pain when you urinate?	¿Alguna vez siente Ud. dolor al orinar?
– How often?	– ¿Con qué frecuencia?
Every time?	¿Cada vez que orina?
Frequently?	¿Con frecuencia?
Occasionally?	¿De vez en cuando?
Where's the pain?	¿Dónde siente Ud. el dolor?
– At the urethral opening?	– ¿En la abertura de la uretra?
– Around the urethral opening?	– ¿Alrededor de la uretra?
– Inside the urethra?	– ¿Dentro de la uretra?
– In the lower abdomen?	– ¿En la parte inferior del abdomen (vientre)?
– In the lower back?	– ¿En la parte inferior de la espalda?
What does the pain feel like?	¿Qué tipo de dolor siente Ud.?
– Burning sensation?	– ¿Una sensación de ardor?
– Squeezing?	– ¿Siente que lo oprime?
– Dull or aching?	– ¿Sordo o intenso?
– Sharp or stabbing?	– ¿Agudo o punzante?
– Sensation of heaviness?	– ¿Una sensación de pesadez?
Do you ever have pain in your side that radiates around to your back or into your lower abdomen?	¿Hay veces que Ud. siente un dolor en el costado que se extiende hasta la espalda o la parte inferior del abdomen?
– Does a change in position relieve the pain or make it worse?	– ¿El cambiar de postura le mitiga el dolor o lo empeora?
Does anything else relieve the pain?	¿Hay alguna otra cosa que mitigue el dolor?
– What?	– ¿Qué?
Do you ever have pain below the ribs near the back?	¿Alguna vez tiene Ud. dolor por debajo de las costillas cerca de la espalda?

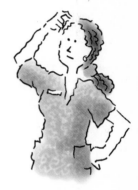

What does the pain feel like?

¿Qué tipo de dolor siente Ud.?

In a hurry

Do you ever feel that you must urinate immediately?	¿Hay veces que Ud. siente que tiene que orinar inmediatamente?
– How often does this occur?	– ¿Con qué frecuencia ocurre esto?
Most of the time?	¿La mayor parte del tiempo?
Frequently?	¿Con frecuencia?
Occasionally?	¿De vez en cuando?
Does this ever happen without urinating afterward?	¿Le ocurre a Ud. esto sin orinar luego?

Do you ever have urine leakage?
– When does it occur?
    When you laugh, sneeze, or cough?

    During exercise?
    When bending to pick something up?
    When you change positions?
    When you strain to move your bowels?
    After you feel the urge to urinate?

– How often does it occur?
    All the time?
    Frequently?
    Occasionally?
– How long have you had this leakage?

Do you wear absorbent pads to prevent soiling your clothes?

Does urine leakage interfere with your activities?
– How?

¿Tiene Ud. pérdida de orina?
– ¿Cuándo la tiene?
    ¿Cuándo Ud. se ríe, estornuda, o tose?

    ¿Cuándo Ud. hace ejercicio?
    ¿Cuándo se agacha Ud. a recoger algo?
    ¿Cuándo Ud. cambia de postura?
    ¿Cuándo se esfuerza Ud. para evacuar?
    ¿Después de sentir urgencia de orinar?
– ¿Con qué frecuencia ocurre esto?
    ¿Todo el tiempo?
    ¿Con frecuencia?
    ¿De vez en cuando?
– ¿Hace cuánto tiempo que Ud. tiene esta pérdida de orina?

¿Usa Ud. una almohadilla absorbente para evitar manchar su ropa?

¿Interfiere la pérdida de orina con sus actividades?
– ¿Cómo?

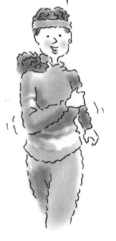

Does urine leakage interfere with your activities?

¿Interfiere la pérdida de orina con sus actividades?

Night watch

Do you awaken at night to urinate?

– How often does this occur?
    Once nightly?
    More than once nightly?
    Every other night?
    A few times weekly?
    Once weekly?

How long has this been happening?

Does this happen only when you drink large amounts of liquid in the evening?

Are your pajamas or sheets ever soiled with urine?

¿Ha notado Ud. que se despierta durante la noche para orinar?

– ¿Con qué frecuencia ocurre esto?
    ¿Una vez por noche?
    ¿Más de una vez por noche?
    ¿Una noche sí y otra no?
    ¿Unas cuantas veces a la semana?
    ¿Una vez a la semana?

¿Hace cuánto tiempo que le pasa esto?

¿Le pasa esto solamente cuando ha bebido grandes cantidades de líquido en la noche?

¿Que sus pijamas o las sábanas están manchadas de orina?

UTI info

Have you ever had a kidney or bladder problem such as a urinary tract infection (UTI)?
– What was the problem?
– When did it first occur?

Do you have a problem now?

Have you ever been hospitalized for a kidney or bladder problem?

– When?
– For how long?
– How was it treated?

Have you ever had kidney or bladder stones?
– When?
– How were they treated?

¿Ha tenido Ud. alguna vez un problema del riñón o de la vejiga tal como una infección en el sistema urinario?
– ¿Cuál fue el problema?
– ¿Cuándo ocurrió por primera vez?

¿Todavía tiene Ud. ese problema?

¿Ha estado Ud. hospitalizado(a) alguna vez a causa de un problema del riñón o de la vejiga?
– ¿Cuándo?
– ¿Por cuánto tiempo?
– ¿Qué tratamiento se le dió?

¿Ha tenido Ud. alguna vez cálculos en el riñón o en la vejiga?
– ¿Cuándo?
– ¿Qué tratamiento se le dió?

Stones and injury

Have you ever had a kidney or bladder injury?
– What kind of injury?
– When did it occur?
– How was it treated?
– Did you pass a kidney stone?

Have you ever worn an external drainage device?
– When?
– Why?

Have you ever had a catheter inserted into your bladder?
– Why?

¿Ha tenido Ud. alguna vez una lesión del riñón o de la vejiga?
– ¿Qué tipo de lesión?
– ¿Cuándo la tuvo?
– ¿Qué tratamiento se le dió?
– ¿Tuvo cálculos?

¿Ha utilizado algúna vez una unidad de drenaje externa?
– ¿Cuándo?
– ¿Por qué?

¿Ya le han colocado un catéter en la vejiga?
– ¿Por qué?

History

Do you have any medical problems, such as diabetes mellitus or high blood pressure?

¿Tiene Ud. algúnos problemas médicos, tal como diabetes melitus o alta presión sanguínea?

How is the problem being treated?

¿Cómo se está tratando el problema?

What medications do you routinely take?
– What are they for?

¿Qué medicamentos toma como rutina?
– ¿Para qué son?

Have you had any surgery?
– What was it for?
– When was it?
– Did you have any complications?
– What were they?

¿Ha tenido alguna cirugía?
– ¿Para qué?
– ¿Cuándo?
– ¿Tuvo alguna complicación?
– ¿Cuáles?

Family medical chart

Has anyone in your family ever been treated for urinary and kidney problems?
– What kind of problem?
    Bladder infection?
    Kidney infection?
    Kidney stones?
    Bladder stones?
    Bladder cancer?
    Kidney cancer?
    Enlarged prostate?
    Prostate cancer?
– When?
– How was the problem treated?
    Surgery?
    Medicine?
    No treatment?

¿Hay algún miembro de su familia que se le haya tratado a causa de un problema del riñón?
– ¿Qué tipo de problema?
    ¿Infección de vejiga?
    ¿Infección renal?
    ¿Cálculos renales?
    ¿Cálculos en la vejiga?
    ¿Cáncer de vejiga?
    ¿Cáncer de riñón?
    ¿Próstata expandida?
    ¿Cáncer de prostata?
– ¿Cuándo?
– ¿Qué tratamiento se le dió?
    ¿Cirugía?
    ¿Medicamentos?
    ¿Ningún tratamiento?

Has anyone in your family ever had:

– high blood pressure?
– diabetes mellitus?
– gout?
– coronary artery disease?
    Who?
    How was it treated?

¿Hay algún miembro de su familia que haya tenido:
– presión sanguínea alta?
– diabetes melitus?
– gota?
– enfermedad de la arteria coronaria?
    ¿Quién?
    ¿Qué tratamiento se le dió?

Food and drink

Do you follow a special diet?
– What kind of diet?
– Who prescribed the diet?
– How long have you been on the diet?

– What's the reason for the diet?

Do you limit your salt intake?
– How much salt do you use, if any?

How many glasses of liquid do you drink daily?

What type of liquid do you drink?

Where's the bathroom in your house?

¿Tiene Ud. una dieta especial?
– ¿Qué clase de dieta?
– ¿Quién le recetó la dieta?
– ¿Hace cuánto tiempo que tiene Ud. esta dieta?

– ¿Por qué razón tiene Ud. esta dieta?

¿Limita Ud. la cantidad de sal que toma?
– ¿Cuánta sal usa Ud., si es que la usa?

¿Cuántos vasos de líquido toma Ud. al día?

¿Qué tipo de líquidos bebe Ud.?

¿Dónde está el baño en su casa?

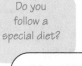

Do you follow a special diet?

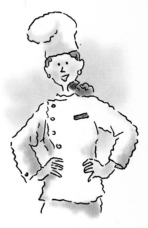

¿Tiene Ud. una dieta especial?

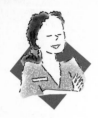

Practice makes perfecto

1. Joy wants to know when the patient's last menstrual period began. Can you finish the question?

_____

_____

_____

_____

> ¿Cuándo fue el primer día de su último _____?

2. Joy wants to ask if the patient is sexually active. Can you fill in the right phrase?

_____

_____

_____

_____

> ¿Tiene Ud. _____ actualmente?

3. A patient has told Joy he feels a burning sensation when he urinates. Can you help Joy ask the patient where he feels the burning sensation?

_____

_____

_____

_____

> ¿Dónde siente Ud. _____?

> ¿Tiene Ud. dificultad a veces cuando _____ a orinar?

4. Joy wants to know if the patient has trouble starting a urine stream. Can you supply the right verb?

_____

_____

_____

_____

Answer key

1. What was the first day of your last menstrual period?
¿Cuándo fue el primer día de su último <u>periodo menstrual</u>?

2. Are you sexually active?
¿Tiene Ud. <u>relaciones sexuales</u> actualmente?

3. Where do you feel the burning sensation?
¿Dónde siente Ud. <u>el ardor</u>?

4. Do you have trouble starting a urine stream?
¿Tiene Ud. dificultad a veces cuando <u>comienza</u> a orinar?

Examining the musculoskeletal system

Health problems

Health problems associated with the musculoskeletal system involve weakness, swelling, pain, and impaired movement. (See *Asking parents about their child's musculoskeletal problems*, page 104.) To learn the Spanish for anatomic terms that may be relevant to your patient's condition, see *Skeletal muscles—Los músculos del esqueleto*, pages 106 and 107, and *Bones of the human skeleton—Los huesos del esqueleto humano*, pages 108 and 109.

Moving slowly

Do you have any trouble moving?

¿Tiene algún problema para moverse?

Do you have a problem with:
– raising your arm?
– turning your head?
– kneeling?
– bending over?
– other?

¿Tiene Ud. problema con:
– levantar el brazo?
– voltear la cabeza?
– arrodillarse?
– agacharse?
– otro?

When did the problem start?

¿Cuándo comenzó el problema?

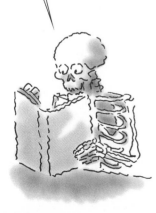

Whaddya know? *Rigidez* (stiffness) looks like *rigidity*.

What's the cause?

Is your movement limited because of pain?
– What else do you think might be causing this problem?

¿Piensa Ud. que el dolor limita alguno de sus movimientos?
– ¿Qué otra cosa piensa Ud. que podría ser la causa de este problema?

Does anything improve your ability to move?
– What?

¿Hay algo que mejora el movimiento?

– ¿Qué?

What makes movement worse?

¿Qué empeora el movimiento?

Have you noticed any other signs or symptoms such as:
– fever?
– rash?

¿Ha notado Ud. algún otro síntoma tal como:
– fiebre?
– erupción?

La clinica

Asking parents about their child's musculoskeletal problems

If you suspect musculoskeletal problems in a child, here are some questions to help you assess the child's history and current symptoms.

Labor and delivery

Were labor and delivery difficult?	¿Fue difícil el parto?
At what age did the child first do the following:	¿A qué edad hizo la criatura lo siguiente?
Hold up his head?	¿Sostener la cabeza levantada?
Sit?	¿Sentarse?
Crawl?	¿Gatear?
Pull himself into a standing position?	¿Pararse?
Walk?	¿Andar?
Have you noticed any lack of coordination?	¿Ha notado Ud. alguna falta de coordinación?
Can the child move about normally?	¿Puede la criatura moverse normalmente?
Would you describe the child's strength as normal for his age?	¿Diría Ud. que la fuerza de la criatura es normal para su edad?
Can the child roll over without help?	¿Puede la criatura darse vuelta sin ayuda?
Can the child hold up his head?	¿Puede la criatura sostener la cabeza le vantada?

Past injuries

Has the child ever broken a bone?	¿El niño/la niña ya se ha fracturado algún hueso?
Which one?	¿Cuál de ellos?
Arm?	¿Brazo?
Leg?	¿Pierna?
Elbow?	¿Codo?
Wrist?	¿Muñeca?
When?	¿Cuándo?
How did the break happen?	¿Cómo ocurrió la fractura?
Did any complications occur during the healing?	¿Se le desarrollaron complicaciones mientras sanaba?
Did the child develop an infection?	¿Tuvo alguna infección?
Did the extremity swell up?	¿Se le hinchó la extremidad?
Did the cast have to be removed?	¿Se le tuvo que quitar el yeso?
How long was the cast on?	¿Por cuánto tiempo llevó puesto el yeso?
Did the broken bone have to be reset?	¿Se le tuvo que volver a encajar el hueso roto?

– numbness?	– adormecimiento?
– inflammation?	– inflamación?
– joint grinding?	– articulaciones que crujen?
– tingling?	– hormigueo?
– swelling?	– hinchazón?
Are you having any joint or muscle pain?	¿Tiene usted dolor en las articulaciones o músculos?

– Can you point to the area where you feel pain?	– ¿Me puede indicar dónde siente Ud. el dolor?
– How long have you had the pain?	– ¿Hace cuánto tiempo que Ud. tiene este dolor?
A day?	¿Un día?
A week?	¿Una semana?
Several months?	¿Varios meses?
Is the pain constant or intermittent?	¿Es constante el dolor o es intermitente?

(See *Talking about pointing.*)

When does it hurt?

Does the pain occur at any specific time?	¿Le empieza el dolor a una hora específica?
– When?	– ¿Cuándo?
In the early morning?	¿Temprano por la mañana?
During the day?	¿Durante el curso del día?
After activities?	¿Después de hacer ciertas actividades?
Which activities?	¿Qué actividades?
At night?	¿Por la noche?
While you're sleeping?	¿Mientras Ud. duerme?
How would you describe the pain?	¿Cómo describiría Ud. el dolor?
– Dull ache?	– ¿Dolor sordo?
– Burning sensation?	– ¿Sensación de ardor?
– Sharp and stabbing, like a knife?	– ¿Agudo y punzante, como una cuchillada?
– Throbbing?	– ¿Palpitante?
– Pressure?	– ¿Presión?

Zip code for pain

When you have this pain, do you also have pain in any other area?	Cuando Ud. siente este dolor, ¿siente al mismo tiempo dolor en otro lugar?
– Can you point to the other area where you feel pain?	– ¿En qué otro lugar le duele?
– Is the pain in this area the same kind of pain?	– ¿Es el dolor de esta región del mismo tipo que el otro?
When did this pain begin?	¿Cuándo comenzó este dolor?
– What were you doing at the time it began?	– ¿Qué hacía Ud. en el momento que le empezó el dolor?
What lessens the pain?	¿Qué disminuye el dolor?
What makes the pain worse?	¿Qué empeora el dolor?
Do you have any unusual sensations along with the pain?	¿Tiene Ud. otras sensaciones anormales al mismo tiempo que el dolor?
– What are they?	– ¿Cuáles son?
Tingling?	¿Hormigeo?

Pump up your pronunciation

Talking about pointing

To help overcome the language barrier, you may want to ask your Spanish-speaking patient to point to the injured area. Here's how to pronounce your request:

¿Me puede indicar dónde siente Ud. el dolor? (Meh <u>pweh</u>-deh een-dee-<u>kar</u> <u>dohn</u>-deh see-<u>ehn</u>-teh oo-<u>sted</u> ehl doh-<u>lohr</u>?)

Skeletal muscles
Los músculos del esqueleto

Anterior view
Vista anterior

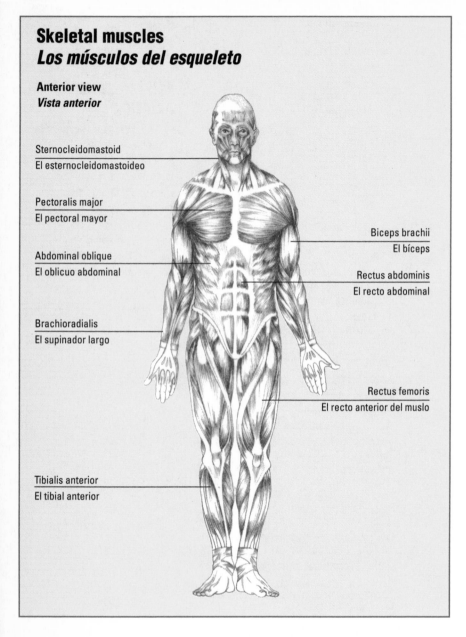

Sternocleidomastoid
El esternocleidomastoideo

Pectoralis major
El pectoral mayor

Biceps brachii
El bíceps

Abdominal oblique
El oblicuo abdominal

Rectus abdominis
El recto abdominal

Brachioradialis
El supinador largo

Rectus femoris
El recto anterior del muslo

Tibialis anterior
El tibial anterior

Burning?	¿Ardor?
Prickling?	¿Comezón?
Numbness?	¿Adormecimiento?

Creaking along

Do you have any joint or muscle stiffness?

¿Tiene rigidez en las articulaciones o músculos?

Skeletal muscles

Los músculos del esqueleto (continued)

Posterior view
Vista posterior

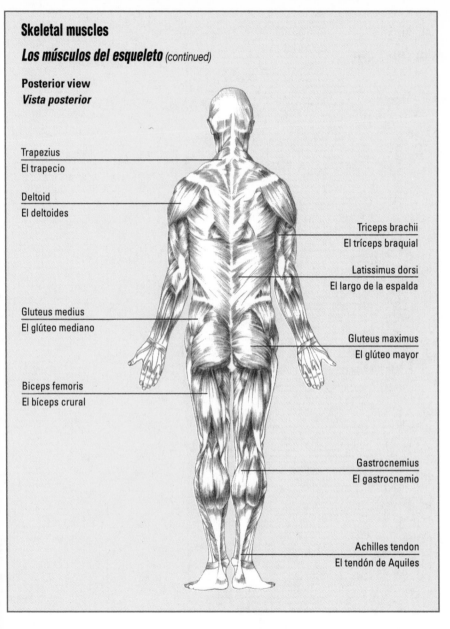

Trapezius
El trapecio

Deltoid
El deltoides

Triceps brachii
El tríceps braquial

Latissimus dorsi
El largo de la espalda

Gluteus medius
El glúteo mediano

Gluteus maximus
El glúteo mayor

Biceps femoris
El bíceps crural

Gastrocnemius
El gastrocnemio

Achilles tendon
El tendón de Aquiles

– When did it begin?	– ¿Dónde comenzó?
– Where is it?	– ¿Dónde?
Arm?	¿Brazo?
Leg?	¿Pierna?
Neck?	¿Cuello?
Hand?	¿Mano?
Jaw?	¿Mandíbula?
How would you describe the stiffness?	¿Cómo describiría Ud. la rigidez?

Bones of the human skeleton
Los huesos del esqueleto humano

Anterior view
Vista anterior

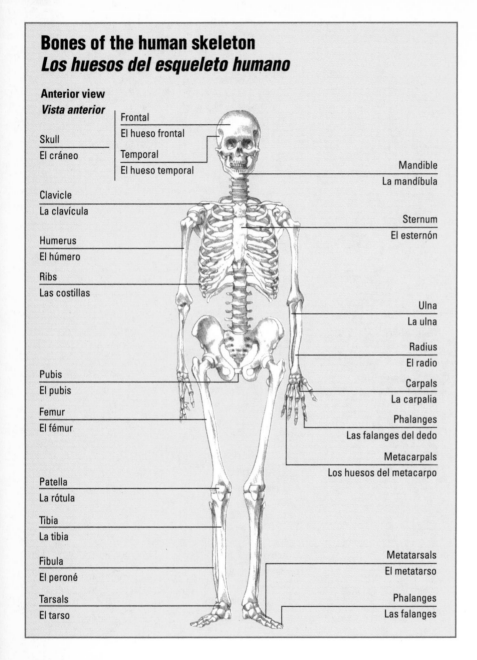

Frontal
El hueso frontal

Skull
El cráneo

Temporal
El hueso temporal

Mandible
La mandíbula

Clavicle
La clavícula

Sternum
El esternón

Humerus
El húmero

Ribs
Las costillas

Ulna
La ulna

Radius
El radio

Pubis
El pubis

Carpals
La carpalia

Femur
El fémur

Phalanges
Las falanges del dedo

Metacarpals
Los huesos del metacarpo

Patella
La rótula

Tibia
La tibia

Fibula
El peroné

Metatarsals
El metatarso

Tarsals
El tarso

Phalanges
Las falanges

– Constant?

– Intermittent?

Does the stiffness occur at any specific time?

– When?

    Early morning?

    During the day?

– ¿Constante?

– ¿Intermitente?

¿Empieza Ud. a sentir la rigidez a una hora en particular?

– ¿Cuándo?

    ¿Por la mañana temprano?

    ¿Durante el curso del día?

Bones of the human skeleton

Los huesos del esqueleto humano (continued)

Posterior view
Vista posterior

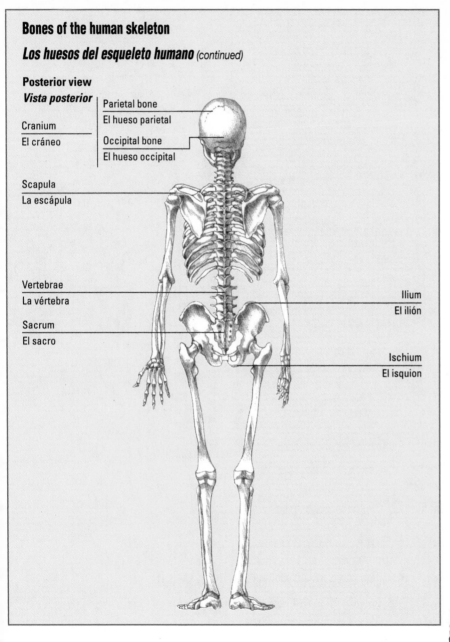

Parietal bone
El hueso parietal

Cranium
El cráneo

Occipital bone
El hueso occipital

Scapula
La escápula

Vertebrae
La vértebra

Sacrum
El sacro

Ilium
El ilión

Ischium
El isquion

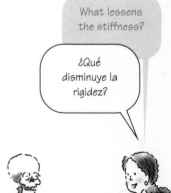

What lessens the stiffness?

¿Qué disminuye la rigidez?

After activities?	¿Después de hacer ciertas actividades?
At night?	¿Por la noche?
While you're sleeping?	¿Mientras Ud. duerme?
What lessens the stiffness?	¿Qué disminuye la rigidez?
What makes it worse?	¿Qué la empeora?

Pain also?

Do you have pain with the stiffness?
– What's the pain like?
  Dull ache?
  Burning sensation?
  Sharp and stabbing, like a knife?

  Throbbing?
  Pressure?

Do you sometimes hear a grating sound or feel a grating sensation as if your bones are scraping together?

Do you ever hear a pop in your joints?

¿Tiene Ud. dolor junto con la rigidez?
– ¿Cómo es el dolor?
  ¿Dolor sordo?
  ¿Sensación de ardor?
  ¿Agudo y punzante, como una cuchillada?
  ¿Palpitante?
  ¿Presión?

¿Hay ocasiones en que Ud. oye un chirrido o siente que los huesos chirrian como si se rozaran los unos con los otros?

¿Alguna vez escucha que le crujen las articulaciones?

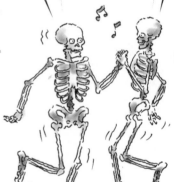

Do you ever hear a pop in your joints?

¿Alguna vez escucha que le crujen las acticulaciones?

Quite often!

¡Muy a menudo!

Home remedies

What methods have you tried to reduce the pain or stiffness?
– Exercise?
– Stretching?
– Over-the-counter medications?
    Which ones?
    How often do you take them?
– Warm baths?
– Heating pads?
– Creams?

¿Qué remedios ha intentado Ud. para aminorar el dolor o la rigidez?
– ¿Hacer ejercicios?
– ¿Extirarse?
– ¿Medicamentos sin receta?
    ¿Cuáles?
    ¿Con qué frecuencia los toma?
– ¿Baños calientes?
– ¿Compresas calientes?
– ¿Pomadas?

Tender skin

Do you ever have swelling in your joints or muscles?

When did you first notice swelling?

Did you injure this area?

Is the area tender?

Does the overlying skin ever look red or feel hot?

What have you tried to reduce the swelling?
– Have you tried applying heat?
– Have you tried applying ice?

¿Se le hinchan las articulaciones o músculos?

¿Cuándo notó Ud. la hinchazón por primera vez?

¿Se lastimó Ud. esta región?

¿Está adolorida esta región?

¿Parece a veces que la epidermis esta enrojecida o caliente?

¿Qué remedio ha intentado Ud. para reducir la hinchazón?
– ¿Ha tratado Ud. de aplicarle calor?
– ¿Ha tratado Ud. de aplicarle hielo?

Not strong, but...

Have you ever felt weak?	¿Se ha sentido débil alguna vez?
How would you describe the weakness?	¿Cómo describiría Ud. la debilidad?
When did you first notice the weakness?	¿Cuándo notó Ud. la debilidad por primera vez?
Did the weakness begin in the muscles where you now notice it?	¿Comenzó la debilidad en los mismos músculos que ahora la tienen?

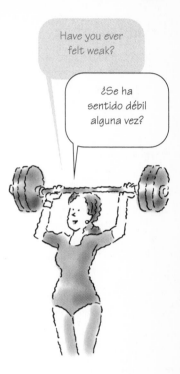

Have you ever felt weak?

¿Se ha sentido débil alguna vez?

Medications

What prescription medications do you take?	¿Qué medicamentos bajo receta toma?
– What are they for?	– ¿Para qué son?
What over-the-counter medications do you take?	¿Qué medicamentos de venta libre toma?
– How often do you take them?	– ¿Con qué frecuencia los toma?
What herbal remedies do you take?	¿Qué medicamentos herbales toma?
– How often do you take them?	– ¿Con qué frecuencia los toma?
What illicit drugs do you use?	¿Qué drogas ilícitas usa?
– How often do you use them?	– ¿Con qué frecuencia las usa?
Are you allergic to any medications?	¿Es alérgico(a) a algún medicamento?

Medical history

For the medical history, ask the patient about past injuries as well as diagnostic tests and treatments to address the injuries.

Even a sprain counts

Have you ever injured a:	¿Se ha lastimado Ud. alguna vez:
– bone?	– un hueso?
– muscle?	– un músculo?
– ligament?	– un ligamento?
– cartilage?	– un cartílago?
– joint?	– una articulación?
– tendon?	– un tendón?
What was the injury?	¿Qué se lastimó?
How did it occur?	¿Cómo se lo lastimó?
When did it occur?	¿Cuándo ocurrió?
How was it treated?	¿Qué tratamiento se le dió?
Have you had any lasting effects? (See *Pronounce these parts*.)	¿Ha tenido Ud. algún efecto duradero?

Pump up your pronunciation

Pronounce these parts

Use this quick pronunciation guide to help you ask about different parts of the musculo-skeletal system:

- bone—*hueso* (<u>hweh</u>-so)
- muscle—*músculo* (<u>moos</u>-kooh-loh)
- ligament—*ligamento* (lee-gah-<u>mehn</u>-toh)
- cartilage—*cartílago* (cahr-<u>tee</u>-lah-goh)
- joint—*articulación* (ahr-tee-koo-lah-see-<u>ohn</u>)
- tendon—*tendón* (tehn-<u>dohn</u>).

Under the knife

Have you had surgery or other treatment involving bone, muscle, joint, ligament, tendon, or cartilage?
– What was the surgery?
– Why was it done?

¿Ha tenido Ud. cirugía u otro tratamiento en un hueso, músculo, ligamento, tendón, cartílago, o articulación?
– ¿Cuál fue el resultado?
– ¿Por qué se realizó?

X marks the injury

Have you had X-rays of your bones?

– What was X-rayed?

– When was it X-rayed?
– What were the results?

Have you had any other tests because of a muscle or bone problem?
– What was it?
– When?
– What were the results of these tests?

¿Se le han tomado radiografías de los huesos?
– ¿De qué hueso se le tomaron las radiografías?
– ¿Cuándo se tomaron las radiografías?
– ¿Cuáles fueron los resultados?

¿Le han hecho algún otro estudio debido a un problema muscular u óseo?
– ¿Cuál?
– ¿Cuándo?
– ¿Cuáles fueron los resultados de estos análisis?

Fluid removed?

Have you had joint fluid removed or a biopsy performed?

– When?
– What were the results?

What immunizations have you had?
– Tetanus?
– Measles?
– Mumps?
– Rubella?
– Diphtheria?
– Hepatitis?

When did you have them?

Do you have any other medical problems?
– Diabetes mellitus?
– High blood pressure?
– Heart disease
– Osteoporosis
– Arthritis
– Other?

¿Se le ha extraído líquido de las articulaciones (coyunturas) o se le ha hecho una biopsia?
– ¿Cuándo?
– ¿Cuáles fueron los resultados?

¿Qué inmunizaciones ha tenido Ud.?
– ¿Tétano?
– ¿Sarampión?
– ¿Paperas?
– ¿Rubeola?
– ¿Difteria?
– ¿Hepatitis?

¿Cuándo las recibió?

¿Tiene algún otro problema médico?

– ¿Diabetes mellitus?
– ¿Presión sanguínea alta?
– ¿Enfermedad cardiaca?
– ¿Osteoporosis?
– ¿Artritis?
– ¿Otro?

Family history

Ask the patient about a family history of osteoporosis, gout, arthritis, and tuberculosis.

A short list

Has anyone in your family had:	¿Hay algún miembro de su familia que tenga:
– osteoporosis?	– osteoporosis?
– gout?	– gota?
– arthritis?	– artritis?
– tuberculosis?	– tuberculosis?
When?	¿Cuándo?
How was it treated?	¿Qué tratamiento se le dió?

Lifestyle

When asking about the patient's lifestyle, inquire about exercise habits, the patient's environment and occupation, and sensitivity to heat or cold.

Work this out

Describe your diet.	Describa su dieta.
Do you eat foods high in calcium?	¿Come alimentos con alto contenido de calcio?
Have you have a recent weight change? How much?	¿Ha tenido un cambio reciente en su peso? ¿Cuánto?
– Gain?	– ¿Aumento?
– Loss?	– ¿Pérdida?
– What type of exercise do you do?	– ¿Qué tipo de ejercicio hace Ud.?

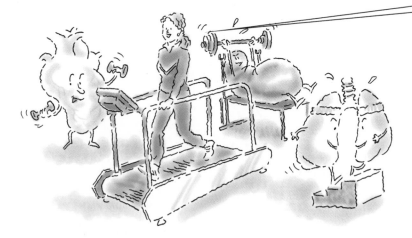

What type of exercise do you do?

¿Qué tipo de ejercicio hace Ud.?

Walking? | ¿Caminar?

Running? | ¿Correr?

Biking? | ¿Montar en bicicleta?

Lifting weights? | ¿Levantar pesas?

Aerobics? | ¿Aerobismo?

Another type? | ¿Otro?

– How often do you exercise? | – ¿Con qué frecuencia hace Ud. ejercicio?

Every day? | ¿Todos los días?

Three times per week? | ¿Tres veces por semana?

Less? | ¿Menos?

More? | ¿Más?

How has your current problem affected your usual exercise routine? | ¿Cómo le ha afectado el problema que Ud. tiene actualmente en su rutina de hacer ejercicio?

Have any of your usual activities become more difficult or impossible? | ¿Se han vuelto difíciles o imposibles algunas de sus actividades usuales?

– Dressing? | – ¿Vestirse?

– Grooming? | – ¿Peinarse?

– Climbing stairs? | – ¿Subir escaleras?

– Rising from a chair? | – ¿Levantarse de una silla?

– Getting out of bed? | – ¿Levantarse de la cama?

Are you now using a cane, walker, or brace? | ¿Usa Ud. actualmente un bastón, un andador o una abrazadera?

– Do you think using a cane, walker, or brace would be helpful? | – ¿Cree que usar un bastón, un andador, o una abrazadera ayudaría?

Do you live in a one- or two-story dwelling? | ¿Vive usted en una vivienda de un piso o de dos pisos?

Do you need to climb steps? | ¿Necesita ayuda para subir escaleras?

How does climbing steps affect your problem? | ¿De qué manera el subir escaleras afecta su problema?

What's the forecast?

Do weather changes seem to affect the problem in any way?
– How?

¿Afecta su problema el cambio de clima?

– ¿Cómo?

Does the problem increase in cold, rainy, or damp weather?

¿Aumenta su problema cuando el clima está húmedo o frío?

What is your occupation?

¿Cúal es su ocupación?

Does your work affect your problem?
– How?

¿Su trabajo afecta su problema?
– ¿De qué manera?

Does your problem affect your work?
– How?

¿Su problema afecta su trabajo?
– ¿De qué manera?

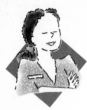

Practice makes perfecto

1. Joy is asking her patient if he has problems raising his arm. Can you finish her question?

_____

_____

_____

_____

¿Tiene Ud. algún problema al _____?

2. Now Joy wants to ask if a patient has problems bending over. Can you supply the correct phrase?

_____

_____

_____

_____

¿Tiene Ud. algún problema _____?

3. Joy notices that her patient's wrist is swollen and wants to know when the swelling began. Can you help her ask the question?

_____

_____

_____

_____

¿Cuándo notó _____?

4. Joy wants to ask if the patient injured that area. Can you supply the right verb?

_____

_____

_____

_____

¿_____ Ud. esta región?

10

Examining the immune and endocrine systems

Fast fact

Key terms for examining the immune and endocrine systems include:

- *sangrado* (bleeding)
- *dolor de las articulaciones* (joint pain)
- *contracción muscular* (muscle twitching)
- *debilidad* (weakness).

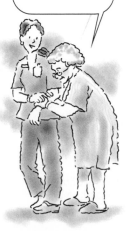

I don't remember getting this bruise.

No recuerdo cuándo recibí esta contusión.

Health problems

Health problems relevant to the immunologic and endocrine systems include bleeding, fatigue, fever, sensory changes, skin changes, swelling, and weakness. To learn the Spanish for anatomic terms that may be relevant to your patient's condition, see *Endocrine system—El sistema endocrino*, page 118.

Anything unusual?

Have you noticed unusual bleeding?
– When did it start?
– How long have you had this?
    A few days?
    Weeks?
    Months?

¿Ha notado Ud. un sangrado anormal?
– ¿Cuándo comenzó?
– ¿Hace cuánto tiempo que lo tiene?
    ¿Unos días?
    ¿Unas semanas?
    ¿Unos meses?

Where's the bleeding?
– Nose?
– Mouth?
– Gums?
– Cuts or lacerations?
– Other?

¿Dónde sangra?
– ¿En la nariz?
– ¿En la boca?
– ¿En las encías?
– ¿En cortadas o laceraciones?
– ¿Otro lugar?

Mystery spots

Have you noticed bruises that you don't remember getting?

¿Tiene Ud. contusiones que no recuerda haber recibido?

Have you ever bled for a long time from a cut?
– When did this happen?
– How did you stop the bleeding?
    Direct pressure?
    Was it sutured in the doctor's office or the emergency department?

¿Ha sangrado Ud. por mucho tiempo a causa de una cortada?
– ¿Cuándo ocurrió esto?
– ¿Cómo paró Ud. el flujo de sangre?
    ¿Aplicando presión directa?
    ¿Se le suturó (cosió) en el consultorio del médico o en la clínica de emergencia?

How long were you bleeding for?

¿Durante cuánto tiempo sangró?

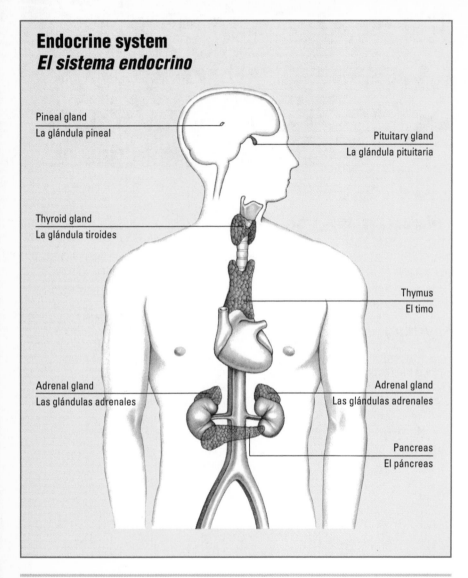

Endocrine system
El sistema endocrino

Pineal gland
La glándula pineal

Pituitary gland
La glándula pituitaria

Thyroid gland
La glándula tiroides

Thymus
El timo

Adrenal gland
Las glándulas adrenales

Adrenal gland
Las glándulas adrenales

Pancreas
El páncreas

Blood where it doesn't belong

Have you vomited recently?	¿Ha vomitado Ud. últimamente?
– What color was it?	– ¿De qué color fue?
Bright red?	¿Rojo vivo?
Brown?	¿Pardo?
Black?	¿Negro?
Other?	¿Otro?

Have you noticed blood with your bowel movements?

¿Ha notado sangre en su materia fecal?

Have you had any black, tarry bowel movements?

¿Ha tenido Ud. defecación negra, alquitranada?

Do you have hemorrhoids?
– If so, do you experience any discomfort when defecating?

¿Tiene hemorroides?
– Si así fue, ¿sintió Ud. alguna molestia al defecar?

Have you noticed blood in your urine?

¿Notó sangre en su orina?

Have you noticed any change in the color of your urine?
– What color was it?
    Pink?
    Bright red?
    Other?
– Was the urine cloudy?
    Clear?

¿Ha notado Ud. algún cambio en el color de la orina?
– ¿De qué color fue?
    ¿Color rosado?
    ¿Rojo vivo?
    ¿Otro?
– ¿Era la orina turbia?
    ¿Clara?

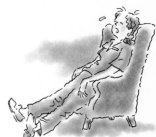

Do you ever feel tired?

¿Se siente Ud. cansado(a) alguna vez?

Talk about being tired

Do you ever feel tired?
– When?
    Morning?
    Afternoon?
    Night?

¿Se siente Ud. cansado(a) alguna vez?
– ¿Cuándo?
    ¿Por la mañana?
    ¿Por la tarde?
    ¿Por la noche?

Are you tired all the time or only after doing something strenuous?

¿Está Ud. cansado(a) todo el tiempo o sólo después de hacer ejercicio?

Do you take naps?
– How often do you nap?

– For how long?

¿Duerme Ud. la siesta?
– ¿Con qué frecuencia duerme Ud. la siesta?
– ¿Por cuánto tiempo?

How many hours do you sleep at night?
– Do you feel rested when you wake up?

¿Cuántas horas duerme a la noche?
– ¿Se siente descansado(a) al despertar?

Burning up

Have you had a fever recently?
– How high was it?

¿Ha tenido Ud. fiebre últimamente?
– ¿A cuánto le subió la fiebre?

How would you describe the fever?
– Constant?
– Intermittent?

¿Cómo describiría Ud. la fiebre?
– ¿Constante?
– ¿Intermitente?

Did it follow any particular pattern?
– What type of pattern?
    Recurs every few days?
    Rises and falls within a day?
    Occurs in the morning?
    Occurs at night?

¿Siguió un patrón en particular?
– ¿Qué tipo de patrón?
    ¿Le volvió a los pocos días?
    ¿Sube y baja dentro del mismo día?
    ¿Otro tipo de cambio?
    ¿Se produce de noche?

Joint pain

Do you ever have joint pain?

¿Tiene Ud. alguna vez dolor en las articulaciones?

> A patient who has a Mexican background may say *calentura* instead of *fiebre* for fever.

– Which joints are affected?

Elbows?
Hands or fingers?
Hips?
Knees?
– How often does it occur?
– How long does it last?
– What makes the pain worse?
– What eases the pain?

Does swelling, redness, or warmth accompany the pain?

Do your bones ache?

– ¿Qué articulaciones (coyunturas) se le afectan?
¿Los codos?
¿Las manos o los dedos?
¿Las caderas?
¿Las rodillas?
– ¿Con qué frecuencia ocurre esto?
– ¿Cuánto tiempo dura?
– ¿Qué es lo que agrava el dolor?
– ¿Qué es lo que mitiga el dolor?

¿Va el dolor acompañado de hinchazón, enrojecimiento, o calor?

¿Le duelen a Ud. los huesos?

Sight and sound

Have you developed any vision problems recently?
– What kind of changes?
Blurred vision?
Flashing lights?
Double vision?
Increased sensitivity to light?
Floating spots?
Other?
– When did you first notice them?
– How long have you had them?

Do your eyes ever burn or feel gritty when you close them?
– When does this occur?
(See *How recent?*)

Has your hearing changed recently?
– Has it decreased?
– Do you have ringing in your ears?
– In both ears or in one ear?
Which one?
– When did you first notice the change?

– How long have you experienced the change?

¿Ha tenido a Ud. problemas de visión últimamente?
– ¿Qué clase de cambios?
¿Visión borrosa?
¿Halos de luz?
¿Visión doble?
¿Mayor sensibilidad a la luz?
¿Ve manchas negras?
¿Otro?
– ¿Cuándo los notó Ud. por primera vez?
– ¿Hace cuánto tiempo que los tiene?

¿Hay veces que los ojos le arden o se sienten arenosos cuando Ud. los cierra?
¿Cuándo ocurre esto?

¿Ha cambiado su audición últimamente?
– ¿Cómo?
– ¿Le zumban los oídos?
– ¿En ambos o en un oído?
¿Cuál?
– ¿Cuándo notó Ud. el cambio por primera vez?
– ¿Por cuánto tiempo ha sentido el cambio?

Spots and sores

Have you noticed changes in your skin?

– Describe the change.

Have you had any sores that heal slowly?

¿Ha notado Ud. algunos cambios en su piel?

– Describa el cambio.

¿Ha tenido Ud. alguna llaga que demora en sanar?

Joy's grammar guide

How recent?

If a patient indicates that he has noticed a particular symptom, it's helpful to know how long ago that symptom occurred. Begin by saying *¿Este síntoma ocurrió___?* (Did the symptom occur___?) and then add one of the following phrases:
• recently—*últimamente*
• 1 week ago—*hace 1 semana*
• 2 weeks ago—*hace 2 semanas*
• 1 month ago—*hace 1 mes*
• 2 months ago—*hace 2 meses*
• 6 months ago—*hace 6 meses*
• 1 year ago—*hace 1 año*
• more than 1 year ago—*hace más de 1 año.*

– Where are the sores?

– When did they develop?

– What measures have you used to help them heal?

Have you noticed any rashes or skin discolorations?

– Point to the areas where you have noticed rashes.

– How long have you had this problem?

– ¿Dónde tiene Ud. las llagas?

– ¿Cuándo se le desarrollaron?

– ¿Qué medidas ha tomado Ud. para aliviarlas?

¿Ha notado Ud. alguna erupción o descoloramiento de la piel?

– Señále las áreas donde haya notado erupciones.

– ¿Hace cuánto tiempo que lo tiene?

You're swell

Have you noticed swelling in any of the following areas?

– Neck?

– Armpits?

– Groin?

Are the swollen areas sore, hard, or red?

Do they appear on one or both sides?

How long have you had the swelling?

– When did you first notice the swelling?

¿Ha notado Ud. algo de hinchazón en alguna de las siguientes áreas?

– ¿El cuello?

– ¿Las axilas?

– ¿La ingle?

¿Están las áreas hinchadas adoloridas, duras, o rojas?

¿Le han aparecido de un lado o de los dos?

¿Hace cuánto tiempo que Ud. tiene la hinchazón?

– ¿Cuándo notó Ud. la hinchazón por primera vez?

Weakly discussion

Do you ever feel weak?

– When?

Are you weak all the time or only at certain times?

Does weakness ever interfere with your ability to perform your usual tasks?

¿Se siente Ud. débil a veces?

– ¿Cuándo?

¿Está Ud. débil todo el tiempo o sólo en ciertas ocasiones?

¿Interfiere la debilidad con su habilidad de hacer sus quehaceres cotidianos?

Not yourself lately?

Have you recently experienced any changes in your normal behavior, such as nervousness, mood swings, or sadness?

– When did you first notice this?

– How long have you experienced this?

    For a few days?

    For a week?

¿Ha notado Ud. últimamente algún cambio en su conducta normal, tal como nerviosismo, o cambios de humor?

– ¿Cuándo notó Ud. esto por primera vez?

– ¿Hace cuánto tiempo que Ud. ha tenido esto?

    ¿Por unos días?

    ¿Por una semana?

Have you recently experienced mood swings?

¿Ha notado Ud. últimamente cambios de humor?

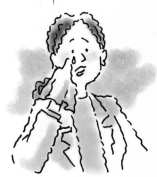

For a month?	¿Por un mes?
For several months?	¿Por varios meses?
How would you rate your memory and attention span?	¿Cómo clasificaría Ud. su memoria y el tiempo que dura su atención?
Have you noticed any muscle twitching?	¿Ha notado Ud. alguna contracción muscular?
– Where?	– ¿Dónde?
– Can you point to where the muscles twitch?	– ¿Puede indicarme dónde le ocurre?
– How long does it last?	– ¿Cuánto tiempo le dura?
– When did you first notice the twitching?	– ¿Cuándo notó Ud. la contracción por primera vez?
How would you describe it?	¿Cómo la describiría Ud.?
– Constant?	– ¿Constante?
– Intermittent?	– ¿Intermitente?
Does the twitching seem to follow a pattern?	¿Sigue un patrón en particular?
– What kind of pattern?	– ¿Qué tipo de patrón?
Do you feel any numbness or tingling in your arms or legs?	¿Siente Ud. algún adormecimiento u hormigueo en los brazos o las piernas?

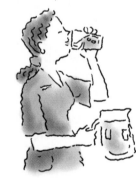

How much liquid do you drink per day?

¿Cuánto líquido bebe Ud. al día?

Increased intake?

Have you noticed feeling unusually thirsty lately?	¿Ha tenido Ud. más sed que de costumbre últimamente?
– When did you first notice feeling unusually thirsty?	– ¿Cuándo fue la primera vez que notó que se sentía inusualmente sediento(a)?
– How long have you felt this way?	– ¿Hace cuánto tiempo que se siente Ud. así?
What types of liquid do you drink?	¿Qué tipode líquidos ingiere?
How much liquid do you drink a day?	¿Cuánto líquido bebe Ud. al día?

More bathroom breaks

How many times do you urinate each day?	¿Cuántas veces al día orina Ud.?
Have you noticed an increase in the amount of urine you pass?	¿Ha notado un aumento en la cantidad de orina?
– How much of an increase?	– ¿Cuánto ha aumentado?
– When did you first notice this?	– ¿Cuándo notó Ud. esto por primera vez?

More or less of you?

Have you recently gained weight unintentionally?	¿Aumentó recientemente de peso sin proponérselo?
– How much?	– Cuánto?
– Over what time period?	– Durante cuánto tiempo?
Have you recently lost weight unintentionally?	¿Ha perdido peso Ud. últimamente sin proponérselo?
– How much?	– ¿Cuánto?
– Over what time period?	– ¿Durante cuánto tiempo?

Medical history

For the medical history, investigate if the patient has ever had a blood transfusion, had an organ transplant, or been rejected as a blood donor. Also investigate if the patient was born with a glandular or endocrine problem. (See *Asking parents or caregivers about a child's endocrine problems*, page 124.)

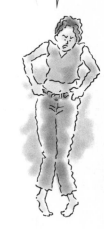

Have you recently gained weight unintentionally?

¿Aumentó recientemente de peso sin proponérselo?

Pins and needles

Have you had any difficulty walking, or do you experience a pins-and-needles sensation?	¿Ha tenido Ud. dificultad al andar, o ha sentido un hormigueo?
– When did it start?	– ¿Cuándo empezó esto?
– How long have you had this?	– ¿Hace cuánto tiempo que ha tenido esto?

Breathing woes

Have you recently developed wheezing?	¿Ha tenido últimamente una respiración jadeante?
– A runny nose?	– ¿Le gotea la nariz?
– Difficulty breathing?	– ¿Dificultad en respirar?
– When did the problem start?	– ¿Cuándo empezó?
Do you ever have heart palpitations?	¿Tiene Ud. alguna vez palpitaciones del corazón?
– When?	– ¿Cuándo?
– What aggravates them?	– ¿Qué es lo que las agrava?
– What relieves them?	– ¿Qué es lo que las mitiga?

Not another cold

Are you bothered by a persistent or recurrent cough or cold?	¿Le molesta un catarro o una tos persistente o recurrente?
– Do you cough up sputum?	– ¿Escupe Ud. esputo al toser?
– How much sputum?	– ¿Cuánto?
– What color is it?	– ¿De qué color es el esputo?
Red?	¿Rojo?

La clinica

Asking parents or caregivers about a child's endocrine problems

When obtaining a health history on a child, remember to ask the parent or caregiver the following questions about possible immune system problems.

Is the infant breast-fed or bottle-fed?	¿Amamnta al bebé ole de la mamila o el biberón?
What type of formula do you use?	¿Qué clase de fórmula usa Ud.?
Does the child ever seem pale or lethargic?	¿Hay veces que la criatura se ve pálida o letárgica?
Does the child sleep too much?	¿Duerme la criatura demasiado?
Has the child gained weight at a normal rate?	¿Ha aumentado de peso la criatura a un ritmo normal?
Did the mother have any obstetric bleeding complications?	¿Tuvo la madre alguna complicación obstétrica o sangrado?
Were the parents' blood types Rh compatible?	¿Era la sangre de los padres de tipo Rh compatible?
Does the child have frequent or continuous severe infections?	¿Tiene la criatura infecciones graves con frecuencia o continuamente?
What kinds of infections?	¿Qué clase de infecciones?
How long do they last?	¿Cuánto tiempo le duran?
How are the infections treated?	¿Qué tratamiento se da a las infecciones?
Does the child have any allergies?	¿Tiene la criatura alguna alergia?
To what?	¿A qué?
Does anyone else in the family have allergies?	¿Hay otro miembro de la familia que tenga alergias?
To what?	¿A qué?
Which immunizations has the child received?	¿Qué inmunizaciones se han puesto a la criatura?

Pink?	¿Color rosado?
Blood-streaked?	¿Con vetas de sangre?
Yellow?	¿Amarillo?
White?	¿Blanco?
Frothy or foamy?	¿Espumoso?
Clear?	¿Claro?
Do you feel chest pain when you cough, breathe deeply, or laugh?	¿Siente Ud. dolor de pecho cuando tose, cuando respira profundamente, o cuando se ríe?
Have you had a sore throat?	¿Tiene dolor de garganta?
Have you had sore throats in the past? – Frequently?	¿Tuvo dolores de garganta antes? – ¿Frecuentemente?
Do you recall being seriously ill as a child or having a long illness requiring frequent visits to a doctor?	¿Recuerda Ud. si de niño(a) estuvo enfermo(a) de gravedad o si tuvo una enfermedad prolongada que requiriera visitas frecuentes al médico?
Has your appetite changed recently?	¿Ha cambiado su apetito últimamente?
Do you experience nausea? – Flatulence? – Diarrhea?	¿Tiene Ud. náuseas? – ¿Flatulencia? – ¿Diarrea?

Has your appetite changed recently?

¿Ha cambiado su apetito últimamente?

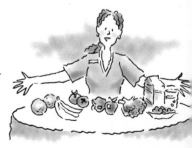

Wheezin' and sneezin'

Do you have allergies?

– What causes them?

– Which symptoms are most bothersome?

Have you ever had asthma?

¿Tiene Ud. alergias?

– ¿Qué es lo que las provoca?

– ¿Qué síntomas le molestan más?

¿Ha tenido Ud. asma alguna vez?

How 'bout a little history?

Do you have an autoimmune disease such as acquired immunodeficiency syndrome?

– Have you tested positive for human immunodeficiency virus?

Have you had any other disorders or health problems?

– Which ones?

Have you ever had surgery?

– What type?

– When?

Have you ever been in military service?

– When?

– Where did you serve?

¿Sufre Ud. de alguna enfermedad autoinmune tal como síndrome de inmunodeficiencia adquirida?

– ¿Ha tenido Ud. un análisis positivo del virus de inmunodeficiencia humana?

¿Ha tenido Ud. otros trastornos o problemas de salud?

– ¿Cuáles?

¿Ha tenido Ud. cirugía alguna vez?

– ¿Qué tipo?

– ¿Cuándo?

¿Ha servido Ud. alguna vez en el ejército?

– ¿Cuándo?

– ¿Dónde hizo Ud. el servicio militar?

Medications

What prescription medications do you take?

– What are they for?

What over-the-counter medications do you take?

– How often do you take them?

What herbal remedies do you take?

– How often do you take them?

What illicit drugs do you use?

– How often do you use them?

Are you allergic to any medications?

¿Qué medicamentos bajo receta toma?

– ¿Para qué son?

¿Qué medicamentos de venta libre toma?

– ¿Con qué frecuencia los toma?

¿Qué medicamentos herbales toma?

– ¿Con qué frecuencia los toma?

¿Qué drogas ilícitas usa?

– ¿Con qué frecuencia las usa?

¿Es alérgico(a) a algún medicamento?

Importing parts

Have you had an organ transplant?

¿Se ha transplantado a Ud. algún órgano?

– When?
– What kind of transplant?
– What follow-up care did you receive?

– ¿Cuándo?
– ¿Qué tipo de transplante?
– ¿Qué tratamiento complementario se le dió?

Have you ever had a blood transfusion?

¿Ha tenido Ud. alguna vez una transfusión de sangre?

– When?
– Why?
– How many units did you receive?

– ¿Cuándo?
– ¿Por qué?
– ¿Cuántas unidades le dieron?

Did you ever have a reaction to a transfusion?
– What happened?

¿Alguna vez tuvo una reacción a una transfusión?
– ¿Qué sucedió?

Have you ever been rejected as a blood donor?
– Do you know why?

¿Lo(a) han rechazado alguna vez como donante de sangre?
– ¿Por qué?

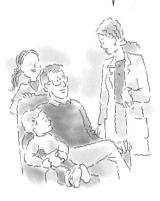

Have you had an organ transplant?

¿Se ha transplantado a Ud. algún órgano?

Hit your head?

Have you ever had a skull fracture or broken bones in other areas of the body?

¿Ha sufrido alguna vez una fractura de cráneo o fracturas de huesos en otras partes del cuerpo?

– When?
– How was it treated?

– ¿Cuándo?
– ¿Qué tratamiento se le dió?

Radical treatment

Have you ever had radiation treatments?

¿Ha tenido Ud. alguna vez tratamienos de radiación?

– Why?

– ¿Por qué?

Have you ever had a brain infection, such as meningitis or encephalitis?

¿Ha tenido Ud. alguna vez una infección del cerebro, tal como meningitis o encefalitis?

– When?
– How was it treated?

– ¿Cuándo?
– ¿Qué tratamiento se le dió?

Tall or short

Were you considered tall or short for your age?
– Did you have any growth spurts?

¿Se consideraba a Ud. alto(a) o bajo(a) para su edad?
– ¿Tuvo Ud. momentos repentinos de crecimiento?

    When?
    To what degree?

    ¿Cuándo?
    ¿En qué grado?

Have you ever been diagnosed as having an endocrine or glandular problem?
– What was the problem?
– When was it diagnosed?
– How was it treated?

¿Se le ha diagnosticado alguna vez un problema endocrino o glandular?
– ¿Cuál fue el problema?
– ¿Cuándo se diagnosticó a Ud.?
– ¿Qué tratamiento se le dió?

Skin shifts

Have you had any changes in your skin such as acne?
– Increased or decreased oiliness?

– Dryness?
– Changes in color?
– When?

¿Ha tenido Ud. algunos cambios de la piel tal como acné?
– ¿Aumento o disminución de la grasa natural de la piel?
– ¿Resequedad?
– ¿Cambio de color?
– ¿Cuándo?

Do you bruise more easily than you used to?

¿Le salen contusiones con mayor facilidad que antes?

Have you noticed any increase in the size of your hands or feet?

¿Ha notado Ud. algún aumento en el tamaño de las manos o de los pies?

Do your fingernails and toenails ever seem brittle?

– Have they thickened or separated from your fingers and toes?

¿Le parece a Ud. que hay veces que las uñas de las manos y de los pies están quebradizas?
– ¿Ha aumentado el espesor de las uñas o se han separado de los dedos de la mano y del pie?

Have you noticed any change in the hair on your body?

¿Ha notado Ud. algún cambio en el cabello de cuerpo?

Describe the change.
– When did you notice the change?
– Have you observed more or less hair?

Describa el cambio.
– ¿Cuándo notó el cambio?
– ¿Ha observado más o menos cabello?

Has your voice changed?
– How?

¿Ha cambiado su voz?
–¿Cómo?

Change in shirt size

Have you ever had neck pain?

¿Ha tenido Ud. alguna vez dolor de cuello?

Does your neck seem larger than normal?
– Have you noticed that your shirts or blouses are tighter at the neck?

¿Le parece a Ud. que su cuello está más ancho de lo normal?
– ¿Ha notado Ud. que sus camisas o blusas le quedan más apretadas en el cuello que antes?

Extra beats

Have you ever felt as though your heart was racing for no reason?

¿Hay veces que Ud. siente que el corazón le late a un ritmo exagerado sin motivo?

Have you ever been told you have high blood pressure?
– When was it diagnosed?
– How was it treated?

¿Se le ha dicho a Ud. alguna vez que tiene la presión sanguínea alta?
– ¿Cuándo se le diagnosticó?
– ¿Qué tratamiento se le dió?

Have you ever had seizures?
– What parts of your body were involved when you had the seizure?
– Under what circumstances did you have the seizure?

¿Ha tenido Ud. alguna vez convulsiones?
– ¿Qué partes de su cuerpo sufrieron las convulsiones?
– ¿En qué circunstancias?

Have you ever had a migraine?
– How often do you have one?

¿Tuvo migrañas alguna vez?
– ¿Con qué frecuencia?

Do you ever have sudden, severe headaches that go away gradually?

¿Tiene Ud. alguna vez dolores de cabeza repentinos que desaparecen gradualmente?

Family history

Investigate if anyone in the patient's family has or ever had an immune or endocrine disorder or other problems. The family history will also help you determine if any of the patient's family members have or ever had a blood disorder, high blood pressure, or elevated blood fats.

Checking the bloodline

How would you describe the health of your blood relatives? (See *All in the family*, page 39.)
– Excellent?
– Good?
– Fair?
– Poor?

¿Cómo describiría Ud. la salud de sus parientes consanguíneos(as)?

– ¿Excelente?
– ¿Buena?
– ¿Regular?
– ¿Mala?

How old are your living relatives?

¿Qué edad tienen sus parientes que aún viven?

How old were those who died?

¿De qué edad murieron los otros?

What caused their deaths?
– Heart problems?
– Diabetes?
– Stroke?
– Cancer?
– Breathing problems, such as lung disease or asthma?
– Infection?

¿Qué fue lo que causó su muerte?
– ¿Problemas cardiacos?
– ¿Diabetes?
– ¿Apoplejía?
– ¿Cáncer?
– ¿Problemas respiratorios, como enfermedad del pulmoñ o asma?
– ¿Infección?

Do or did any of them have immune, blood, or other problems?

¿Tienen o tuvieron algunos de ellos problemas inmunológicos, sanguíneos o otros?

Consulting the charts

Does anyone in your family have any of the following?
– Diabetes mellitus?
– Thyroid disease?

– High blood pressure?
– High cholesterol?
    When was it diagnosed?
    How was it treated?

¿Hay algún miembro de su familia que sufra de alguno de los siguientes?
– ¿Diabetes melitus?
– ¿Mal funcionamiento de la glándula tiroides?
– ¿Presión sanguínea alta?
– ¿Colesterol alto?
    ¿Cuándo se le diagnosticó?
    ¿Qué tratamiento se le dió?

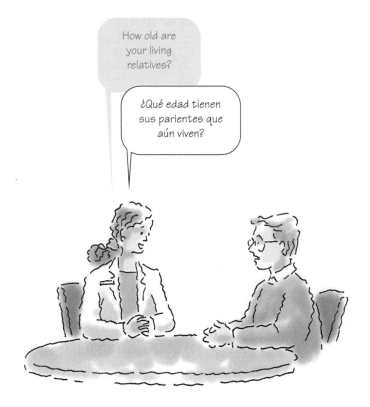

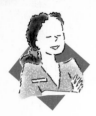

Practice makes perfecto

1. Joy wants to ask the patient if he has joint pain. Can you finish her question?

_____

_____

_____

_____

> ¿Tiene Ud. dolor en _____?

2. Now Joy wants to know how often the joint pain occurs. Can you supply the right phrase?

_____

_____

_____

_____

> ¿_____ ocurre esto?

3. Joy wants to know if a patient has noticed any muscle twitching. Can you help?

_____

_____

_____

_____

> ¿Ha notado Ud. alguna _____?

4. Joy wants to ask how long the twitching lasts. Can you give Joy the correct verb?

_____

_____

_____

_____

> ¿Cuánto tiempo le _____?

Answer key

1. Do you have joint pain?
¿Tiene Ud. dolor en <u>las articulaciones</u>?

2. How often does this occur?
<u>¿Con qué frecuencia</u> ocurre esto?

3. Have you noticed any muscle twitching?
¿Ha notado Ud. alguna <u>contracción muscular</u>?

4. How long does it last?
¿Cuánto tiempo le <u>dura</u>?

Examining the skin, hair, and nails

Fast fact

Key terms for examining the skin, hair, and nails include:

- *problemas de piel* (skin problems)
- *pérdida de cabello* (hair loss)
- *problemas con las uñas* (nail problems).

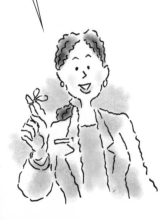

Remember *pérdida de apetito* (loss of appetite) from chapter 7? Then you'll remember *pérdida de cabello* (hair loss).

Health problems

Health problems relevant to the skin, hair, and nails include skin problems, such as rashes, sores, flaking, and dryness; hair loss; scalp infections and infestations; and nail problems, such as breakage, splitting, and discoloration. To learn the Spanish for anatomic terms that may be relevant to your patient's condition, see *Skin and hair— La piel y el cabello*, page 132.

Hair and nail history

Have you noticed any unusual overall or patchy hair loss?
– Where?

¿Ha notado Ud. pérdida de cabello en general o en ciertas partes?
– ¿Dónde?

Have you noticed any unusual overall or patchy hair growth?

¿Ha notado un crecimiento inusual del vello a nivel general o en zonas?

Have you had any recent exposure to any of the following?
– Radiation?
– Chemotherapy?
– Chemicals?
– Scalp infections?
– Infestations?
    When?
    Did you receive treatment?
    How was it treated?

¿Ha estado Ud. expuesto(a) a uno de los siguientes?
– ¿Radiación?
– ¿Quimioterapia?
– ¿Productos químicos?
– ¿Infecciones del cuero cabelludo?
– ¿Infestaciones?
    ¿Cuándo?
    ¿Recibió Ud. tratamiento?
    ¿Cómo se le trató?

Have you had an illness recently?

– What was it?
– How was it treated?

¿Ha tenido Ud. alguna enfermedad recientemente?
– ¿Qué fue?
– ¿Cómo se le trató?

Have you ever had itching or flaking in your scalp?
– How long did it last?

¿Le ha picado o se ha descamado alguna vez el cuero cabelludo?
– ¿Cuánto duró?

Skin and hair
La piel y el cabello

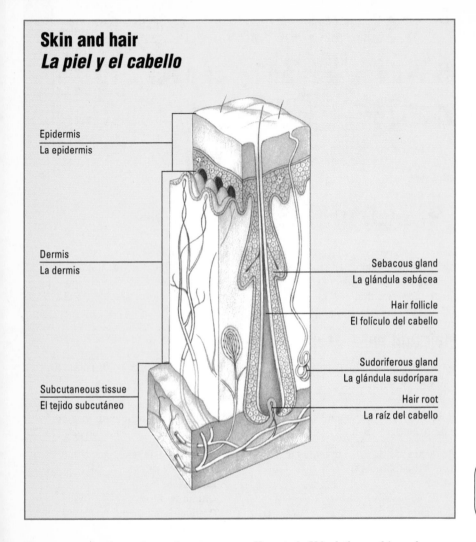

Epidermis
La epidermis

Dermis
La dermis

Subcutaneous tissue
El tejido subcutáneo

Sebacous gland
La glándula sebácea

Hair follicle
El folículo del cabello

Sudoriferous gland
La glándula sudorípara

Hair root
La raíz del cabello

Have you noticed any change in your nails?
– What type of change?
   Breakage?
   Splitting?
   Discoloration?
   Change in shape?
   Other?

When did you first notice the problem?

Has the problem gotten worse or better?

¿Ha notado Ud. algún cambio en las uñas?
– ¿Qué tipo de cambio?
   ¿Se le quiebran?
   ¿Se le agrietan?
   ¿Descoloramiento?
   ¿Un cambio en la forma?
   ¿Otra cosa?

¿Cuándo notó Ud. este problema por primera vez?

¿Se ha empeorado o mejorado el problema?

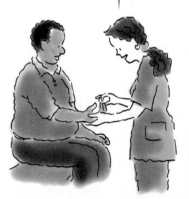

Have you noticed any change in your nails?

¿Ha notado Ud. algún cambio en las uñas?

What makes the problem worse?	¿Qué es lo que empeora el problema?
What makes the problem get better?	¿Qué es lo que alivia el problema?
How do you cut your nails?	¿Cómo se corta Ud. las uñas?
Do you bite your nails?	¿Se come las uñas?
Do you go to a podiatrist?	¿Va Ud. a un podólogo?
Do you see a dermatologist regularly?	¿Consulta un dermatólogo regularmente?

Skin deep

What about your skin problem bothers you the most?	¿Qué aspecto de su problema con la piel le molesta más?
Where on your body did the skin problem begin?	¿En qué parte del cuerpo le comenzó su problema de la piel?
When did you first notice the problem?	¿Cuándo se dió Ud. cuenta por primera vez de este problema?
Has the problem spread to other areas?	¿Se le ha extendido el problema a otras partes?
– Where?	– ¿Dónde?
– In what order?	– ¿En qué orden?

Let's talk about it

How would you describe your skin problem?	¿Cómo describiría Ud. su problema de la piel?
– Sore?	– ¿Llaga?
– Rash?	– ¿Erupción?
– Dryness?	– ¿Sequedad?
– Flaking?	– ¿Escamosidad?
– Discoloration?	– ¿Decoloración?
– Itching?	– ¿Picazón (comezón)?
– Other?	– ¿Otra cosa?
What color is the skin problem?	¿De qué color es el problema en la piel?
Do you have other symptoms?	¿Tiene Ud. otros síntomas?
– What are they?	– ¿Cuáles son?
(See *What's that spot?*)	

Mole matters

Do you have any moles?	¿Tiene lunares?
– Where?	– ¿Dónde?
– Have they changed?	– ¿Han cambiado?
Changed color?	¿Cambiaron de color?
Changed size?	¿Cambiaron de tamaño?
Changed shape?	¿De forma?

Started bleeding?	¿Comenzaron a sangrar?
– How long have you had the moles?	– ¿Cuánto hace que tiene los lunares?

Talking texture

How does your skin feel?	¿Cómo se ve su piel?
Have you noticed skin changes in other areas?	¿Ha notado Ud. cambios en la piel en otras partes?
Can you relate the skin problem to any of the following?	¿Puede Ud. relacionar el problema de la piel con cualquiera de los siguientes?
– Stress?	– ¿Tensión?
– Contact with a particular substance?	– ¿Contacto con alguna sustancia en particular?
– Change in activities?	– ¿Cambio de actividades?

Better or worse

Has the problem gotten better or worse?	El problema, ¿ha mejorado o empeorado?
Does anything make the problem better?	¿Existe algo que mejore el problema?
– Medications?	– ¿Medicamentos?
– Compresses?	– ¿Compresas?
– Lotions?	– ¿Lociones?
– Creams?	– ¿Pomadas?
– Ointments?	– ¿Ungüentos?
Does anything make the problem worse?	¿Hay algo que agrave el problema?
– Food?	– ¿La comida?
– Heat?	– ¿El calor?
– Cold?	– ¿El frío?
– Exercise?	– ¿El ejercicio?
– Sunlight?	– ¿La luz del sol?
– Stress?	– ¿La tensión?
– Pregnancy?	– ¿El embarazo?
– Menstruation?	– ¿La menstruación?

> Does sunlight make your skin problem worse?
>
> ¿Le empeora el problema de la piel la luz del sol?

Medical history

In the medical history, investigate if the patient has a history of allergies or other illnesses. (See *Asking parents and caregivers about a child's skin problems.*)

Fever, malaise, and other issues

Have you had any fever, discomfort, or breathing or stomach problems?	¿Ha tenido fiebre, molestias, o problemas respiratorios o estomacales?
– When?	– ¿Cuándo?
– How was the problem treated?	– ¿Qué tratamiento tuvo?

La clinica

Asking parents or caregivers about a child's skin problems

Remember to ask the parent or caregiver these questions about the child's skin problems:

Is the infant breast-fed or formula-fed?

¿Le da Ud. de mamar o lo (la) alimenta con fórmula?

Has the child had any skin problems related to a particular formula or food added to the diet?

¿Ha tenido el (la) niño(a) algún problema de la piel relacionado con una fórmula en particular o algún comestible que se haya añadido a su dieta?

Has the infant had any diaper rashes that didn't clear up readily with over-the-counter skin preparations?

¿Ha tenido el (la) niño(a) alguna erupción de la piel que no se le haya quitado fácilmente con alguna preparación para la piel sin necesidad de receta?

What kind of diapers do you use?

¿Qué clase de pañales usa Ud.?

How do you wash cloth diapers?

¿Cómo lava Ud. los pañales de tela?

How often do you bathe the infant?

¿Con qué frecuencia baña Ud. al niño (la niña)?

What products do you use on the infant's skin?

¿Qué productos usa Ud. en la piel de su criatura?

How do you dress the infant in hot weather and in cold weather?

¿Cómo viste Ud. a la criatura cuando hace calor y cuando hace frío?

Is the child attending nursery school?

¿Va la criatura a una guardería de niños?

Do you have an older child in kindergarten or elementary school?

¿Tiene Ud. un hijo mayor en párvulos o en la escuela primaria?

Do you have pets in your home?

¿Tiene Ud. animales en casa?

What type of pets?

¿Qué clase de animales?

Does the child sleep with stuffed animals?

¿Duerme la criatura con animales de juguete?

Has the child been scratching his scalp?

¿Se rasca la criatura el cuero cabelludo?

Does the skin or scalp scale in circular patterns?

¿La piel o el cuero cabelludo se escama en forma circular?

Has the child lost an unusual amount of hair?

¿Ha perdido la criatura una cantidad grande de cabello?

Has the child been pulling his hair?

¿El niño o la niña se jala el cabello?

Has the child ever had warts?

¿Ha tenido la criatura verrugas alguna vez?

Where?

¿Donde?

How were the warts treated?

¿Qué tratamiento se les dió?

Does the child play where he might come in contact with bugs, weeds, or other plants?

¿Juega donde puede estar en contacto con insectos, hierbas, o arbustos?

How often does the child play there?

¿Con qué frecuencia juega allí?

What does the child usually eat each day, including junk food?

¿Qué come usualmente cada día, incluyendo comida chatarra?

Has the child had any bad cuts or scrapes from falls or other accidents?

¿Ha tenido algunas heridas serias o raspaduras a causa de caídas u otros accidentes?

How long did it take the injuries to heal?

¿Cuánto tiempo tardó en sanar?

Does the child bite his nails?

¿Se muerde las uñas?

Does the child twirl or otherwise play with his hair?

¿Se enrosca o juega de otra manera con el cabello?

Does the child's face, upper back, or chest ever break out?

¿Le sale alguna vez erupción en la cara, la parte superior de la espalda, o en el pecho?

Have you recently had any other illnesses, such as heart problems, muscle aches, or infections?

¿Ha tenido Ud. recientemente cualquier otra enfermedad, tal como problemas del corazón, dolor de músculos, o infecciones?

Reading reactions

Are you allergic to any foods or other substances?
– Fruits?
– Oranges, bananas, strawberries, or mangos?
– Other foods?
– Cosmetics?
– Cleaning agents?
– Something else?
– What reaction occurred?
   Rash?
   Hives?
   Itching?
   Redness?
   Swelling?

¿Es alérgico(a) a algún alimento u otras sustancias?
– ¿Frutas?
– ¿Naranjas, plátanos, fresas o mangos?

– ¿Otras comidas?
– ¿Cosméticos?
– ¿Agentes de limpieza?
– ¿Algo más?
– ¿Qué reacción tuvo?
   ¿Erupción?
   ¿Ronchas?
   ¿Picazón (comezón)?
   ¿Enrojecimiento?
   ¿Hinchazón?

Medications

What prescription medications do you take?
– What are they for?

¿Qué medicamentos bajo receta toma?
– ¿Para qué son?

What over-the-counter medications do you take?
– How often do you take them?

¿Qué medicamentos de venta libre toma?
– ¿Con qué frecuencia los toma?

What herbal remedies do you take?
– How often do you take them?

¿Qué medicamentos herbales toma?
– ¿Con qué frecuencia los toma?

What illicit drugs do you use?
– How often do you use them?

¿Qué drogas ilícitas usa?
– ¿Con qué frecuencia las usa?

Are you allergic to any medications?

¿Es alérgico(a) a algún medicamento?

Family history

In the family history, investigate if anyone in the patient's family has or has ever had skin problem or allergies.

The skin(ny) on the family

Has anyone in your family had a skin problem?
– What was it?
   Acne?

¿Ha tenido algún miembro de su familia un problema de piel?
– ¿Cuál fue?
   ¿Acné?

Skin cancer?	¿Cáncer de piel?
Rash?	¿Erupción?
Tumor?	¿Tumor?
Allergic reaction?	¿Reacción alérgica?
Lupus?	¿Lupus?
Psoriasis?	¿Soriasis?

Has anyone in your family had an allergy?
– What was it?
– What reaction did they have?
– How was it treated?

¿Hay alguien de su familia que haya tenido alguna alergia?
– ¿Cuál fue?
– ¿Qué reacciones le provocaban?
– ¿Qué tratamiento recibió?

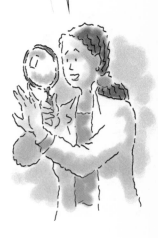

Do you try to keep your skin healthy?

¿Se cuida la piel?

Lifestyle

Ask the patient about skin and hair care habits, exposure to the sun, exposure to possible irritants, and how he copes with his health problems.

Lotions and creams

How do you clean your skin?
– What kind of soap do you use?

¿Cómo se lava la piel?
–¿Qué tipo de jabón usa?

Do you use skin creams or lotions?

¿Usa Ud. pomadas o lociones para el piel?

– How often do you use them?
  Every day?
  Twice a day?

– ¿Con qué frecuencia os usa?
  ¿Todos los días?
  ¿Dos veces por día?

Points for style

Do you use styling products on your hair?
– What do you use?
– How often do you use them?

¿Usa Ud. algún producto de belleza para el cabello?
– ¿Qué usa Ud.?
– ¿Con qué frecuencia los usa?

How often do you shampoo?

¿Con qué frecuencia se lava Ud. el cabello?

– What product do you use?

– ¿Qué productos usa?

Do you use cosmetics or perfumes?
– What type?

¿Usa Ud. cosméticos o perfumes?
– ¿Qué clase?

Do you shave with a blade or an electric razor?
Do you use creams to remove unwanted hair?
– Where?

¿Se rasura Ud. con navaja o con máquina de afeitar eléctrica?
¿Usa Ud. crema depilatoria?
– ¿Dónde?

Do you color your hair?
– How often?
– What products do you use?

¿Se tiñe Ud. el cabello?
–¿Con cuánta frecuencia?
–¿Qué productos usa?

Do you perm your hair? | ¿Se hace la permanente en el cabello?
– How often? | –¿Con cuánta frecuencia?
– What products do you use? | –¿Qué productos usa?

Fun in the sun?

Are you in the sun a lot? | ¿Pasa mucho tiempo en el sol?
– Do you wear a sunblock or cover your skin with clothing before going out in the sun? | – ¿Usa Ud. una loción para proteger su piel contra los rayos del sol o se cubre Ud. la piel con ropa antes de salir al sol?

Do you tan in tanning salons? | ¿Se broncea Ud. en salones de belleza?
– How often? | – ¿Con cuánto frecuencia?

Do you use tanning creams or lotions? | ¿Usa cremas o lociones bronceadoras?

More time at home?

Has your skin problem affected your daily activities? | ¿Ha afectado su problema de la piel sus activdades diarias?
– How? | – ¿Cómo?

What do you do for leisure activities? | ¿Cuáles son sus actividades recreacionales?

Do these activities expose you to any of the following? | ¿Lo(a) exponen estas actividades a cualquiera de los siguientes?
– Sun or other light? | – ¿El sol u otra luz?
– Chemicals or other toxins? | – ¿Productos químicos u otros tóxicos?
– Animals? | – ¿Animales?
– Outdoors? | – ¿Al aire libre?
– Foreign travel? | – ¿Viajes al extranjero?

Focus on feelings

How does the affected area look to you? | ¿En su opinión cómo se ve el area afectada?

How does your skin problem make you feel? | ¿Cómo le hace sentir el problema de su piel?

Do you have concerns about your skin problem and its treatment? | ¿Qué preocupaciones tiene Ud. con relación a su problema de la piel y su tratamiento?

Have you been upset lately? | ¿Ha sufrido algún disgusto recientemente?

Reading relationships

How has your skin problem affected your relationships with others? | ¿Cómo le ha afectado su problema de la piel en su relación con otras personas?

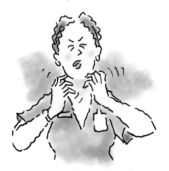

How does your skin problem make you feel?

¿Cómo le hace sentir el problema de su piel?

How do you feel about going out socially?

¿Qué sientes con respecto a salir socialmente?

Has your skin problem interfered with your role as a spouse (or student, parent, or other) or with your sexuality?

¿Ha interferido su problema de la piel con su papel de esposo(a) (o de estudiante, de padre, de madre u otro) o con su sexualidad?

Work hazards

What are your current and past occupations?

¿Cuál es su empleo actual? ¿Y los anteriores?

Does your work expose you to any of the following?
– Sun or other light?
– Chemicals or other toxins?
– Animals?
– Outdoors?
– Foreign travel?

¿Su trabajo lo(a) expone a cualquiera de los siguientes?
– ¿El sol u otra luz?
– ¿Productos químicos u otros tóxicos?
– ¿Animales?
– ¿Al aire libre?
– ¿Viajes al extranjero?

Practice, practice, practice. Try the exercises on the next page, and soon your Spanish will be *perfecto!*

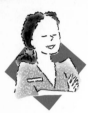

Practice makes perfecto

1. Joy wants to ask the patient if he has noticed any change in his nails. Can you supply the correct phrase?

_____

_____

_____

_____

> ¿Ha notado Ud. algún cambio _____?

2. Joy notices that a patient has a rash on his arm and wants to know if it has spread to other areas. Can you help her ask the question?

_____

_____

_____

_____

> ¿Se le ha _____ el problema a otras partes?

3. Joy's patient says that a dry area sometimes appears on her back. Joy wants to know how big the area is. Can you give Joy the right word?

_____

_____

_____

_____

> ¿De qué _____ es?

> ¿Estas actividades la exponen _____?

4. Joy wants to know if her patient's activities expose her to the sun. Can you finish her question?

_____

_____

_____

Examining the eyes, ears, nose, and throat

Eyes and health problems

Health problems associated with the eyes include blurred vision and vision changes. To learn the Spanish for anatomic terms that may be relevant to your patient's eye condition, see *Eye—El ojo*, page 142.

Blurry lines

Do you have blurred vision?
– When did you first notice it?
– How long have you had it?

¿Tiene Ud. visión borrosa?
– ¿Cuándo la notó Ud. por primera vez?
– ¿Hace cuánto tiempo que la tiene?

What things in your line of vision appear blurred?

¿Qué objetos en su campo visual parecen estar borrosos?

Is it associated with any activity, such as:
– sitting?
– standing?
– walking?
– changing positions?
– reading?
– working at the computer?
– other?
(See *Part pronunciation*, page 143.)

¿Está esto relacionado con cualquier actividad, como por ejemplo:
– estar sentado(a)?
– estar parado(a)?
– caminar?
– cambiar de posición?
– leer?
– trabajar frente a la computadora?
– otra?

Do you have a history of high blood pressure or diabetes?

¿Tiene Ud. un historial de presión sanguínea alta o de diabetes?

Do you have any other illnesses?

¿Tiene alguna otra enfermedad?

What else happens?

Do you experience other signs or symptoms, such as:
– headache?
– dizziness?
– nausea?
– fainting?

¿Tiene Ud. otros síntomas, tales como:
– dolor de cabeza?
– mareo?
– náuseas?
– desmayo?

Eye
El ojo

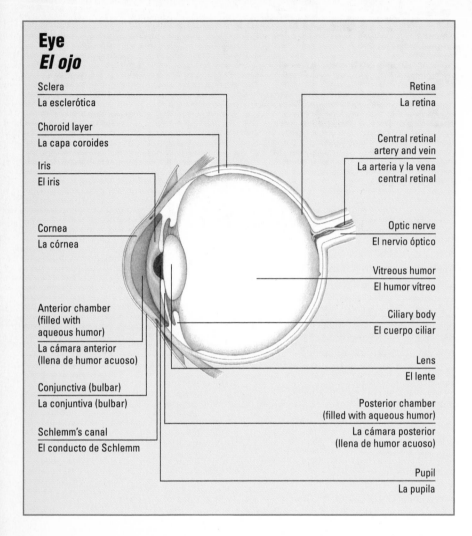

Sclera
La esclerótica

Choroid layer
La capa coroides

Iris
El iris

Cornea
La córnea

Anterior chamber
(filled with
aqueous humor)
La cámara anterior
(llena de humor acuoso)

Conjunctiva (bulbar)
La conjuntiva (bulbar)

Schlemm's canal
El conducto de Schlemm

Retina
La retina

Central retinal
artery and vein
La arteria y la vena
central retinal

Optic nerve
El nervio óptico

Vitreous humor
El humor vítreo

Ciliary body
El cuerpo ciliar

Lens
El lente

Posterior chamber
(filled with aqueous humor)
La cámara posterior
(llena de humor acuoso)

Pupil
La pupila

Does anything accompany the blurred vision?	¿Va la visión borrosa acompañada de algo más?
– Spots?	– ¿Manchas?
– Floaters?	– ¿Puntos negros?
– Halos around lights?	– ¿Halos alrededor de las luces?
– Stars?	– ¿Estrellas?
– Flashes of light?	– ¿Destellos de luz?
– Loss of vision?	– ¿Pérdida de visión?
– Pain?	– ¿Dolor?

Something sudden?

Was this a sudden change or has it occurred for a while?	¿Fue éste un cambio súbito o lo ha tenido Ud. por algún tiempo?
– How long?	– ¿Cuánto tiempo?

Does anything make the problem worse?	¿Hay algo que egrava el problema?
– What?	– ¿Qué?
Does anything make it better?	¿Hay algo que lo alivia?
– What?	– ¿Qué?

Part pronunciation

The words *ojo* (eye) and *oído* (inner ear) can be difficult to pronounce. Here's a quick guide to help you pronounce these words as well as some other parts of the body used in this chapter:

- eye—*ojo* (<u>oh</u>-hoh)
- ear—*oído* (oh-<u>ee</u>-doh)
- mouth—*boca* (<u>boh</u>-kah)
- neck—*cuello* (<u>kweh</u>-yoh).

Too close, too far

Do you have problems seeing?	¿Tiene Ud. problemas en la vista?
– What problems?	– ¿Qué problemas?
Seeing objects far away?	¿No puede ver objetos a distancia?
Seeing objects close?	¿No puede ver objetos de cerca?
Other?	¿Otros?
Have you noticed a change in your vision?	¿Ha notado Ud. algún cambio en su vista?
– What change have you noticed?	– ¿Qué cambio ha notado?
– When did you first notice the change?	– ¿Cuándo notó Ud. este cambio por primera vez?
– How long have you had the change?	– ¿Hace cuánto tiempo que lo tiene?
Does anything make it better?	¿Existe algo que mejore el problema?
Does anything make it worse?	¿Existe algo que empeore el problema?

Glasses and contacts

Do you wear glasses or contact lenses?	¿Usa gafas o lentes de contacto?
– How long have you worn them?	– ¿Hace cuánto tiempo que los usa?
– Why do you wear them?	– ¿Por qué los usa Ud.?
When was your last eye appointment?	¿Cuándo fue su última cita con el oculista?
When did you last have your glasses or contacts changed?	¿Cuándo fue la última vez que cambió sus gafas o lentes de contacto?

Dryness, colors, glare

Do your eyes feel dry?	¿Siente Ud. sus ojos secos?
Do you have difficulty seeing to the side but not in front of you?	¿Tiene Ud. dificultad en ver a los costados pero no de frente?
Do you have problems with glare?	¿Un resplandor le causa problemas?
Do you have any problems seeing colors?	¿Tiene problemas para ver diferentes colores?
Do you have difficulty seeing at night?	¿Tiene Ud. dificultad en ver de noche?
– What improves this?	– ¿Qué es lo que mejora esto?
Do you suffer from frequent eye infections or inflammation?	¿Sufre Ud. de frecuentes infecciones o inflamación de los ojos?
– How often?	– ¿Con qué frecuencia?

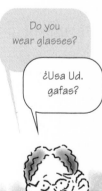

Do you wear glasses?

¿Usa Ud. gafas?

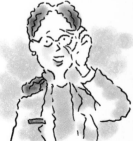

La clinica

Asking parents or caregivers about a child's eye problems

Remember to ask the parent or caregiver these questions about the child's eye problems:

Does the infant look at you or other objects and blink at bright lights or quick, nearby movements?	¿La criatura lo(a) mira fijamente a Ud. o a otros objetos y parpadea al ver luces brillantes o movimientos rápidos de objetos cercanos?
Are the child's eyes ever crossed?	¿Hay veces que la criatura tiene bizquera?
Do both eyes ever move in different directions?	¿Hay ocasiones en que los dos ojos se mueven en direcciones diferentes?
–Which directions?	–¿En qué direcciones?
Does the child often rub the eyes?	¿La criatura se frota los ojos con frecuencia?
Does the child squint frequently?	¿El niño (la niña) mira con frecuencia con los ojos entrecerrados?
Does the child often bump into or have difficulty picking up objects?	¿Se da el niño (la niña) golpes contra objetos con frecuencia o tiene dificultad en recoger objetos?
Does the child sit close to the television at home?	¿Se sienta el niño (la niña) muy cerca de la televisión?
How is the child's progress in school?	¿Ha hecho progreso el niño (la niña) en el colegio?
Does the child have to sit at the front of the classroom to see the chalkboard?	¿Se tiene que sentar la criatura en la parte delantera de la clase para poder ver la pizarra?

– How is the infection or inflammation treated?	– ¿Cómo se trata la infección o la inflamación?

(See *Asking parents or caregivers about a child's eye problems.*)

Asking about injury

Have you ever had eye surgery?	¿Ha requerido de alguna cirugía en los ojos?
– When?	– ¿Cuándo?
– For what reason?	– ¿Por qué razón?
– What kind of surgery?	– ¿Qué clase de cirugía?
Have you ever had an eye injury?	¿Ha tenido Ud. alguna vez una herida en el ojo?
– What kind of injury?	– ¿Qué clase de herida?
– When did it happen?	– ¿Cuándo la tuvo?
– How was it treated?	– ¿Qué tratamiento recibió?

Eye spy a stye?

Do you often have styes?	¿Le salen orzuelos con frecuencia?
– How often?	– ¿Con qué frecuencia?
– How are they treated?	– ¿Qué tratamiento se les da?

Do you have cysts? (See *Styes and cysts.*)	¿Tiene quistes?

Medications

What prescription medications do you take?	¿Qué medicamentos bajo receta toma?
– What are they for?	– ¿Para qué son?
What over-the-counter medications do you take?	¿Qué medicamentos de venta libre toma?
– How often do you take them?	– ¿Con qué frecuencia los toma?
What herbal remedies do you take?	¿Qué medicamentos herbales toma?
– How often do you take them?	– ¿Con qué frecuencia los toma?
What illicit drugs do you use?	¿Qué drogas ilícitas usa?
– How often do you use them?	– ¿Con qué frecuencia las usa?
Are you allergic to any medications?	¿Es alérgico(a) a algún medicamento?

Family facts

Has anyone in your family ever been treated for:	¿Hay algún miembro de su familia que haya tenido alguna enfermedad:
– cataracts?	– cataratas?
– glaucoma?	– glaucoma?
– blindness?	– ceguera?
– diabetes?	– diabetes?
– retinopathy?	– retinopatía?
– macular degeneration?	– degeneración macular?
Who was it?	¿Quién fue?
How was the problem treated?	¿Cómo se trató el problema?
Does anyone in your family wear glasses?	¿Hay alguien en su familia que use gafas?
– Who wears them?	– ¿Quién los usa?
– How long have they worn them?	– ¿Hace cuánto tiempo que los usa?
– Why do they wear them?	– ¿Por qué los usa?

Going with goggles

Do you play any sports?	¿Participa Ud. en algún deporte?
Do you wear goggles when playing such sports as swimming, fencing, or racquetball?	¿Usa gafas protectoras cuando practica deportes como natación, esgrima, o racquetball?
Does your poor eyesight affect your social activities?	Sus problemas de visión, ¿afectan sus actividades sociales?
– To what extent?	– ¿Hasta qué punto?

Styes and cysts

Here are key terms you can use to explain the difference between a stye and a cyst.

Stye
- Infección bacteriana—bacterial infection
- Aparece como una pequeña protuberancia en el borde del párpado—appears as a small bump at the edge of the eyelid
- Puede hincharse, ponerse colorado, y ser doloroso—may be swollen, red, and painful

Cyst
- Edema en el párpado producido por las glándulas sebáceas bloqueadas—swelling in the eyelid from blocked oil glands
- Puede ser un bulto duro, enrojecido, y doloroso—may be a hard, red, and painful lump
- La mayor parte del nódulo común está en el párpado—most common lump in the eyelid.

Take a look at this—the words *cataratas* (cataracts) and *glaucoma* (glaucoma) are almost exactly like their English counterparts.

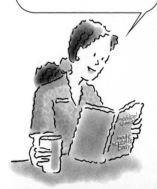

Eye irritants

Does the air where you work or live contain eye irritants, such as:
– cigarette smoke?
– chemicals?
– glues?
– formaldehyde insulation?
    What problems do you notice?

Do you take birth control pills?
– Have your eyes bothered you since you've been taking them?

El aire del lugar en que trabaja o vive, ¿contiene irritantes oculares como:
– humo de cigarrillos?
– productos químicos?
– pegamento, cola?
– insulación de formaldehído?
    ¿Qué problemas ha notado?

¿Toma pastillas anticonceptivas?
– ¿Le han molestado sus ojos de contacto desde que los ha estado tomando?

Eyeing work

How does wearing glasses or contact lenses make you feel about yourself?

Are your glasses or contact lenses a problem for you?

Does your health insurance cover eye examinations and lenses?

Does your job require close use of your eyes, such as long-term reading or prolonged use of a computer monitor?

Do you wear goggles when working with power tools, chain saws, or table saws?

Do vision problems make it difficult to fulfill home or work obligations?

¿Cómo le hace sentirse el usar lentes correctivos o lentes de contacto?

¿Le causan los lentes correctivos o de contacto algún problema?

¿Su seguro médico cubre exámenes de la vista y lentes correctivos?

¿Su trabajo requiere el uso minucioso de sus ojos, tal como leer mucho tiempo o el uso prolongado de una computadora?

¿Usa Ud. gafas protectoras cuando trabaja con herramientas mecánicas, sierras de cadena, o sierras de mesa?

¿Tiene Ud. dificultad en cumplir con sus obligaciones en casa o en el trabajo debido a sus problemas de la vista?

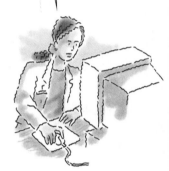

Does your occupation require prolonged use of a computer screen?

¿Su trabajo le requiere mirar la pantalla de una computadora por largo rato?

Examining the ears

Health problems related to the ears include hearing loss and tinnitus. To learn the Spanish for anatomic terms that may be relevant to your patient's ear condition, see *Ear—El oído,* page 148.

Should I speak up?

Have you recently noticed a change in your hearing?
– What is the change?
– When did you first notice it?
– How long have you had it?

Is the change only in one ear?
– Which ear?

¿Ha notado Ud. últimamente un cambio en audición?
– ¿Cuál es el cambio?
– ¿Cuándo lo notó Ud. por primera vez?
– ¿Hace cuánto tiempo que lo tiene?

¿Es el cambio sólo en un oído?
– ¿Cuál oído?

Did the change come on suddenly?	¿Fue súbito este cambio?
– When?	– ¿Cuándo ocurrió?
When does the change in hearing occur?	¿Cuándo ocurre el cambio en la audición?
– With all sounds?	– ¿Con todos los sonidos?
– High-pitched sounds only?	– ¿Sólo con sonidos agudos?
– Low-pitched sounds only?	– ¿Sólo con sonidos de tono grave?
Is the change always present? (See *Communicating clearly*.)	¿Está el cambio siempre presente?

Muffling, ringing, crackling

How would you describe the change?	¿Cómo describiría Ud. el cambio?
– Muffling?	– ¿Amortiguado?
– Ringing?	– ¿Zumbido?
– Crackling?	– ¿Crujiente?
– Sounds of the ocean?	– ¿Sonidos del oceáno?
– Hard to hear?	– ¿Problemas de audición?
– Other?	– ¿Otro?

Added issues

Do you have other symptoms, such as:	¿Tiene Ud. otros síntomas, tales como:
– pain?	– dolor?
– headache?	– dolor de cabeza?
– pressure?	– presión?
– dizziness?	– mareo?
What aggravates the change?	¿Qué es lo que lo agrava?
What improves it?	¿Qué es lo que lo alivia?
Have you been taking any prescription medications, over-the-counter medications, or home remedies for your ears?	¿Toma Ud. actualmente medicamentos de receta, medicamentos que no necesitan receta o remedios caseros para el oído?
– What?	– ¿Cuál (Cuáles)?
– How often do you use remedies?	– ¿Con qué frecuencia?

The school bell rings

Have you noticed a ringing in your ears?	¿Ha notado Ud. un zumbido en los oídos?
– When did you first notice it?	– ¿Cuándo lo notó por primera vez?
– How long have you had it?	– ¿Hace cuánto tiempo que lo tiene?
Is the ringing only in one ear?	¿Es el zumbido sólo en un oído?
– Which ear?	– ¿En qué oído?
Did the ringing come on suddenly?	¿Empezó el zumbido de repente?
– When?	– ¿Cuándo?

Is the ringing only in one ear?

¿Es el zumbido sólo en un oído?

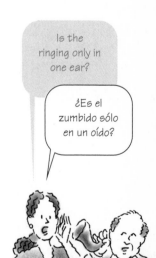

Ear
El oído

External ear
El oído externo

Middle ear
El oído medio

Inner ear
El oído interno

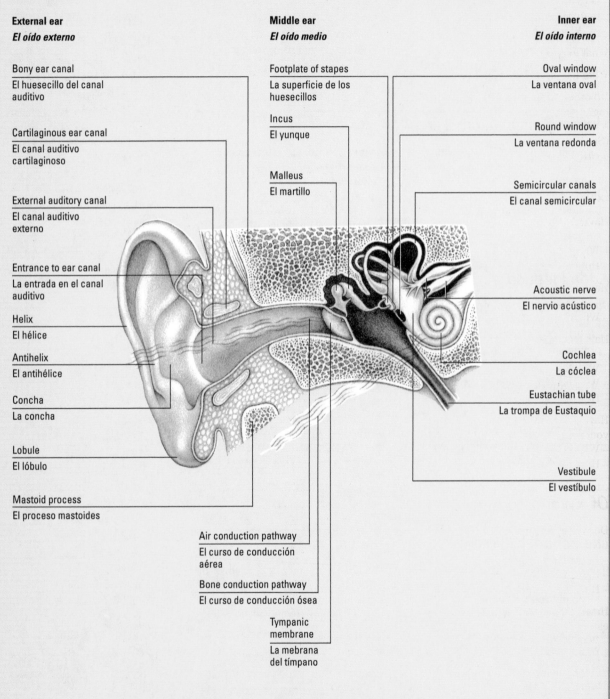

Bony ear canal
El huesecillo del canal
auditivo

Footplate of stapes
La superficie de los
huesecillos

Oval window
La ventana oval

Incus
El yunque

Round window
La ventana redonda

Cartilaginous ear canal
El canal auditivo
cartilaginoso

Malleus
El martillo

Semicircular canals
El canal semicircular

External auditory canal
El canal auditivo
externo

Entrance to ear canal
La entrada en el canal
auditivo

Acoustic nerve
El nervio acústico

Helix
El hélice

Antihelix
El antihélice

Cochlea
La cóclea

Concha
La concha

Eustachian tube
La trompa de Eustaquio

Lobule
El lóbulo

Vestibule
El vestíbulo

Mastoid process
El proceso mastoides

Air conduction pathway
El curso de conducción
aérea

Bone conduction pathway
El curso de conducción ósea

Tympanic
membrane
La mebrana
del tímpano

Does the ringing occur all the time?
– How often does it occur?
– How long does it last?
– Is there anything that seems to occur before the ringing starts?
    What?

¿Tiene Ud. el zumbido todo el tiempo?
– ¿Con qué frecuencia le ocurre?
– ¿Cuánto tiempo le dura?
– ¿Le ocurre algo antes de comenzar el zumbido?
    ¿Qué?

What makes the ringing worse?

¿Qué agrava el zumbido?

What lessens the ringing?

¿Qué alivia el zumbido?

Do other symptoms accompany the ringing?
– What?
(See *Asking parents or caregivers about a child's ear problems*, page 150.)

¿Va acompañado el zumbido de algunos otros síntomas?
– ¿Cuáles?

Q-tip questions

Have you ever had trouble with earwax?

– When?
– How was it treated?

¿Ha tenido Ud. problemas de cerilla en los oídos?
– ¿Cuándo?
– ¿Qué tratamiento se le dió?

Have you ever had a ruptured eardrum?

– When?

¿Alguna vez ha tenido una rotura de tímpano?
– ¿Cuándo?

Have you ever had an ear injury?

– When?
– What type of injury?
– How was it treated?

¿Ha tenido Ud. alguna vez una herida en el oído?
– ¿Cuándo?
– ¿Qué tipo de herida?
– ¿Qué tratamiento se le dió?

Have you ever had a foreign body in your ear?
– When?
– How was it treated?

¿Ha tenido Ud. alguna vez un objeto extraño en el oído?
– ¿Cuándo?
– ¿Qué tratamiento se le dió?

Often infected?

Do you suffer from frequent ear infections?
– How often?
– How long do they last?
– How are they treated?

¿Sufre Ud. de frecuentes infecciones del oído?
– ¿Con qué frecuencia?
– ¿Cuánto tiempo le duran a Ud.?
– ¿Qué tratamiento se les ha dado?

Have you ever had drainage from your ears?
– When?
– How was it treated?

¿Ha tenido Ud. drenaje de los oídos?

– ¿Cuándo?
– ¿Qué tratamiento se les dió?

Do you suffer from frequent ear infections?

¿Sufre Ud. de frecuentes infecciones del oído?

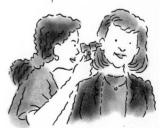

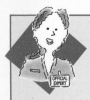

La clinica

Asking parents or caregivers about a child's ear problems

Remember to ask the parent or caregiver these questions about a child's ear problems:

Does the infant respond to loud or unusual noises?	¿Responde la criatura a ruidos fuertes o extraños?
Does the infant babble?	¿Balbucea el (la) niño(a)?
Does the toddler try to make sounds?	¿El (la) pequeño(a) tratade responder consonidos?
Is the toddler talking appropriately for his or her age?	¿Habla el (la) pequeño(a) adecuadamente para su edad?
Have you noticed the child tugging at either ear?	¿Ha notado Ud. si la criatura tira de una oreja?
Which ear?	¿De cuál oreja?
Have you noticed any coordination problems?	¿Ha notado Ud. problemas de coordinación?
What?	¿Cuáles?
When did you first notice the problem?	¿Cuándo notó Ud. el problema por primera vez?
Has the child had any of the following:	¿Ha tenido la criatura cualquiera de las siguientes enfermedades:
Meningitis?	Meningitis?
Recurrent ear infections?	Recurrentes infecciones de oído?
Mumps?	Parotiditis (paperas)?
Encephalitis?	Encefalitis?
When?	¿Cuándo?
How was the illness treated?	¿Qué tratamiento se le dió?
Does the child sleep well?	¿Duerme bien el niño/la niña?
Is the child frequently irritable?	El niño, ¿se irrita frecuentemente?

Staying straight up?

Have you ever had problems with:	¿Alguna rez ha tenido problemas de:
– balance?	– falta de equilibrio?
– dizziness?	– mareo?
– vertigo?	– vértigo?
When?	¿Cuándo?
How was the problem treated?	¿Qué tratamiento se le dió?

Eager for exams?

When was your last ear examination and hearing test?	¿Cuándo se hizo Ud. su último examen del oído?
– What were the results?	– ¿Cúales fueron los resultados?
– Why did you get the exam and test?	– ¿Por qué se le hizo el examen?
How do you routinely care for your ears?	¿Cómo se cuida Ud. sus oídos y orejas de costumbre?

Outside aid

Do you wear a hearing aid?
– In which ear?

¿Usa Ud. algún tipo de audífono?
– ¿En que oído?

How long have you had it?

¿Hace cuánto tiempo que lo tiene?

How do you care for it?

¿Cómo lo cuida Ud.?

Focus on family

Has anyone in your family ever had a hearing problem?
– Who was it?
– When did it occur?
– How was it treated?
    Surgery?
    Hearing aid?

¿Hay algún miembro de su familia que haya tenido problemas del oído?
– ¿Quién fue?
– ¿Cuándo ocurrió esto?
– ¿Qué tratamiento se le dió?
    ¿Cirugía?
    ¿Audífono?

Does your hearing difficulty interfere with your daily activities?
– How?

¿Su problema de audición interfiere en su vida cotidiana?
– ¿Cómo?

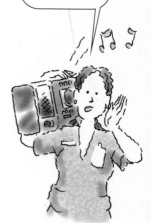

Do you listen to loud music?

¿Escucha Ud. la música a un volumen muy alto?

Pump up the volume?

Do you listen to loud music or turn up the television volume?

– How often?
– For how long each time?

¿Escucha Ud. la música a un volumen muy alto o le sube el volumen a su televisión?
– ¿Con qué frecuencia?
– ¿Por cuánto tiempo cada vez?

Loud sounds

Are you around loud equipment, such as heavy machinery, airguns, or airplanes?

– How long are you exposed to the noise each day?
– Do you wear protective ear coverings when you are exposed to the noise?

¿Está Ud. alrededor de equipos ruidosos, tales como maquinaria pesada, pistolas de aire, o aviones?
– ¿Durante cuánto tiempo por día está expuesto al ruido?
– ¿Usa protección para los oídos cuando está expuesto al ruido?

Daily doings

Does your hearing problem interfere with your daily work?
– How?

¿Su problema de audición interfiere con su trabajo diario?
– ¿Cómo?

Has your hearing problem affected the way you feel about yourself?
– How?

¿Su problema de audición ha afectado la opinión de sí mismo(a)?
– ¿Cómo?

Does your hearing problem affect your relationships with other people? – How?	¿Su problema de audición afecta sus relaciones con otras personas? – ¿Cómo?

Examining the head and neck

Health problems related to the head and neck include difficulty swallowing, facial swelling, hoarseness, nasal discharge, neck stiffness, nosebleed, and ulcers. To learn the Spanish for anatomic terms that may be relevant to your patient's condition, see *Mouth—La boca*.

Chew and swallow

Do you have difficulty swallowing? – How would you describe it?	¿Tiene Ud. alguna dificultad al tragar? – ¿Cómo la describiría Ud.?
Do you have any pain when you chew or swallow? – Where?	¿Alguna vez tiene dolor al masticar o tragar? – ¿Dónde?
Do you have problems swallowing food? – What foods?	¿Tiene Ud. problemas para tragar la comida? – ¿Qué comidas?
Do you have a problem swallowing fluids?	¿Tiene Ud. problemas para tragar líquidos?
Do you have difficulty chewing? – How would you describe this difficulty? – Does it occur all the time or only when you eat or drink?	¿Tiene dificultad para masticar? – ¿Cómo describiría Ud. esta dificultad? – ¿Ocurre todo el tiempo o sólo cuando come y bebe?

Do you have problems swallowing food?

¿Tiene Ud. problemas para tragar la comida?

Face facts

Do you have swelling on your face? – When did you first notice the swelling?	¿Tiene Ud. la cara algo inflamada? – ¿Cuándo notó Ud. la inflamación por primera vez?
– How long have you had it? – Have you noticed a change in the swelling? Is the swelling worse? Is the swelling better?	– ¿Hace cuánto tiempo que la tiene? – ¿Ha notado Ud. algún cambio en la inflamación? ¿Ha empeorado la inflamación? ¿Ha mejorado la inflamación?
Is there swelling in other areas, such as: – the jaw? – behind the ear? When did it occur?	¿Tiene Ud. inflamación en otras partes, tales como: – la mandíbula (quijada)? – detrás de la oreja? ¿Cuándo ocurrió?

Mouth
La boca

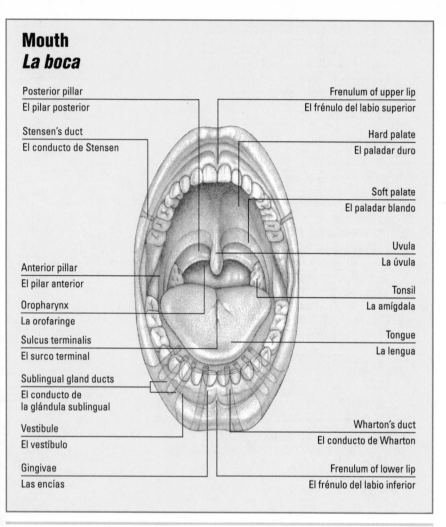

Posterior pillar
El pilar posterior

Stensen's duct
El conducto de Stensen

Anterior pillar
El pilar anterior

Oropharynx
La orofaringe

Sulcus terminalis
El surco terminal

Sublingual gland ducts
El conducto de
la glándula sublingual

Vestibule
El vestíbulo

Gingivae
Las encías

Frenulum of upper lip
El frénulo del labio superior

Hard palate
El paladar duro

Soft palate
El paladar blando

Uvula
La úvula

Tonsil
La amígdala

Tongue
La lengua

Wharton's duct
El conducto de Wharton

Frenulum of lower lip
El frénulo del labio inferior

Pain, tenderness, warmth

Do other signs or symptoms accompany the swelling, such as:
– pain?
– tenderness?
– redness?
– warmth?
– impaired movement?
　　Where?

What makes the swelling worse?

What lessens the swelling?

¿Tiene Ud. otros síntomas que acompañan la inflamación, tales como:
– dolor?
– sensibilidad?
– enrojecimiento?
– calor moderado?
– impedimento del movimiento?
　　¿Dónde?

¿Qué es lo que empeora la inflamación?

¿Qué alivia la inflamación?

Losing your voice?

Have you noticed any changes in the sound of your voice?
– What kind of change?

What makes it worse?

What makes it better?

¿Ha notado Ud. algún cambio en el sonido de su voz?
– ¿Qué clase de cambio?

¿Qué lo empeora?

¿Qué lo mejora?

Have you noticed any changes in the sound of your voice?

¿Ha notado Ud. algún cambio en el sonido de su voz?

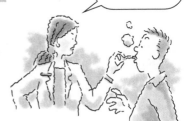

The nose knows

Do you have a runny nose?
– When did you first notice it?
– How long have you had it?
– When does it occur?
    All the time?
    In the morning?
    At night?
    Other?
– Does it seem to follow a pattern?
    What kind of pattern?

How would you describe the fluid?
– Thick?
– Thin?
– Watery?
– Like pus?

What color is the fluid?
– Clear?
– White?
– Yellow?
– Green?
– Other?

¿Le gotea la nariz?
– ¿Cuándo la notó Ud. por primera vez?
– ¿Hace cuánto tiempo que la tiene?
– ¿Cuándo ocurre?
    ¿Todo el tiempo?
    ¿Por la mañana?
    ¿Por la noche?
    ¿En otro momento?
– ¿Parece seguir un patrón?
    ¿Qué patrón?

¿Cómo describiría el fluido?
– ¿Espesa?
– ¿No densa?
– ¿Acuosa?
– ¿Parecida a pus?

¿De qué color es el fluido?
– ¿Transparente?
– ¿Blanco?
– ¿Amarillo?
– ¿Verde?
– ¿Otros?

Assessing allergies

Do you have any allergies?
– To what?

What happens?

Do you have hayfever?

Do you have other signs or symptoms, such as:
– fever?
– headache?
– cough?
– wheezing?
– runny nose?
– other?

¿Tiene Ud. alergias?
– ¿A qué?

¿Qué sucede?

¿Tiene Ud. fiebre de heno?

¿Tiene Ud. otros síntomas, tales como:

– fiebre?
– dolor de cabeza?
– tos?
– respiración jadeante?
– goteo de nariz?
– otros?

When are they worse?	¿Cuándo empeoran?
– Spring?	– ¿Primavera?
– Summer?	– ¿Verano?
– Fall?	– ¿Otoño?
– Winter?	– ¿Invierno?
Has the discharge improved or worsened since it started?	¿Ha mejorado o empeorado la descarga desde que le comenzó?
What aggravates it?	¿Qué es lo que la agrava?
What relieves it?	¿Con qué se mejora?

Head turns

Do you have any neck stiffness or pain?	¿Tiene agarrotado o adolorido el cuello?
When did the discomfort begin?	¿Cuándo comenzó la molestia?
How would you describe the discomfort?	¿Cómo describiría la molestia?
– Constant?	– ¿Constante?
– Intermittent?	– ¿Intermitente?
Does the discomfort occur at a specific time?	La molestia, ¿se produce en un momento específico?
– When?	– ¿Cuándo?
Early morning?	¿Temprano por la mañana?
During the day?	¿Durante el día?
After activities?	¿Después de hacer actividades?
At night?	¿Por la noche?
While you're sleeping?	¿Mientras Ud. duerme?
– What makes it better?	– ¿Qué la mejora?
– What makes it worse?	– ¿Qué la empeora?

Pain problems

Do you sometimes hear a grating sound or feel a grating sensation as if your bones are scraping together?	¿Hay veces que Ud. oye un chirrido o siente Ud. como si los huesos se rasparan los unos con los otros?

Nosey questions

Do you have nosebleeds?	¿Tiene Ud. hemorragia nasal?
– How often?	– ¿Con qué frecuencia?
– When do they occur?	– ¿Cuándo se producen?
How long do the nosebleeds last?	¿Cuánto tiempo duran las hemorragias?
– Less than a minute?	– ¿Menos de un minuto?
– A few minutes?	– ¿Unos cuantos minutos?
– Longer?	– ¿Más tiempo?
What do you usually do to stop the nosebleed?	¿Qué hace Ud. para mitigar la hemorragia?
Have the nosebleeds gotten worse since they first started?	¿Se han empeorado las hemorragias desde que tuvo la primera?

Sore points

Do you have ulcers?	¿Tiene Ud. llagas?
– Where?	– ¿Dónde?
In your nose?	¿En la nariz?
In your mouth?	¿En la boca?
On your tongue?	¿En la lengua?
On your lips?	¿En los labios?
Other?	¿En otra parte?

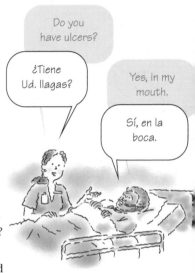

Do you
have ulcers?

¿Tiene
Ud. llagas?

Yes, in my
mouth.

Sí, en la
boca.

How would you describe them?	¿Cómo las describiría Ud.?
– Soft?	– ¿Blandas?
– Hard?	– ¿Duras?
– Crusty?	– ¿Costrosas?
– Moist?	– ¿Húmedas?
Are they painful?	¿Son dolorosas?
How long have you had them?	¿Hace cuánto tiempo que las tiene?
– Do they recur?	– ¿Vuelven a aparecer?
Do you notice that the ulcers are associated with any activity or event?	¿Ha notado Ud. si las úlceras están relacionadas con alguna actividad o evento?
– What?	– ¿Cuál?
Do the ulcers interfere with eating or drinking?	¿Las úlceras interfieren con su habilidad de comer y beber?
– How?	– ¿Cómo?

Thoughts about the throat

Have you ever had any allergy that caused breathing difficulty and the feeling that your throat was closing?	¿Ha tenido Ud. alguna vez alguna alergia que le haya causado dificultad en respirar y que le haya dado la sensación de que la garganta se le cerraba?
– What caused the reaction?	– ¿Qué la causó?
– When did these symptoms typically occur?	– ¿En qué ocasiones ocurrían estos síntomas generalmente?
– How did you treat the symptoms?	– ¿Cómo los trató Ud.?

Sudden jolts

Have you ever had a neck injury or had trouble moving your neck in any direction?	¿Ha tenido Ud. alguna vez una lesión o dificultad en mover el cuello en cualquier dirección?
– What direction?	– ¿Cuál?
– What caused the problem?	– ¿Qué causó el problema?
– What type of injury did you have?	– ¿Qué tipo de lesión tuvo?
– When did it occur?	– ¿Cuándo ocurrió?
– How was the problem treated?	– ¿Cómo se trató el problema?
Have you ever had neck surgery?	¿Ha tenido Ud. cirugía en el cuello?
– When?	– ¿Cuándo?
– Why?	– ¿Por qué razón?

Serious stuff

Have you ever had:
– head trauma?
– skull surgery?
– jaw surgery?
– facial fractures?
    When?
    What happened before?
    What happened afterward?

¿Ha tenido Ud. alguna vez:
– un trauma en la cabeza?
– cirugía del cráneo?
– cirugía de la mandíbula (quijada)?
– fracturas de la cara?
    ¿Cuándo?
    ¿Qué pasó antes?
    ¿Qué pasó después?

Seeing about sinus

Have you ever had a sinus infection or tenderness?
– When?
– How was it treated?

¿Alguna vez ha tenido una infección o molestia sinusal?
– ¿Cuándo?
– ¿Qué tratamiento se le dió?

Have you ever had surgery on your nose or sinuses?
– Why?
– When?

¿Alguna vez le operaron la nariz o senos nasales?
-¿Por qué?
-¿Cuándo?

Do you ever have headaches or tightness in the neck or jaw?
– When?

¿Alguna vez tiene dolor de cabeza o tensión en el cuello o la mandíbula?
– ¿Cuándo?

Is headache or neck or jaw tightness related to:

– lack of sleep?
– missed meals?
– stress?

¿El dolor de cabeza o la rigidez del cuello o de la mandíbula (quijada) se relaciona con alguno:

– la falta de sueño?
– el saltearsé comidas?
– elestrés?

What lessens it?

¿Qué hace que se alivie?

What makes it worse?

¿Qué hace que se empeore?

Family photo

Do any of your family members have a neurologic disease?

¿Tiene algún miembro de su familia una enfermedad neurológica?

What is it?
– Which relative?
– How was it treated?

¿Cuál?
– ¿Qué pariente?
– ¿Qué tratamiento recibió?

Have any of your family members had:

– high blood pressure?
– diabetes?
– stroke?
– heart disease?
– headaches?

¿Hay algún miembro de su familia que haya tenido:

– presión sanguínea alta?
– diabetes?
– un derrame cerebral?
– una enfermedad cardiaca?
– dolores de cabeza?

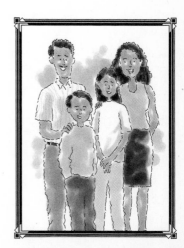

– arthritis?

    When?

    How was it treated?

– artritis?

    ¿Cuándo?

    ¿Qué tratamiento se le dió?

Brush and floss?

Do you grind your teeth?

¿Cruje Ud. sus dientes?

How often do you brush and floss your teeth?

¿Con qué frecuencia se lava Ud. los dientes o usa seda dental?

When was your last dental examination?

¿Cuándo fue la última vez que tuvo Ud. un reconocimiento dental?

– What were the results?

– ¿Cuáles fueron los resultados?

Do your teeth hurt?

¿Le duelen los dientes?

Do your gums hurt or bleed?

¿Le sangran o duelen las encías?

Did you ever have braces?

¿Alguna vez usó aparatos en los dientes?

Did you ever have an injury that affected your teeth?

¿Alguna vez tuvo una lesión que haya afectado sus dientes?

Daily living

Do you wear a seatbelt when you are in an automobile?

¿Usa Ud. cinturón de seguridad cuando va en un automóvil?

Has your head or neck problem interfered with your regular activities?

Su problema en la cabeza o el cuello, ¿ha interferido con sus actividades cotidianas?

– How?

– ¿Cómo?

Do you do exercises to help with your head or neck problem?

¿Hace Ud. algún ejercicio para mejorar su problema de la cabeza o el cuello?

Do you play a sport that requires a helmet?

¿Practica un deporte que requiera el uso de un casco?

– Which sport?

– ¿Qué deporte?

– How often do you participate in this sport?

– ¿Con qué frecuencia participa Ud. en este deporte?

Has your head or neck problem affected your ability to eat or drink?

Su problema e de la cabeza o el cuello, ¿ha afectado su capacidad de comer o beber?

– How?

– ¿Cómo?

Which foods are difficult for you to eat?

¿Con qué clase de comestibles tiene Ud. dificultad?

Which foods are easy for you to eat?

¿Qué comestibles puede Ud. comer con facilidad?

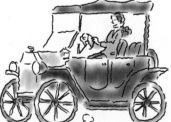

Do you wear a seatbelt when you are in an automobile?

¿Usa Ud. cinturón de seguridad cuando va en un automóvil?

What about weather?

Do weather changes seem to affect your head or neck problem?

– How?

Does your head or neck problem affect the way you feel about yourself or the way you relate to your family?

– How?

¿Su problema de la cabeza o el cuello se afecta de alguna forma con los cambios de clima?
– ¿Cómo?

¿Afecta el problema de su cabeza o cuello la opinión que tiene sobre sí mismo(a) o la manera en que se relaciona con su familia?
– ¿Cómo?

Long time sitting?

Does your job require sitting at a computer terminal?
– How long?

Does your job put you at risk for head injury?
– Do you wear a hard hat?

Su trabajo, ¿requiere que esté sentado en una terminal de computadoras?
– ¿Por cuánto tiempo?

¿Existe el riesgo de lastimarse la cabeza en su trabajo?
– ¿Usa Ud. un casco protector?

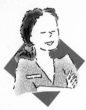

Practice makes perfecto

1. Joy wants to ask if the patient has noticed a ringing in his ears. Can you give Joy the correct word?

_____

_____

_____

_____

> ¿Ha notado Ud. _____ en los oídos?

2. Now Joy wants to know if the ringing is only in one ear. Can you supply the right phrase?

_____

_____

_____

_____

> ¿Es el zumbido _____?

3. Joy wants to know if the patient wears contact lenses. Can you help Joy?

_____

_____

_____

_____

> ¿Usa Ud. _____?

4. Joy wants to ask if the patient has neck stiffness. Can you finish the question?

_____

_____

_____

_____

> ¿Tiene Ud. _____?

Answer key

1. Have you noticed a ringing in your ears?
¿Ha notado Ud. <u>un zumbido</u> en los oídos?

2. Is the ringing only in one ear?
¿Es el zumbido <u>sólo en un oído</u>?

3. Do you wear contact lenses?
¿Usa Ud. <u>lentes de contacto</u>?

4. Do you have neck stiffness?
¿Tiene Ud. <u>rigidez en el cuello</u>?

13 Evaluating mental health

Health problems

Effective patient care requires consideration of the psychological and physiologic aspects of health. A patient who seeks medical help for chest pain, for example, may also need to be assessed for anxiety and depression. Knowing the brain's basic function and structures will help you perform a comprehensive mental health assessment and recognize abnormalities. (See chapter 6, Examining the nervous system.) Be sure to utilize therapeutic communication techniques to obtain the most in-depth responses. (See *Therapeutic communication techniques*, page 162.)

Jogging memories

Have you had any trouble remembering things lately?	¿Ha tenido problemas para recordar las cosas últimamente?
– When did your trouble with remembering start?	– ¿Cuándo comenzó su problema para recordar?
– How often do you have trouble remembering?	– ¿Con cuánta frecuencia tiene problemas para recordar?
Do you know what day today is?	¿Sabe qué día es hoy?
– What day is it?	– ¿Qué día es hoy?
Do you know the current year?	¿Sabe en qué año estamos?
– What is today's date?	– ¿En qué fecha estamos?
Do you know where you are?	¿Sabe dónde está?
Have you had any trouble concentrating?	¿Ha tenido problemas para concentrarse?
– Describe your trouble concentrating.	– Describa sus problemas para concentrarse.
Have you had any periods of confusion?	¿Ha tenido períodos de confusión?
– How often are you confused?	– ¿Con cuánta frecuencia se confunde?
– How long does the confusion last?	– ¿Cuánto dura la confusión?

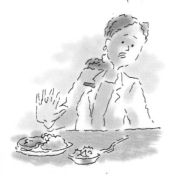

Has your appetite changed recently?

¿Ha sufrido cambios en su apetito recientemente?

Food facts

How is your appetite?	¿Cómo es su apetito?
– Good?	– ¿Bueno?

Therapeutic communication techniques

Therapeutic communication is the foundation for any good nurse-patient relationship. Here are some effective techniques for developing that relationship.

Listening
Listening intently to the patient enables you to hear and analyze everything the patient is saying, alerting you to your patient's communication patterns.

Rephrasing
Succinct rephrasing of key patient statements helps ensure that you understand and emphasize important points in the patient's message. For example, you might say, "You're feeling angry, and you say your anger is because of the way your friend treated you yesterday." ("Estás enfadado[a] y dices que tu enojo se debe a la manera en que te trató tu amigo[a] ayer.")

Using broad openings and general statements
Using broad openings and general statements to initiate conversation encourages the patient to talk about any subject that comes to mind. These openings allow him to focus the conversation while you demonstrate your willingness to interact. An example of this technique is: "Is there something you would like to talk about?" ("¿Hay algo sobre lo que quieras hablar?")

Clarifying
Asking the patient to clarify a confusing or vague message demonstrates your desire to understand what he's saying. It can also elicit precise information crucial to his recovery. An example of clarification is: "I'm not sure I understood what you said." ("No estoy seguro[a] de haber entendido lo que dijiste.")

Focusing
In this technique, you help the patient redirect attention toward something specific. Focusing fosters the patient's self-control and helps him avoid vague generalizations so that he can accept the responsibility of facing his problems. "Let's go back to what we were just talking about," ("Volvamos al asunto sobre el que estábamos hablando antes,") is one example of this technique.

Silence
Silence has several benefits. It gives the patient time to talk, think, and gain insight into problems. It also allows you to gather more information. You must use this technique judiciously, however, to avoid giving the impression of disinterest or judgment.

Suggesting collaboration
When used correctly, suggesting collaboration gives the patient an opportunity to explore the pros and cons of a suggested approach. It must be used carefully to avoid directing the patient. An example of this technique is: "Perhaps we can meet with your parents to discuss the matter." ("Tal vez podamos reunirnos con tus padres para conversar sobre el tema.")

Sharing impressions
In this technique, you attempt to describe the patient's feelings and then seek his corrective feedback. Doing so allows the patient to clarify any misperceptions and gives you a better understanding of his true feelings. For example, you might say, "Tell me if my perception of what you're saying agrees with yours." ("Dime si mi impresión de lo que dices concuerda con la tuya.")

– Poor?	– ¿Malo?
Has your appetite changed recently?	¿Ha sufrido cambios en su apetito recientemente?
– When did it change?	– ¿Cuándo se produjeron los cambios?
Describe your typical diet.	Describa su dieta habitual.

Rest assured

Lately, have you been more tired than usual?

Últimamente, ¿ha estado más cansado que de costumbre?

How many hours a day do you sleep?
– Do you feel rested when you get up?

¿Cuántas horas por día duerme?
– ¿Se siente descansado(a) al levantarse?

Do you nap?
– How often do you nap?

¿Duerme la siesta?
– ¿Con cuánta frecuencia duerme la siesta?

– How long is your nap?

– ¿Por cuánto tiempo duerme la siesta?

Do you have any trouble moving around?
– In what way is moving difficult?

¿Tiene algún problema para trasladarse?
– ¿En qué sentido le resulta difícil moverse?

Have you ever had a seizure?
– When did you have the seizure?
– How was the seizure treated?
– How often do you have seizures?

¿Alguna vez ha tenido un ataque?
– ¿Cuándo tuvo el ataque?
– ¿Cómo se trató el ataque?
– ¿Con cuánta frecuencia tiene ataques?

Do you ever feel weak?
– When do you feel weak?
– Do you feel weak all the time, or just sometimes?

¿Alguna vez se siente débil?
– ¿Cuándo se siente débil?
– ¿Se siente débil todo el tiempo o solo a veces?

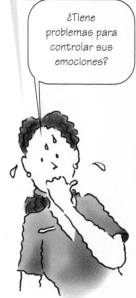

Do you have trouble controlling your emotions?

¿Tiene problemas para controlar sus emociones?

Focus on feelings

Do you have any trouble performing daily activities?
– What type of trouble?
– Which activities?

¿Tiene problemas para realizar actividades cotidianas?
– ¿Qué tipo de problemas?
– ¿Con qué actividades?

Do you have trouble controlling your emotions?
– In what way?

¿Tiene problemas para controlar sus emociones?
– ¿De qué manera?

Have you had any recent feelings of uncontrolled anger or sadness?
– When did you first feel this anger or sadness?
– Describe what happened.

¿Ha tenido recientemente sentimientos descontrolados de ira o dolor?
– ¿Cuándo fue la primera vez que sintió esta ira o este dolor?
– Describa lo que sucedió.

Have you had any recent stressful events in your life, such as:
– death of a family member?
– loss of a job?
– divorce?
– household move?
– marriage?
– birth of a child?
– purchase of a house?

¿Ha tenido recientemente algún suceso estresante en su vida, como:
– muerte de un familiar?
– pérdida de un trabajo?
– divorcio?
– mudanza?
– casamiento?
– nacimiento de un hijo?
– compra de una casa?

– starting a new school or college?

– empezar las clases en una nueva escuela o universidad?

Describe how you respond to stress.

Describa cómo responde ante el estrés.

Passive or active voice

Do you ever hear voices?
– When do you hear these voices?
– For how long have you been hearing voices?
– How often do you hear the voices?

¿A veces oye voces?
– ¿Cuándo oye estas voces?
– ¿Durante cuánto tiempo ha oído voces?
– ¿Con cuánta frecuencia oye estas voces?

Do you participate in any type of therapy or counseling?
– What type of therapy or counseling?
– How often do you participate?
– For what reason are you in therapy or counseling?
– Has participation helped?

¿Se somete a algún tipo de terapia u orientación?
– ¿Qué tipo de terapia u orientación?
– ¿Con cuánta frecuencia participa?
– ¿Qué lo(a) llevó a recurrir a la terapia o la orientación?
– ¿Le ha ayudado?

Do you follow a particular faith?
– Which faith?
– Do you participate in beliefs?

¿Tiene una religión determinada?
– ¿Qué religión?
– ¿Coincide con las creencias?

Medications

What prescription medications do you take?
– What are they for?

¿Qué medicamentos bajo receta toma?
– ¿Para qué son?

What over-the-counter medications do you take?
– How often do you take them?

¿Qué medicamentos de venta libre toma?
– ¿Con qué frecuencia los toma?

What herbal remedies do you take?
– How often do you take them?

¿Qué medicamentos herbales toma?
– ¿Con qué frecuencia los toma?

What illicit drugs do you use?
– How often do you use them?

¿Qué drogas ilícitas usa?
– ¿Con qué frecuencia las usa?

Are you allergic to any medications?

¿Es alérgico(a) a algún medicamento?

Have you ever taken medication for depression?
– What was the medication?
– Did the medication help?
– When did you stop taking it?
– Why did you stop taking it?

¿Ha tomado alguna vez un medicamento para la depresión?
– ¿Qué medicamento era?
– ¿Le ayudó?
– ¿Cuándo dejó de tomarlo?
– ¿Por qué dejó de tomarlo?

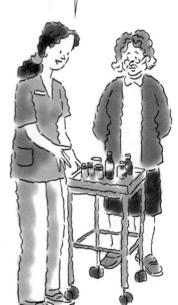

Which medications do you take?

¿Qué medicamentos toma?

Medical history

In the medical history, investigate if the patient suffers from any chronic or terminal illness. Also ask about recent illness, childbirth, and depression. (See *Asking parents or caregivers about a child's emotional health*, page 166.)

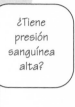

Do you have high blood pressure?

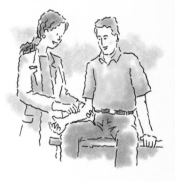

¿Tiene presión sanguínea alta?

Illness, injury, and other concerns

Have you had a recent illness?
– What was it?
– When did you have it?
– How was the illness treated?

¿Ha estado enfermo(a) recientemente?
– ¿Qué enfermedad tuvo?
– ¿Cuándo?
– ¿Cómo se trató la enfermedad?

Do you have any chronic illness, such as:

– diabetes?
– heart disease?
– emphesema?
– high blood pressure?
– kidney disease?

¿Tiene alguna enfermedad crónica como:

– diabetes?
– enfermedad cardiaca?
– enfisema?
– presión sanguínea alta?
– enfermedad renal?

Do you have a history of cancer?
– What kind?
– When did you have the cancer?
– How was it treated?

¿Tiene un historial de cáncer?
– ¿De qué tipo?
– ¿Cuándo tuvo el cáncer?
– ¿Cómo fue tratado?

Have you ever had a head injury?

– When was your head injured?
– How was the injury treated?

¿Alguna vez ha tenido una lesión en la cabeza?
– ¿Cuándo se lesionó la cabeza?
– ¿Cómo se trató la lesión?

Have you ever given birth to a child?
– How many children do you have?
– When were your children born?

¿Ha dado alguna vez a luz?
– ¿Cuántos hijos tiene?
– ¿Cuándo nacieron sus hijos?

Sadness and other emotions

Have you ever been treated for depression?
– When?

¿Ha recibido algún tratamiento para la depresión?
– ¿Cuándo?

– How was the depression treated?

– ¿Cómo se trató la depresión?

Have you ever been treated for any emotional or behavioral problem?
– What was the problem?
– How was the problem treated?

¿Ha recibido algún tratamiento por un problema emocional o de conducta?
– ¿Cuál era el problema?
– ¿Cómo se trató el problema?

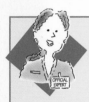

La clinica

Asking parents or caregivers about a child's emotional health

Remember to ask the parent or caregiver these questions about a child's emotional status:

Has the child had any recent change in behavior?	El niño, ¿ha tenido algún cambio reciente en la conducta?
Has the child has any recent change in school grades?	El niño, ¿ha tenido algún cambio reciente en las calificaciones de la escuela?
Does the child interact with family members?	¿Interactúa con sus familiares?
Does the child interact with others his own age?	¿Interactúa con otros niños de su edad?
Does the child have any repetitive behaviors?	¿Posee alguna conducta repetitiva?
– What are the behaviors?	– ¿Cuáles son esas conductas?
Does the child display any irrational fears disproportionate to an object or a situation?	El niño, ¿da señales de miedos irracionales que no corresponden al objeto o la situación?
– What is the fear?	– ¿Cuál es el miedo?
Does the child display uncontrolled anger or other emotion?	El niño, ¿da señales de ira u otra emoción descontrolada?
– How often is the anger or emotion displayed?	– ¿Con qué frecuencia se observan las señales de ira o emoción?
Does the child demonstrate obsession with thoughts or behavoirs?	¿Da muestras de obsesión con ideas o conductas?
– What are the thoughts or behaviors?	– ¿Cuáles son esas ideas o conductas?
Has the child had any unexplained recent weight loss?	¿Ha tenido recientemente una pérdida de peso sin explicación?
– How much of a loss?	– ¿Cuán grande fue la pérdida?
Does the child have any unusual eating tendencies, such as binge eating?	¿Tiene alguna tendencia alimentaria inusual, como atracones?
How does the child usually respond to stress?	¿Cómo responde habitualmente al estrés?
Has the child ever participated in counseling or therapy?	¿Se ha sometido alguna vez a una orientación o terapia?
Does the child display any suicidal tendencies?	¿Da señales de tendencias suicidas?
Does the child hurt himself intentionally?	¿Se lastima a sí mismo de manera intencional?
– How does he hurt himself?	– ¿Cómo se lastima?
– How often does this happen?	– ¿Con cuánta frecuencia?

Family history

Investigate if anyone in the patient's family has or ever had a mental health problem and how the problem was treated. The family history will help you obtain a more accurate evaluation of your patient's mental health problem.

All in the family

Has anyone in your family ever suffered from depression?	¿Alguno de sus familiares ha tenido depresión alguna vez?
– Which family member?	– ¿Qué familiar?
– How was the depression treated?	– ¿Cómo se trató la depresión?

Has anyone in your family ever been diagnosed with a mental health disorder?

– Which family member?
– What was the disorder?
– How was it treated?

Has anyone in your family been treated in a mental health facility?

– Which family member?
– When was the family member treated?
– What was the reason?

Does anyone in your family display uncontrolled anger?
– Which family member?
– How often is the anger displayed?

– Describe what happens.

Are all your immediate family members still living?
– Who has died? (if the answer is "no")

– What did they die from?

¿A alguno de sus familiares le han diagnosticado un desorden en la salud mental alguna vez?

– ¿Qué familiar?
– ¿Qué desorden era?
– ¿Cómo fue tratado?

¿Alguno de sus familiares ha sido tratado en un establecimiento de salud mental?

– ¿Qué familiar?
– ¿Cuándo fue tratado su familiar?
– ¿Por qué motivo?

¿Algún miembro de su familia da señales de ira descontrolada?
– ¿Qué familiar?
– ¿Con qué frecuencia se observan las señales de ira?
– Describa lo que sucede.

¿Se encuentran con vida todos sus familiares directos?
– ¿Quién ha fallecido? (si la respuesta es "no")
– ¿De qué fallecieron?

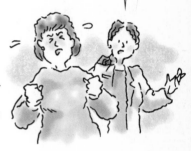

Does anyone in your family display uncontrolled anger?

¿Algún miembro de su familia da señales de ira descontrolada?

Lifestyle

Ask the patient about occupation, social activities, and alcohol consumption. Determine if he has any financial burdens causing increased stress, and whether he has a support network.

Work-related

Are you currently employed?

What is your job?
– What type of responsibilites do you have at your job?
– Are your responsibilities stressful?

– How many hours a day do you work?
– How many hours a week do you work?

Are you unemployed?
– How long have you been unemployed?

Do you have time to do things that you enjoy?

What are your usual family responsibilities?

¿Tiene un empleo actualmente?

¿Cuál es su trabajo?
– ¿Qué tipo de responsabilidades tiene en su trabajo?
– Sus responsabilidades, ¿son estresantes?

– ¿Cuántas horas por día trabaja?
– ¿Cuántas horas por semana trabaja?

¿Está desocupado?
– ¿Hace cuánto que está desocupado?

¿Tiene tiempo para hacer cosas que le dan placer?

¿Cuáles son sus responsabilidades familiares habituales?

– Can you fulfill your responsibilities?

– What interferes with these responsibilities?

Do you have any financial concerns?

– ¿Puede cumplir con sus responsabilidades?

– ¿Qué interfiere con estas responsabilidades?

¿Tiene algún problema financiero?

Liquid matters

Do you drink alcohol?
– How often do you have alcohol?
– How many drinks per day do you have?
– What type of alcohol do you drink?

Did you drink more frequently in the past?

Did you quit drinking?
– When did you quit?

¿Bebe alcohol?
– ¿Con cuánta frecuencia bebe alcohol?
– ¿Cuántos tragos por día bebe?

– ¿Qué tipo de alcohol ingiere?

¿Bebía con mayor frecuencia anteriormente?

¿Dejó de beber?
– ¿Cuándo dejó de beber?

Daily routines

Describe your typical day.

Do you exercise?
– How often do you exercise?
– What type of exercise?
– Has the type or frequency of exercise changed recently?
– What caused the change?

Do you participate in any recreational activities?
– What do you do?
– How often do you participate?
– Has the frequency changed recently?

Describa un día habitual en su vida.

¿Se ejercita?
– ¿Con cuánta frecuencia se ejercita?
– ¿Qué tipo de ejercicio?
– ¿Ha cambiado recientemente el tipo o la frecuencia del ejercicio?
– ¿Qué provocó el cambio?

¿Participa de alguna actividad recreativa?
– ¿Qué hace?
– ¿Con cuánta frecuencia?
– ¿Se ha modificado la frecuencia recientemente?

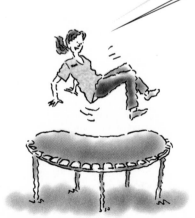

Do you exercise?

¿Se ejercita?

– What caused the change? | – ¿Qué provocó el cambio?

Stressing out

How often do you experience stress? | ¿Con qué frecuencia siente estrés?
– Rarely? | – ¿Casi nunca?
– Once in awhile? | – ¿De vez en cuando?
– Often? | – ¿A menudo?

Are you ever overwhelmed by stress? | ¿Alguna vez se siente abrumado(a) por el estrés?

What causes you to feel stress? | ¿Qué le provoca estrés?
– Work? | – ¿El trabajo?
– School? | – ¿La escuela?
– Family? | – ¿La familia?
– Marriage? | – ¿El matrimonio?
– Finances? | – ¿Las finanzas?
– Illness? | – ¿La enfermedad?
– Relationships? | – ¿Las relaciones?

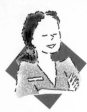

Practice makes perfecto

1. Joy wants to ask her patient if he was ever depressed. Help her finish her question.

_____

_____

_____

_____

> ¿Ha tenido _____?

2. Joy wants to know if her patient has ever participated in therapy or counseling. Help her ask about participation.

_____

_____

_____

_____

> ¿Ha ido a _____?

3. Joy wants to know about recent changes that may be causing stress. Help Joy ask the patient if she has experienced any recent loss, such as a divorce.

_____

_____

_____

_____

> ¿Ha sufrido _____?

> ¿Qué _____?

4. Joy is asking about the medication the patient is taking. Can you help her?

_____

_____

_____

_____

Answer key

1. Have you ever suffered from depression?
¿Ha tenido <u>depresión alguna vez</u>?

2. Have you ever gone to therapy or counseling?
¿Ha ido a <u>terapia u orientación alguna vez</u>?

3. Have you had a recent loss, such as a divorce, that is causing you stress?
¿Ha sufrido <u>una pérdida reciente, como un divorcio, que le esté provocando estrés</u>?

4. What medication you are taking?
¿Qué <u>medicamentos toma</u>?

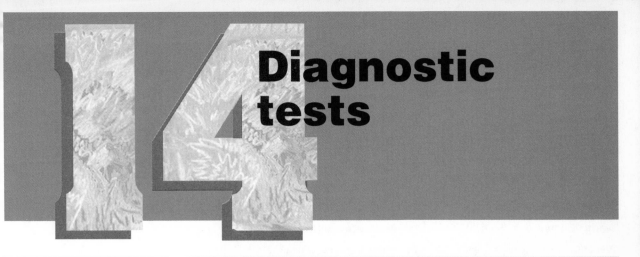

Diagnostic tests

Positioning and preparation

This section presents words and phrases you can use to position your patient and prepare him for possible procedures.

Rollin', rollin', rollin'

Bend backward.	Inclínese hacia atrás.
Bend forward.	Inclínese hacia adelante.
Lean backward.	Recuéstese.
Lean forward.	Inclínese hacia adelante.
Lie down.	Acuéstese.
Lie on your back.	Acuéstese boca arriba.
Lie on your: – side. – left side. – right side. – stomach.	Acuéstese: – del lado. – del lado izquierdo. – del lado derecho. – boca abajo.
Roll over.	Dé una vuelta.
Sit down.	Siéntese.
Sit up.	Enderécese.
Stand up.	Párese.
Turn to the side.	Voltéese hacia un lado.
Keep your feet together.	Mantenga los pies juntos.
Tighten your muscle.	Tense el músculo.
Turn to the right.	Voltéese hacia la derecha.
Turn to the left.	Voltéese hacia la izquierda.
Don't move your head.	No mueva la cabeza.

Don't move your head and follow my finger with your eyes.	Deje la cabeza quieta y siga mi dedo con los ojos.
Make a fist.	Cierre el puño.
Don't move.	No se mueva.

Respiratory rap

When I tell you, hold your breath.	Cuando le diga, contenga Ud. el aliento.
Take a deep breath and hold it.	Inspire profundo y contenga el aire.
Don't breathe (hold your breath).	No respire (contenga el aire).
Breathe. – Once more.	Respire. – Una vez más.

By the way

Are you pregnant?	¿Está Ud. embarazada?
Is there a possibility that you could be pregnant?	¿Es posible que ésta embarazada?

Speak softly

Don't talk.	No hable.
Say "AAHH."	Diga "AAAA."
Whisper.	Murmure.

What to expect, what to do

I need to put a tourniquet on your arm.	Tengo que ponerle un torniquete en el brazo.
You'll feel pain like a pinprick.	Ud. sentirá un dolor como un pinchazo de alfiler.
Don't drink anything before the test.	No beba nada antes del estudio.
Don't eat anything before the test.	No coma nada antes del estudio.
You must drink this liquid before the test.	Ud. tiene que tomarse este líquido antes de la prueba.
You must drink this liquid during the test.	Ud. tiene tomarse este líquido durante la prueba.
I must give you an enema before the test.	Tengo que ponerle una enema (lavativa) antes de la prueba.
You must hold the fluid in until we're finished with the test.	Ud. tiene que retener la enema (la lavativa) hasta que terminemos con la prueba.

You may go to the bathroom when we tell you.	Ud. puede ir al baño cuando le digamos.
Do you need to go to the bathroom?	¿Necesita ir al baño?
You'll need to empty your bladder before the test.	Deberá vaciar su vejiga antes de la prueba.
You can't empty your bladder until the test is finished.	Ud. no puede vaciar la vejiga hasta que la prueba se termine.

Physical examination

These terms and phrases will aid in the physical examination of your patient.

First things first

I'm going to check your:	Le voy a reconocer:
– skin.	– la piel.
– hair.	– el cabello.
– nails.	– las uñas.
– head.	– la cabeza.
– nose.	– la nariz.
– mouth.	– la boca.
– throat.	– la garganta.
– neck.	– el cuello.
– eyes.	– los ojos.
– ears.	– los oídos.
– chest.	– el pecho.
– lungs.	– los pulmones.
– heart.	– el corazón.
– pulse.	– el pulso.
– abdomen.	– del abdomen.
– rectum.	– el recto.
– bladder.	– la vejiga.
– kidneys.	– los riñones.
– breasts.	– las mamas or los senos.
– pelvis.	– la pelvis.
– penis.	– el pene.
– testicles.	– los testículos.
– reflexes.	– los reflejos.
– arms.	– los brazos.
– legs.	– las piernas.
I'm going to check your:	Voy a medirle:
– blood pressure.	– la presión sanguínea.
– heart rate.	– ritmo cardíaco.
– temperature.	– la temperatura.
I'm going to take a blood sample.	Voy a tomarle a Ud. una muestra de sangre.

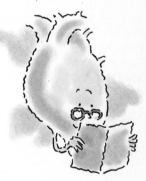

Important words to remember: *el corazón* for the heart and *el pulso* for pulse.

You need to give a urine specimen.	Tiene Ud. que darnos un espécimen de orina.
I'm going to look at your _____.	Le voy a examinar _____.
I'm going to listen to your _____.	Le voy a auscultar _____.
I'm going to touch your _____.	Tocaré su(s) _____.
I'm going to tap and listen to your _____.	Le(s) daré un golpecito y escucharé su(s) _____.
Are you comfortable?	¿Está Ud. cómodo?
Does this hurt?	¿Le duele esto?
– Where does it hurt?	– ¿Dónde le duele?

> You may also hear the word *una muestra* used for "specimen."

> I'm going to check your blood pressure.

> Voy a medirle la presión sanguínea.

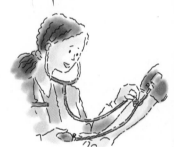

Tooling around with medical instruments

I'm going to:	Voy a:
– measure your:	– medirle:
arm.	el brazo.
leg.	la pierna.
belly.	el vientre.
hand.	la mano.
head.	la cabeza.
chest.	el pecho.
– look in your eyes.	– mirar en sus ojos.
– look in your ears.	– mirar en sus oídos.
– shine a light in your eyes.	– apuntar una luz en sus ojos.
– measure your eye pressure.	– medir su presión ocular.
– weigh you.	– pesarlo(a).
– listen to your:	– eschuchar:
lungs and breathing.	sus pulmones y su respiración.
– do a pelvic examination.	– hacer un examen pélvico.
– test your eyesight.	– medir su agudeza visual.

Test terms

These terms and phrases will help you inform your patient about diagnostic tests.

Jive for general tests

Your doctor has ordered:	El médico ha pedido que se le haga:
– a biopsy.	– una biopsia.
– a blood test.	– un análisis de la sangre.
– a blood culture.	– un cultivo de la sangre.
– a computed tomography scan.	– una tomografía computarizada.
– an endoscopy.	– una endoscopia.
– a magnetic resonance imaging scan.	– una resonancia magnética.
– an ultrasound.	– un ultrasonido.
– a urinalysis.	– un urinálisis (*or* un análisis de orina).
– an X-ray.	– una radiografía.
Do you know how this test is done?	¿Sabe cómo se realiza este estudio?

More tests: Heady stuff

Your doctor has ordered:
– allergy tests.
– a neck X-ray.
– a nose culture.
– a skull X-ray.
– a throat culture.
– a glaucoma test.
– a vision test.
– a hearing test.

Do you know how this test is done?

El médico ha pedido que se le haga:
– pruebas de alergia.
– una radiografía del cuello.
– un cultivo de la nariz.
– una radiografía del cráneo.
– un cultivo de la garganta.
– un examen de glaucoma.
– un examen de la vista.
– un examen de la audición.

¿Sabe cómo se realiza este estudio?

In some Spanish dialects, *prueba auditiva* may be used for "hearing test" and *pruebas* may be used for "tests."

Huff and puff

Your doctor has ordered:
– an arterial blood gas test.
– a bronchoscopy.
– a chest X-ray.
– a lung scan.
– pulmonary function tests.
– a pulse oximetry.

Do you understand what this test is looking for and how it's done?

El médico ha pedido que se le haga:
– gases de la sangre arterial.
– una broncoscopia.
– una radiografía del tórax.
– un ultrasonido pulmonar.
– una prueba de la función pulmonar.
– una oximetría del pulso.

¿Comprende lo que busca este estudio y cómo se realiza?

Pulmonary function tests measure how well I breathe.

Las pruebas de la función pulmonar miden cuán bien funcióno yo.

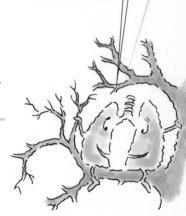

Lubba dub dub—cardiovascular tests

Your doctor has ordered:
– an arteriogram.
– a blood test for:
    cardiac enzymes.
    cholesterol.
    bleeding time.
    triglycerides.
– a cardiac catheterization.
– an electrocardiogram.
– an echocardiogram.
– a Holter monitor.
– a stress test.
– a venogram.

El médico ha pedido que se le haga:
– un arteriograma.
– un análisis de la sangre para:
    enzimas cardiacas.
    colesterol.
    tiempo de sangrado.
    triglicéridos.
– un cateterismo cardiaco.
– un electrocardiograma.
– un ecocardiograma.
– monitoreo Holter.
– un examen de estrés.
– un venograma.

Digest this!

Your doctor has ordered:
– an abdominal ultrasound.
– a barium enema.
– a barium swallow.

El médico ha pedido que se le haga:
– un ultrasonido abdominal.
– una enema de bario.
– tragar bario.

– a blood test for: – un análisis de la sangre para:
  amylase.   amilasa.
  liver enzymes.   enzimas del hígado.
– a cholangiogram. – un colangiograma.
– a cholecystogram. – un colecistograma.
– a colonoscopy. – una colonoscopia.
– a gastric analysis. – un análisis gástrico.
– a gastroscopy. – una gastroscopia.
– a liver biopsy. – una biopsia del hígado.
– a sigmoidoscopy. – una sigmoidoscopia.
– an endoscopy. – una endoscopia.
– a spleen scan. – una visualización del bazo por ecos de ultrasonidos.

– a stool culture. – un cultivo de la defecación.
– an upper GI series. – una serie gastrointestinal superior.

The water works: Urology

Your doctor has ordered: El médico ha pedido que se le haga:
– a blood test for: – un análisis de la sangre para:
  blood urea nitrogen.   nitrógeno y urea sanguínea.
  creatinine.   creatinina.
  electrolytes.   electrolitos.
– a cystoscopy. – una cistoscopia.
– an excretory urography. – una urografía excretora.
– a renal biopsy. – un cultivo renal.
– a retrograde pyelogram. – un pielograma retrógrado.
– a urine culture. – un cultivo de la orina.
– a renal ultrasound. – un ultrasonido renal.

Reproductive system

Your doctor has ordered a: El médico ha pedido que se le haga:
– breast biopsy. – una biopsia de la mama.
– breast examination. – un reconocimiento de los senos.
– cervical biopsy. – una biopsia cervical.
– mammogram. – un mamograma.
– Pap smear. – estudio de Papanicolau.
– pelvic examination. – un reconocimiento pélvico.
– pregnancy test. – un análisis de embarazo.
– prostate examination. – un reconocimiento de la próstata.
– prostatic biopsy. – una biopsia de la próstata.
– rectal examination. – un reconocimiento del recto.
– semen analysis. – un análisis del semen.
– vaginal culture. – un cultivo vaginal.

Mind games: Testing the brain

Your doctor has ordered:
– a brain scan.
– a cerebral arteriogram.
– a computed tomography scan of the brain.
– an electroencephalogram.
– a lumbar puncture.
– a myelogram.

El médico ha pedido que se le haga:
– un ultrasonido cerebral.
– un arteriograma cerebral.
– una tomografía computarizada del cerebro.
– un electroencefalograma.
– una punción lumbar.
– un mielograma.

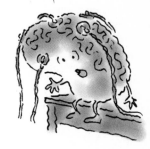

I'm going to undergo an electroencephalogram.

Me harán un electroencefalograma.

Boning up on bones and muscles

Your doctor has ordered:
– an arthroscopy.
– a bone biopsy.
– an electromyogram.
– a muscle biopsy.
– an X-ray of the:
    ankle.
    arm.
    back.
    elbow.
    foot.
    hand.
    hip.
    knee.
    leg.
    shoulder.
    wrist.

El médico ha pedido que se le haga:
– una artroscopia.
– una biopsia del hueso.
– un electromiograma.
– una biopsia del músculo.
– una radiografía de:
    el tobillo.
    el brazo.
    la espalda.
    el codo.
    el pie.
    la mano.
    la cadera.
    la rodilla.
    la pierna.
    el hombro.
    la muñeca.

A plate full of platelets

Your doctor has ordered:
– a blood test for:
    blood cell count.
    red blood cell count.

    white blood cell count.

    prothrombin time/International Normalized Ratio.
    clotting times.
    hematocrit.
    hemoglobin.
    hepatitis B.

El médico ha pedido que se le haga:
– un análisis de la sangre para:
    recuento sanguíneo.
    recuento de los glóbulos rojos de la sangre.
    recuento de los glóbulos blancos de la sangre.
    tiempo de protrombina/Deficiente Normalizado Internacional.
    el tiempo de coagulación.
    hematócrito.
    de hemoglobina.
    hepatitis tipo B.

human immunodeficiency virus.

platelet count.
– bone marrow biopsy.

virus de inmunodeficiencia humana.
recuento de plaquetas.
– una biopsia de la médula ósea del hueso.

Haven for hormones

Your doctor has ordered:
– an analysis of:
    adrenal function.
    ovarian function.
    parathyroid function.
    pancreatic function.
    pituitary function
    testicular function.
    thyroid function.
– a blood test for:
    serum calcium level.
    serum glucose level.
    fasting glucose level.
    glucose tolerance.
    glycosylated hemoglobin level.

    2-hour postprandial glucose level.
    serum hormone levels.
    serum phosphorus concentration.

El médico ha pedido que se le haga:
– un análisis de:
    la función adrenal.
    la función ovárica.
    la función paratiroidea.
    la función pancreática.
    la función de la pituitaria.
    la función testicular.
    la función de la tiroides.
– un análisis de sangre para revisar:
    el nivel de calcio.
    el nivel de glucosa.
    el nivel de glucosa en abstención.
    la tolerancia a la glucosa.
    el nivel de hemoglobina glucosilatada.
    el nivel de glucosa dos-horas posprandial.
    niveles hormonales.
    niveles de fósforo.

Just don't do it

Don't eat or drink anything after midnight before the test.

No coma ni beba nada después de medianoche antes de la prueba (*or* del examen).

Don't eat or drink anything after _____ a.m.

No coma ni beba nada después de las _____ de la mañana.

Don't eat or drink anything after _____ p.m.

No coma ni beba nada después de las _____ de la tarde (*or* la noche).

You may take your usual medicine in the morning with a small amount of water.

Ud. puede tomarse todas sus medicinas habituales en la mañana con una cantidad pequeña de agua.

You may take all of your usual medicine in the morning with a small amount of water except _____.

Ud. puede tomarse todas sus medicinas habituales en la mañana con una cantidad pequeña de agua con la excepción de _____.

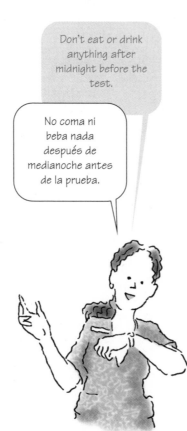

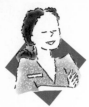

Practice makes perfecto

1. Help Joy tell the patient that her doctor has ordered a blood test.

_____

_____

_____

_____

> Su médico ha pedido que _____.

2. Joy needs to tell this patient not to eat or drink anything after midnight before the test. Can you help?

_____

_____

_____

_____

> No coma ni beba nada después de _____.

> Acuéstese _____.

3. Joy needs to position a patient for examination of his spine. Help Joy tell the patient to lie on his stomach.

_____

_____

_____

_____

Answer key

1. Your doctor has ordered a blood test.
Su médico ha pedido que <u>se le haga un análisis de la sangre</u>.

2. Don't eat or drink anything after midnight before the test.
No coma ni beba nada después de <u>la medianoche antes de la prueba</u>.

3. Lie on your stomach.
Acuéstese <u>boca abajo</u>.

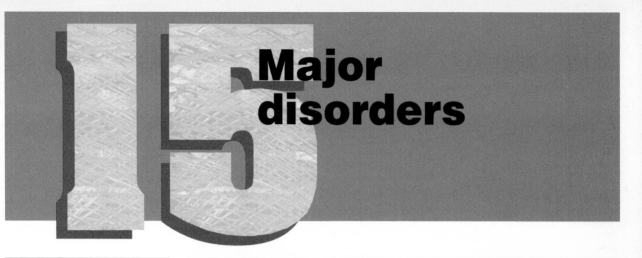

Major disorders

15

Basic phrases

These statements may be used to teach your patient about his disorder.

Here's the scoop

The doctor has diagnosed you with:
– an aneurysm.
– a blockage in your artery.
– a blood clot.
– a damaged or diseased area.
– a growth or tumor.
– a hemorrhage.
– an infection.
– a muscle spasm.
– a narrowing.
– an ulcer.
– anemia.
– cancer.
– a heart attack.
– heart disease.

As a result, your _____ is (are): (See *Body parts*.)
– not working or functioning properly.

– not working efficiently.
– not working at all.
– working too hard.
– not producing enough _____.
– producing too much _____.
– not receiving an adequate oxygen or blood supply.

Here's some written information about _____ for you to read.

We don't know what causes this condition.

El doctor le ha diagnosticado:
– un aneurisma.
– una obstrucción arterial.
– un coágulo de sangre.
– una región dañada o enferma.
– una formación anormal o tumor.
– una hemorragia.
– una infección.
– un espasmo muscular.
– un estrechamiento.
– una úlcera.
– anemia.
– cáncer.
– un ataque cardiaco.
– una enfermedad cardiaca.

Como consecuencia, el órgano _____ de su cuerpo o sistema:
– no funciona o no funciona debidamente.
– no funciona eficientemente.
– no funciona en absoluto.
– funciona con demasiada dificultad.
– no produce suficiente _____.
– produce demasiado(a) _____.
– no recibe una cantidad adecuada de oxígeno o sangre.

Aquí tiene información escrita acerca de _____ para que la lea.

No se sabe qué provoca este problema.

Common disorders

Here's an overview of some common disorders you may encounter and phrases to help you explain them to your patients. (See *AIDS and Latinos.*)

Acquired immunodeficiency syndrome

Acquired immunodeficiency syndrome (AIDS) is called *síndrome de inmunodeficiencia adquirida* (*SIDA*) in Spanish. These phrases will help you explain AIDS.

What it is

Acquired immunodeficiency syndrome (AIDS) is a weakening of the immune system that makes you vulnerable to infection.

El síndrome de inmunodeficiencia adquirida (SIDA) es el debilitamiento del sistema inmune que hace que Ud. sea vulnerable a infecciones.

How it happens

AIDS is caused by a virus and may have been transmitted by unprotected contact with infected blood or body fluids.

El virus que causa el SIDA puede ser transmitido por el contacto con sangre o líquidos infectados.

You may have contracted the disease through:
– I.V. drug use with a dirty, infected needle
– unprotected sexual contact
– blood products or blood transfusions.

Ud. se puede haber contagiado al usar drogas por:
– medio intravenoso con una aguja sucia e infectada
– contacto sexual no protejido
– productos de sangre o una transfusión de sangre.

How we can find it

To determine if you have AIDS, a blood test is done.

Para determinar si usted tiene SIDA, se realiza un análisis de sangre.

How we can treat it

You'll need many different medications, and you must take them all as instructed.

Necesitará tomar muchos medicamentos diferentes, y debe tomarlos todos como se indica.

Results with AIDS treatment are improving all the time.

Los resultados del tratamiento del SIDA son cada vez mejores.

It's a sexually transmitted disease, so anyone with whom you have had sexual intercourse should be informed of your illness.

Es una enfermedad de transmisión sexual, por lo que es necesario informar a todas las personas con las que usted ha tenido relaciones sexuales.

You'll need many medications and you must take them all as instructed.

Necesitará tomar muchos medicamentos, y debe tomarlos todos como se indica.

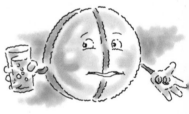

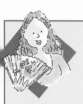

La cultura

AIDS and Latinos

The incidence of new cases of acquired immunodeficiency syndrome (AIDS) among Latinos is a serious threat to both men and women. In 2005, HIV/AIDS was the fourth leading cause of death among Latinos ages 35 to 44.

Looking at demographics
As in past years, the number of new cases among men far outnumbered that among women. Among Latino men, 24% of cases were attributed to injecting illegal drugs, and 55% were attributed to same-sex sexual contact. Among women, about 29% of cases were attributed to injecting illegal drugs, and 69% were related to high-risk heterosexual contact.

Communication is key
A key factor in reducing the incidence of AIDS among your Latino patients is the ability to communicate with them in Spanish and to approach them with knowledge of and respect for their cultural perspective. (Latino women, for example, are reluctant to discuss condom use with their partners.) You need to provide education on both the prevention and treatment of injected illegal drug use, and the importance of safer sex practices.

Addictive disease

Addictive disease is called *adicción* in Spanish. These phrases will help you explain what addictive disease is and its effects, diagnosis, and treatment.

What it is

Addictive disease is a physical disease associated with the ingestion of psychoactive substances.

Una adicción es una enfermedad física vinculada con la ingestión de sustancias psicoactivas.

A psychoactive substance is anything that affects your mind or the way you act.

Una sustancia psicoactiva es algo que afecta su mente o su manera de actuar.

How it happens

It occurs when you can't stop taking a drug on your own.

Ocurre cuando Ud. no puede dejar de tomar una droga por su cuenta.

Examples of addictive substances include alcohol, opioids, stimulants, antidepressants, antianxiety drugs, hallucinogens, and marijuana.

Algunos ejemplos de sustancias adictivas son el alcohol, los opiáceos, las drogas estimulantes, antidepresivas, contra la ansiedad, los alucinógenos, y la marihuana.

Experimentation with psychoactive substances commonly begins in adolescence or earlier, in some cases.

In many cases, substance abuse leads to addictive disease, which may involve physical dependence, psychological dependence, or both.

Dependence means you crave a substance and don't think you can get along without it.

What it does

Addictive disease can lead to life-threatening complications, such as:

– heart and lung infections
– heart attack
– AIDS
– hepatitis
– depression
– increased risk of suicide
– serious mental problems
– brain damage or stroke.

How we can find it

To evaluate the extent of addictive disease or assess for complications, these tests may be ordered:
– laboratory blood testing
– blood or urine drug screening.

How we can treat it

Treatment of addictive disease depends on the substance you're addicted to and complications.

Treatments may include:
– symptomatic treatment for acute intoxication
– detoxification
– rehabilitation
– psychotherapy
– exercise
– relaxation techniques
– nutritional support.

You may be prescribed sedatives and tranquilizers temporarily to help with insomnia, anxiety, and depression.

La experimentación con sustancias psicoactivas comienza comúnmente en la adolescencia o antes, en algunos cases.

En muchos casos, el consumo de sustancias conduce a una adicción que puede incluir una dependencia física, psicológica, o ambas.

Tener dependencia significa desear con desesperación una sustancia y no pensar que se puede vivir sin ella.

La adicción puede conducir a complicaciones que ponen en riesgo la vida, como:
– infecciones cardiacas y pulmonares
– ataque cardiaco
– SIDA
– hepatitis
– depresión
– mayor riesgo de suicidio
– problemas mentales graves
– daño cerebral o derrame cerebral.

Para evaluar el grado de adicción o evaluar complicaciones, se podrá ordenar pruebas de:
– análisis de sangre en laboratorio
– análisis de drogas en sangre u orina.

El tratamiento de las adicciones depende de la sustancia al cual Ud. está adicto y sus complicaciones.

Los tratamientos pueden incluir:
– tratamiento sintomático por intoxicación grave
– destoxificación
– rehabilitación
– psicoterapia
– ejercicio
– técnicas de relajación
– apoyo dietético.

Se le puede ordenar sedantes y tranquilizantes provisionalmente para ayudarle con el insomnio, ansiedad, y depresión.

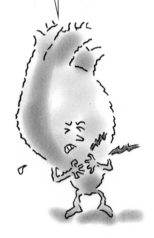

Addictive disease can lead to life-threatening complications such as heart attack.

La adicción puede conducir a complicaciones que ponen en riesgo la vida como un ataque cardiaco.

Alzheimer's disease

Alzheimer's disease is called *mal de Alzheimer* or *demencia mental progresiva* in Spanish. Here are some phrases to help you explain Alzheimer's disease and its effects, diagnosis, and treatment.

What it is

Alzheimer's disease is a type of dementia or brain disease.

El Alzheimer es un tipo de demencia o enfermedad cerebral.

Alzheimer's disease is marked by gradual worsening of mental deterioration.

El mal de Alzheimer se caracteriza por desorientación mental.

How it happens

The cause of Alzheimer's disease is unknown.

No se conoce la causa del mal de Alzheimer.

Several factors are thought to contribute to this condition, including a shortage of certain chemicals in the brain.

Se cree que varios factores contribuyen a este mal, incluido(a) la falta de ciertas sustancias químicas en el cerebro.

What it does

At first the patient may develop:
– forgetfulness.
– inability to recall recent events.

– difficulty learning and remembering new information.
– inability to concentrate.
– declining personal hygiene and appearance.

Al principio, el paciente podrá presentar:
– problemas de memoria.
– incapacidad para recordar eventos recientes.
– dificultad para aprender y recordar información nueva.
– falta de concentración.
– falta de higiene y cuidado del aspecto personal.

Gradually, tasks that require abstract thinking and judgment become more difficult.

Gradualmente, las tareas que requieren pensamiento abstracto y decisión se vuelven más difíciles.

The patient experiences progressive difficulty communicating with others as well as severe deterioration in memory, language ability, and coordination.

El paciente experimenta dificultad progresiva en comunicarse con los demás, así como un grave deterioro de la memoria y de la habilidad del habla y la coordinación.

The patient becomes disoriented and is susceptible to infection and accidents.

El paciente se vuelve desorientado y es susceptible a infecciones y accidentes.

How we can find it

There's no specific test for Alzheimer's disease.

No existe un análisis específico para detectar el Alzheimer.

Tests may be ordered to rule out other disorders or problems.

Se pueden llegar a indicar análisis para descartar otras afecciones o problemas.

Diagnosis is based on history from a reliable family member and examination of physical and mental status.

El diagnóstico se basa en la historia precisa proveniente de un pariente confiable y el examen del estado físico y mental.

How we can treat it

No cure or specific treatment exists.

No existe una cura o un tratamiento específico.

Drugs may be prescribed to try to improve the brain's circulation.

Se pueden llegar a prescribir drogas para tratar de mejorar la circulación en el cerebro.

Drugs may be prescribed to try to improve the patient's mood.

Se pueden llegar a prescribir drogas para tratar de mejorar el ánimo del paciente.

Drugs may be prescribed to treat memory and sleep problems.

Se pueden llegar a prescribir drogas para tratar problemas de memoria y de sueño.

Anthrax

Anthrax is called *ántrax* in Spanish. Here are some phrases to help you explain what anthrax is and its effects, diagnosis, and treatment.

What it is

Anthrax results from exposure to the bacteria *Bacillus anthracis*.

El ántrax resulta de la exposición a las bacterias *Bacillus anthracis*.

Anthrax has three forms in humans:

El ántrax tiene tres formas en los seres humanos:

– inhalation (lung)
– cutaneous (skin)
– digestive or GI (stomach or intestines).

– inhalación (pulmones)
– cutánea (piel)
– digestivo o gastrointestinal (estómago o intestinos).

How it happens

Inhalation anthrax is the most serious and is caused by breathing anthrax into the lungs.

El ántrax por inhalación es el más grave y es provocado al inspirar ántrax en los pulmones.

Cutaneous anthrax occurs when the bacteria comes in contact with skin that has been cut or broken.

El ántrax cutáneo se produce cuando las bacterias entran en contacto con la piel desgarrada o cortada.

GI anthrax occurs when you eat meat from an infected animal or from eating or drinking contaminated food.

El ántrax gastrointestinal ocurre cuando Ud. come carne de un animal infectado o come o bebe comidas contaminadas.

What it does

Inhalation anthrax causes initial flulike symptoms such as:
– tiredness
– fever
– headache
– chills
– muscle aches
– sore throat.

It usually progresses to severe respiratory difficulties, such as:
– difficulty breathing
– obstruction of air passages
– chest pain
– shock or death.

Cutaneous anthrax causes a small, elevated, itchy lesion that resembles an insect bite.

It develops into a blister, and finally becomes a small, painless ulcer with a black center.

It causes enlarged lymph glands.

GI anthrax causes nausea, vomiting, fever, stomach pains, and bloody diarrhea.

How we can find it

To determine if you have anthrax, these tests may be ordered:
– cultures of the blood, skin lesions, or sputum
– laboratory studies for specific antibodies.

How we can treat it

Treatment includes antibiotics and antimicrobials.

Inhalation and GI anthrax aren't contagious.

El ántrax por inhalación causa sintomas iniciales parecidos a la gripe, como:
– cansancio
– fiebre
– dolor de cabeza
– escalofríos
– dolores musculares
– dolor de garganta.

Progresa usualmente a complicaciones respiratorias graves, como:
– dificultad para respirar
– obstrucción de vías aéreas
– dolor de pecho
– estado de shock o fallecimiento.

El ántrax cutáneo causa una lesión pequeña, hinchada, y con comezón que se parece a la picadura de un insecto.

Se convierte en una ampolla y por último, en una llaga pequeña, sin dolor, con un centro negro.

Provoca una expansión de las glándulas linfáticas.

El ántrax gastrointestinal provoca náuseas, vómitos, fiebre, dolores estomacales, y diarrea con sangre.

Para determinar si Ud. tiene ántrax, se podrá ordenar estas pruebas:
– cultivos de sangre, lesiones de piel, o esputo
– análisis de laboratorio para detectar anticuerpos específicos.

El tratamiento incluye antibióticos y antibacterianos.

El ántrax por inhalación y gastrointestinal no son contagiosos.

Arthritis

Arthritis is called *artritis* in Spanish. Here are some phrases to help you explain the different types of arthritis and their effects, diagnosis, and treatment.

What it is

Arthritis is pain and swelling of the joints.

Artritis es dolor e inflamación en las articulaciones.

There are many types of arthritis.

Hay muchos tipos de artritis.

Osteoarthritis and rheumatoid arthritis are the most common types.

Osteoartritis y artritis reumatoide son los tipos más comunes.

What we're looking for

I believe you may have:
– osteoarthritis.
– rheumatoid arthritis.

Creo que Ud. puede tener:
– osteoartritis.
– artritis reumatoide.

In osteoarthritis, the cartilage that covers the ends of the bones wears away.
– This makes the bones change shape and rub together, causing pain.

En la osteoartritis, el cartílago que cubre los extremos de los huesos se desgasta.
– Este produce cambios en la forma de los huesos y fricción, ocasionando dolor.

Rheumatoid arthritis is inflammation of the joints of the hands, arms, and feet as well as the surrounding muscles, tendons, and ligaments.

La artritis reumatoide es la inflamación de las articulaciones de las manos, los brazos y los pies, así como también de los músculos, tendones y ligamentos adyacentes.

How we can find it

To determine if you have arthritis, these tests may be ordered:

Para determinar si Ud. tiene artritis, voy a pedir que se le hagan unas pruebas, incluido(a):

– blood test
– test of fluid around the joint

– X-rays.

– un análisis de sangre.
– análisis de fluidos alrededor de la articulación
– radiografías.

How we can treat it

Treatment for osteoarthritis and rheumatoid arthritis includes such medications as aspirin and other anti-inflammatory drugs.

El tratamiento de la osteoartritis y la artritis reumatoide incluye medicamentos como la aspirina y otros medicamentos antiinflamatorios.

Asthma

Asthma is called *asma* in Spanish. Here are some phrases to help you explain what asthma is and its effects, diagnosis, and treatment.

What it is

Asthma is a reversible lung disease that causes obstruction or narrowing of the airways, which are typically inflamed and hyperresponsive and produce thick secretions.

El asma es una enfermedad pulmonar reversible que produce la obstrucción o el angostamiento de las vías aéreas, que generalmente están inflamadas e hipersensibles y producen secreciones densas.

Asthma may go away on its own with or without treatment.

El asma puede desaparecer naturalmente con o sin tratamiento.

Symptoms range from mild wheezing and difficulty breathing to life-threatening respiratory failure.

Los síntomas van desde resuellos leves y dificultad para respirar hasta una insuficiencia respiratoria que pone en riesgo la vida.

How it happens

Allergic or extrinsic asthma results from inhaling allergens, which may trigger an attack.

El asma alérgico o extrínseco surge de la inhalación de alérgenos, que pueden provocar un ataque.

It may be triggered by:
– pollen
– animal dander
– house dust or mold
– kapok or feather pillows
– food additives containing sulfites.

Puede ser causada por:
– polen
– epitelio de animales
– polvo o moho de la casa
– almohadas de capoc o plumas
– aditivos alimenticios que contienen sulfitos.

Non-allergic or intrinsic asthma is the term used when an allergen isn't obvious.

Asma no alérgico o intrínseco es el término usado cuando no es evidente la presencia de un alérgeno.

It may be triggered by:
– a severe respiratory infection
– irritants
– emotional stress
– fatigue
– noxious fumes
– changes in the weather.

Puede ser causada por:
– una infeccíon respiratoria grave
– irritantes
– estrés emocional
– fatiga
– vahos tóxicos
– cambios climáticos.

Many patients have both intrinsic and extrinsic asthma.

Muchos pacientes tienen asma tanto intrínseco como extrínseco.

What it does

An asthma attack may involve progressively worsening shortness of breath, coughing, wheezing, and chest tightness.

Un acceso de asma puede consistir en la falta de respiración que se agrava progresivamente, tos, respiración jadeante, y rigidez en el pecho.

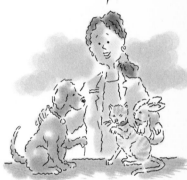

Extrinsic asthma results from allergens such as animal dander.

El asma extrínseca es causada por alergenos, como epitelio de animales.

How we can find it

To determine if you have asthma, these tests may be ordered:
– a review of symptoms and triggers

– lung function studies
– chest X-ray
– allergy testing
– nasal examination.

Para determinar si Ud. tiene asma, se podrá ordenar estas pruebas:
– una revisión de síntomas y desencadenantes
– análisis de función pulmonar
– radiografías de tórax
– pruebas de alergia
– examen nasal.

How we can treat it

Treatment of asthma may involve:

– avoiding or removing allergens
– desensitization to specific allergen

– drugs to dilate the air passages and decrease inflammation.

Treatment during an acute asthma attack or status asthmaticus may include:

– medication
– oxygen administration
– I.V. fluids
– using a ventilator to breathe.

Be sure to have follow-up visits with your doctor.

El tratamiento del asma puede comprender:
– evitar o eliminar alérgenos
– la desensibilización al alergeno especifico
– drogas para dilatar las vías aéreas y disminuir la inflamación.

El tratamiento durante un acceso de asma grave o estado asmático puede incluir:
– medicamentos
– adminstración de oxigeno
– fluidos intravenosos
– uso de un respirador artificial para respirar.

Asegúrese de programar citas de seguimiento con su médico.

> To determine if you have asthma, a chest X-ray may be ordered.
>
> Para determinar si Ud. tiene asma, se podrá ordenar una radiografía de tórax.

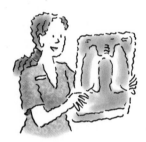

Cancer

Cancer is called *cáncer* in Spanish. Here are some phrases to help you explain what cancer is, the different types of cancer, and their effects, diagnoses, and treatments. (See *Prostate cancer and Latino men.*)

What it is

Cancer is a general term to describe an abnormal and malignant growth or tumor in the body.

Cáncer es untérmino general utilizado paca describir un vulto o tumor anormal o maligno en el cuerpo.

How it happens

Cancer cells were once normal cells that changed into abnormal cells.

Cancer cells continue to grow and divide and can spread to other parts of the body.

Las células cancerígenas son células que alguna vez fueron normales y se convirtieron en células anormales.

Sin embargo, las células del cáncer siguen creciendo y dividiéndose y pueden extenderse a otras partes del cuerpo.

La cultura

Prostate cancer and Latino men

Prostate cancer is the most common form of cancer that occurs in American men. After lung cancer, it's the leading cause of cancer-related death.

Factors and risks

While Latino men are generally at less risk than Whites for developing prostate cancer, certain factors have been tentatively linked with the disease that may place some Latino men at increased risk. It has been reported that men who have been treated for nonmelanoma skin cancers—long known to be associated with exposure to ultraviolet radiation—have a 28% higher risk of death from prostate cancer. It's likely, therefore, that men who work outdoors, such as farmers, may be at greater risk for developing prostate cancer. In addition, men who are employed in work that involves heavy labor may be at higher risk. More than 36% of Latino men living in the United States are employed in such vocations.

Prevention and cultural perspectives

Cultural attitudes toward diet, exercise, educational awareness, and employment will play a significant role in your treatment of Latino men at risk for prostate cancer. Familiarizing yourself with your patients' cultural perspectives and with Spanish will allow you to address the issues of prevention, diagnosis, and treatment more effectively.

These cells accumulate and form tumors (lumps) that may compress, invade, and destroy normal tissue.

If cells break away from such a tumor, they can travel through the bloodstream or lymph system to other areas of the body.

The spread of a tumor to a new site is called *metastasis*.

What we're looking for

I believe you may have cancer of the:
– breast.
– brain.
– bowel.
– bladder.
– liver.
– lung.
– ovary.
– uterus.
– pancreas.
– prostate.

Estas células se acumulan y forman tumores (pellas) que pueden comprimir, invadir y destruir el tejido normal.

Si dichas células se desprenden del tumor, pueden viajar por la corriente sanguínea o el sistema linfático a otras partes del cuerpo.

La extensión de un tumor a una parte nueva se llama *metástasis*.

Creo que Ud. puede tener cáncer:
– de pecho.
– del cerebro.
– del intestino.
– de la vejiga.
– hígado.
– pulmón.
– ovario.
– útero.
– del páncreas.
– de la próstata.

– cervix.

– del cuello uterino.

– blood.

– de la sangre.

– bone.

– de huesos.

How we can find it

To determine if you have cancer or if the cancer has spread to other areas of your body, these tests may be ordered:

Para determinar si Ud. tiene cáncer o si el cáncer se ha extendido a otras partes de su cuerpo, voy a pedir que se le hagan análisis (pruebas) de diagnóstico, incluido(a):

– blood test

– un análisis de sangre

– X-rays

– radiografías

– CT scan

– tomografía computada

– mammogram

– una mamografía

– ultrasound

– un ultrasonido

– biopsy

– una biopsia

– proctoscopy

– una proctoscopia

– colonoscopy

– una colonoscopia

– test of bowel movements for blood.

– control de sangre en materia fecal.

How we can treat it

Treatment depends on the site and stage of the cancer and can include:

El tratamiento depende del lugar y del estado en que se encuentra el cáncer y podrá incluir:

– radiation

– radiación

– chemotherapy

– quimioterapia

– medications to control the adverse effects of the cancer therapy

– medicamentos para controlar los efectos adversos de la terapia del cáncer

– surgery.

– cirugía.

Cataract

A cataract is called *cataratas* in Spanish. Here are some phrases to help you explain what a cataract is and its effects, diagnosis, and treatment.

What it is

A cataract is a gradually developing cloudiness of the lens or lens capsule of the eye.

Las cataratas son una opacidad que se desarrolla gradualmente en el lente cristalino del ojo.

Cataracts commonly occur in both eyes, with each progressing independently.

Las cataratas por lo general se producen en ambos ojos y cada una de las cataratas tiene un progreso independiente.

How it happens

Senile cataracts are caused by degenerative changes related to aging.

Las cataratas seniles son causadas por cambios degenerativos relacionados con el envejecimiento.

Congenital cataracts are from genetic defects or occur as a result of maternal rubella infection in the first trimester.

Las cataratas congénitas surgen de defectos genéticos u ocurren a raíz de una infección de rubéola en la madre durante el primer trimestre de gestación.

Traumatic cataracts develop from foreign body injury to the eye or blunt trauma to the eye.

Las cataratas traumáticas se desarrollan por una lesión ocular por un cuerpo extraño o un traumatismo contuso en el ojo.

Complicated cataracts develop because of other diseases, such as diabetes or glaucoma.

Las cataratas complicadas surgen a raíz de otra enfermedad, como la diabetes o el glaucoma.

Toxic cataracts result from chemical or drug toxicity, or extended exposure to ultraviolet rays.

Las cataratas tóxico-medicamentosas resultan de una toxicidad química o de medicamentos, o una exposición prolongada a rayos ultravioletas.

What it does

A cataract causes the normally black pupil to become hazy.

Las cataratas hacen que la pupila normalmente negra se vuelva opaca.

A patient with a cataract experiences painless, gradual blurring and loss of vision.

Un paciente con cataratas experimenta una opacidad indolora y gradual y la pérdida de visión.

Some patients complain of blinding glare from headlights when driving at night.

Algunos pacientes se quejan de las luces altas de los veheiculos los enceguece cuando manejan por la noche.

Others complain of an unpleasant glare and poor vision in bright sunlight.

Otros se quejan de un resplandor molesto y mala visión con la luz brillante del sol.

How we can find it

To determine if a cataract is present, these tests may be ordered:

Para determinar si una persona teine cataratas, se puede ordenar estas pruebas:

– eye examination
– vision test.

– examen ocular
– examen de visión.

How we can treat it

Treatment of a cataract involves surgically removing it from the eye.

El tratamiento de las cataratas consiste en extirparlas quirúrgicamente del ojo.

Sometimes a lens implant is put in the eye after the cataract is removed.

A veces se implanta un lente en el ojo después de que se elimina la catarata.

After surgery, you must protect your eye(s) from injury by wearing a shield or glasses.

Después de la cirugía, Ud. debe proteger su(s) ojo(s) para que no se lastime(n) usando un protector para ojos o gafas.

Treatment of a cataract involves surgically removing it from the eye.

El tratamiento de las cataratas consiste en extirparlas quirúrgicamente del ojo.

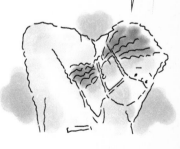

You may need to wear glasses or contact lenses after surgery to improve vision.

Es posible que usted deba usar gafas o lentes de contacto después de la cirugía para mejorar la visión.

Chronic obstructive pulmonary disease

Chronic obstructive pulmonary disease (COPD) is called *enfermedad crónica obstructiva del pulmón* (ECOP) in Spanish. Here are some phrases to help you explain the different types of COPD and their effects, diagnoses, and treatments.

What it is

Chronic obstructive pulmonary disease (COPD) is a group of lung conditions that results in inflamed and narrowed airways in the lungs that make breathing difficult.

La enfermedad crónica obstructiva del pulmón (ECOP) es un grupo de afecciones pulmonares que provoca la inflamación y el angostamiento de las vías aéreas en los pulmones, lo que dificulta la respiración.

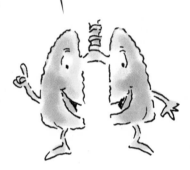

Chronic obstructive pulmonary disease is called *enfermedad crónica obstructiva del pulmón* in Spanish.

What it does

It can cause you to have an increased amount of mucus and be short of breath, especially when you exercise.

Puede causar un aumento de la mucosidad y la falta de aire, principalmente al hacer ejercicio.

It can also cause wheezing, coughing, and trouble breathing.

Además, puede provocar resuellos, tos, y problemas para respirar.

It can include such disorders as bronchitis, asthma, and emphysema.

Puede incluir trastornos como bronquitis, asma, y enfisema.

What we're looking for

I believe you may have:
– asthma.
– emphysema.
– bronchitis.

Creo que Ud. puede tener:
– asma.
– enfisema.
– bronquitis.

How we can find it

To determine if you have COPD, these tests may be ordered:

– chest X-ray
– lung function tests
– blood tests
– pulse oximetry.

Para determinar si Ud. tiene ECOP, voy a pedir que se le hagan unos análisis de diagnóstico, incluidos(as):

– una radiografía del tórax
– exámenes de función pulmonar
– análisis de sangre
– oximetría del pulso.

How we can treat it

Treatment of COPD may include:
– drugs to open passageways in your lungs
– antibiotics to treat infection
– inhaled steroids

El tratamiento de la ECOP podrá incluir:
– medicamentos para abrir los conductos de los pulmones
– antibióticos para tratar la infección
– inhalación de esteroides

– oxygen.

– oxígeno.

You'll need to stop smoking and avoid other lung irritants.

Usted deberá dejar de fumar y evitar otros irritantes pulmonares.

To help remove secretions, learn how to cough effectively.

Para ayudar a eliminar secreciones, aprenda cómo toser correctamente.

If your secretions are thick, drink six 8-ounce glasses of fluid per day.

Si sus secreciones son espesas, tome seis vasos de 8 onzas de líquido por día.

To strengthen your breathing muscles, take slow, deep breaths and exhale through pursed lips.

Para fortalecer sus músculos respiratorios, respire hondo y lentamente y exhale por la boca, frunciendo los labios.

Coronary artery disease

Coronary artery disease (CAD) is called *enfermedad de las arterias coronarias (EAC)* in Spanish. Here are some phrases to help you explain the causes of CAD and its effects, diagnosis, and treatment.

What it is

In coronary artery disease (CAD), the arteries that supply blood to the heart are blocked, slowing or blocking the flow of blood to the heart muscle.

En la enfermedad de las arterias coronarias (EAC), las arterias que suministran sangre al corazón disminuyen o interrumpen el flujo de la sangre al corazón.

Arteriosclerosis is the most common cause of CAD.

La arteriosclerosis es la causa más común de la EAC.

How it happens

In arteriosclerosis, fatty plaques slowly accumulate in the arteries, making blood flow difficult.

En la arteriosclerosis, se acumulan placas de grasa lentamente en las arterias.

What it does

If the accumulation isn't stopped, the fatty plaques will completely block the artery and cause a heart attack.

Si no se detiene dicha acumulación, las placas de grasa bloquearán completamente la arteria, provocando un ataque cardiaco.

Chest pain is a symptom of CAD.

El dolor del tórax es un síntoma de EAC.

How we can find it

To determine if you have CAD, these tests may be ordered:

Para determinar si Ud. tiene EAC, voy a pedir que se le hagan unos análisis (pruebas), incluido(a):

– blood tests
– electrocardiogram
– exercise stress test
– echocardiogram
– cardiac catheterization

– análisis de sangre
– un electrocardiograma
– una prueba de estrés físico
– ecocardiograma
– un cateterismo de corazón

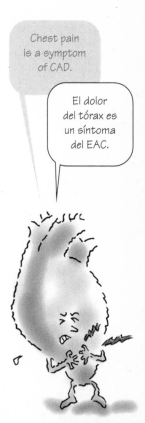

Chest pain is a symptom of CAD.

El dolor del tórax es un síntoma del EAC.

How we can treat it

Treatment for CAD may include drugs to improve blood flow and oxygen supply to your heart.

Blocked arteries may require:
– coronary artery bypass surgery.
– angioplasty
    (a procedure in which a catheter is used to compress fatty deposits and relieve blockages).

– percutaneous transluminal coronary angioplasty with placement of a stent to keep the artery open.

Be sure to follow the prescribed drug therapy and diet.

Get regular, moderate exercise.

You'll need to stop smoking.

El tratamiento de la EAC podrá incluir medicamentos para mejorar el flujo sanguíneo y el suministro de oxígeno al corazón.

Las arterias bloqueadas pueden requerir:
– cirugía de bypass de arteria coronaria.
– angioplastía
    (procedimiento en el que se utiliza un catéter para comprimir los depósitos de grasa y eliminar los bloqueos).

– angioplastía coronaria transluminal percutánea con la colocación de un stent para mantener abierta la arteria.

Es importante que efectúe la terapia de medicamentos recetada y la dieta.

Haga ejercicios regularmente y moderadamente.

Tendrá que dejar de fumar.

Depression

Depression is called *depresión* in Spanish. Here are some phrases to help you explain what depression is and its effects, diagnosis, and treatment.

What it is

Depression is a syndrome of a persistent feeling of unhappiness or being unwell.

It's usually accompanied by problems with sleep and appetite, feeling sluggish, and an inability to feel pleasure.

Depression affects both sexes but is more common in women.

La depresión es un síndrome con una sensación persistente de infelicidad o malestar.

Por lo general viene acompañada de problemas de sueño y apetitito, una sensación de letargo, y la incapacidad de sentir placer.

La depresión afecta a ambos sexos, pero es más común en las mujeres.

How it happens

The causes of depression aren't completely understood.

Depression may be affected by:
– genetics
– medications
– physical environment
– psychological causes
– social causes.

No se comprenden completamente las causas de la depresión.

La depresión puede ser afectada por:
– la genética
– medicamentos
– el entorno físico
– causas psicológicas
– causas sociales.

Depression may also be related to specific medical conditions or medications.

La depresión también puede estar relacionada con afecciones médicas o medicamentos específicos.

What it does

The primary features of depression include a sad mood and a loss of interest or pleasure in daily activities.

Las características principales de la depresión incluyen tristeza y una pérdida de interés o placer en las actividades diarias.

Other signs and symptoms of depression include:
– self-doubt
– difficulty coping
– feelings of anger or anxiety
– difficulty concentrating or thinking clearly
– being easily distracted
– problems making decisions
– fatigue
– increase or decrease in appetite
– inability to sleep (insomnia)
– lack of interest in sexual activity
– constipation or diarrhea.

Otros signos y síntomas de la depresión incluyen:
– falta de autoconfianza
– dificultades para autoabastecerse
– sentimientos de ira o ansiedad
– dificultad para concentrarse o pensar claramente
– distraerse con facilidad
– problemas para tomar decisiones
– fatiga
– mayor o menor apetito
– incapacidad para dormir (insomnio)
– falta de interés en la sexualidad
– constipación o diarrea.

Suicidal thoughts, a preoccupation with death, or previous suicide attempts may also be present in someone with depression.

Tambien pueden estar presentes pensamientos suicidas, una obsesión con la muerte, o intentos suicidas previos en algunas personas depresivas.

How we can find it

To determine if you're suffering from depression, these tests may be ordered:
– psychological evaluation
– blood tests to see if drugs are causing your depression.

Para determinar si Ud. sufre depresión, se puede ordenar estas pruebas:
– evaluación psicológica
– análisis de sangre para ver si las drogas le están provocando la depresión.

How we can treat it

Depression is difficult to treat.

La depresión es dificil de tratar.

Primary treatment methods include:

– drug therapy
– electroconvulsive therapy
– psychotherapy.

Los métodos de tratamiento primario incluyen:
– terapia con medicamentos
– terapia electroconvulsiva
– psicoterapia.

You need to report any thoughts of death or suicide immediately.

Usted debe reportar inmediatamente cualesquier pensamientos de muerte o suicidio.

The primary features of depression include a sad mood and a loss of interest or pleasure in daily activities.

Las características principales de la depresión incluyen tristeza y pérdida de interés o placer en las actividades diarias.

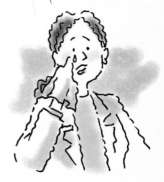

Diabetes mellitus

Diabetes mellitus is called *diabetes melitus* in Spanish. Here are some phrases to help you explain the different types of diabetes and their effects, diagnoses, and treatments. (See *Type 2 diabetes and Latinos.*)

What it is

Diabetes mellitus is a chronic disorder in which the body produces little or no insulin or resists the insulin it does produce.

La diabetes melitus es un trastorno crónico en el que el cuerpo produce poca o ninguna insulina o crea resistencia a la insulina que produce.

What it does

When a person lacks insulin, body tissues have less access to essential nutrients for fuel and storage.

Cuando una persona tiene falta de insulina, los tejidos del cuerpo tienen menos acceso a nutrientes esenciales para uso como combustible y para su almacenaje.

Having diabetes may require you to take regular doses of medicine.

La diabetes puede requerir que usted tome dosis regulares de medicamento.

If your diabetes isn't controlled by diet or taking medicine, you could develop complications that could be life-threatening.

Si su diabetes no está controlada mediante una dieta o la ingesta de medicamentos, usted podría tener complicaciones que pueden poner en riesgo su vida.

How we can find it

To determine if you have diabetes these tests may be ordered:
– blood sugar test
– urinalysis
– eye tests.

Para determinar si usted tiene diabetes, se pueden pedir los siguientes estudios:
– análisis de azúcar en sangre
– urinálisis
– pruebas oftalmológicas.

La cultura

Type 2 diabetes and Latinos

Latinos have a higher risk of developing type 2 diabetes—twice the risk of non-Latino Whites. Dietary factors, such as fat and caloric intake, are key elements in the occurrence of this disease.

Dietary habits and diabetes

In order to effectively address the issue of type 2 diabetes among your Latino patients, you should be familiar with the dietary habits of this population. By tailoring your guidelines for dietary changes to include foods that are staple ingredients of an individual's cultural cuisine, you demonstrate an understanding of his culture that will help your patient feel more comfortable about, and capable of, compliance.

How we can treat it

Type 1 diabetes requires that you take insulin shots, eat a good diet, and exercise.

Type 2 diabetes requires you to eat a good diet, exercise, and perhaps lose some weight.

If these measures don't work, you may require an oral antidiabetic drug or insulin therapy.

You may need to adjust your treatment if you have a cold, the flu, or an upset stomach.

In case your blood sugar becomes low, you should carry a fast-acting carbohydrate such as hard candy to eat.

Wear medical identification jewelry or carry a medical identification card that says you have diabetes.

La diabetes del Tipo 1 requiere que tome inyecciones de insulina, haga una dieta apropiada, y ejercicio.

La diabetes del Tipo 2 requiere que haga una dieta apropiada, ejercicio, y tal vez pierda un poco de peso.

Si dichas medidas no funcionan, podrá necesitar un medicamento antidiabético oral o terapia de insulina.

Es posible que usted deba modificar su tratamiento si tiene un resfrío, gripe, o malestares estomacales.

Si su nivel de azúcar en sangre está bajo, usted debe tener un carbohidrato de acción rápida como un caramelo duro para comer.

Use alhajas de identificación médica o lleve una tarjeta de identificación médica con usted que aclare que usted tiene diabetes.

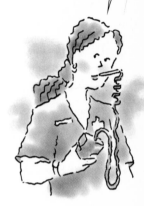

You may need to adjust your treatment if you have a cold, the flu, or an upset stomach.

Es posible que usted deba modificar su tratamiento si tiene un resfrío, gripe, o malestares estomacales.

Glaucoma

Glaucoma is called *glaucoma* in Spanish. Here are some phrases to help you explain what glaucoma is and its effects, diagnosis, and treatment.

What it is

Glaucoma is an eye disorder that causes inceased pressure in the eye that can damage the optic nerve.

If untreated, glaucoma can lead to gradual loss of vision and, eventually, blindness.

Un glaucoma es una afección ocular que provoca un incremento en la presión ocular que puede dañar el nervio óptico.

Si no se lo trata, el glaucoma puede provocar la pérdida gradual de la visión y eventualmente la ceguera.

How it happens

Chronic open-angle glaucoma results from overproduction of eye fluid or obstruction of its outflow.
– Diabetes and high blood pressure have been associated with this form of glaucoma.

Acute angle-closure glaucoma results from obstruction of the outflow of the fluid of the eye.

El glaucoma crónico de ángulo abierto surge de la superproducción de fluido ocular o la obstrucción de su flujo.
– La diabetes y la alta presión sanguínea se han vinculado con esta forma de glaucoma.

El glaucoma agudo de ángulo cerrado surge de la obstrucción del flujo del fluido del ojo.

Congenital glaucoma may result from infection or other problems at birth.

Secondary glaucoma can result from inflammation of the middle layer of the eye, trauma, or drugs (such as steroids).

What it does

Chronic open-angle glaucoma causes:

– mild aching in the eyes
– loss of peripheral vision
– seeing halos around lights
– reduced visual acuity not corrected by glasses.

Acute angle-closure glaucoma causes:

– acute pain in one inflamed eye
– moderate pupil dilation that's nonreactive to light
– cloudy cornea
– blurring and decreased visual acuity
– sensitivity to light
– seeing halos around lights
– nausea and vomiting related to increased pressure inside the eye.

Unless treated promptly, acute angle-closure glaucoma causes blindness in 3 to 5 days.

How we can find it

Diagnosis of glaucoma is made by:
– testing pressure in the eye
– measuring the visual field
– observing changes in the cup-to-disk ratio.

To determine if you have glaucoma, these tests may be ordered:
– tonometry to measure pressure in the eye
– eye examination
– test to measure the angle inside the eye
– vision tests.

El glaucoma congénito puede surgir de una infección u otros problemas en el momento del nacimiento.

El glaucoma secundario puede surgir de la inflamación de la capa media del ojo, un traumatismo, o drogas (como esteroides).

El glaucoma de ángulo abierto crónico causa:
– picazón moderada en los ojos
– pérdida de la visión periférica
– visión de halos alrededor de las luces
– agudeza visual reducida no corregida por gafas.

El glaucoma de ángulo cerrado grave causa:
– dolor agudo en un ojo inflamado
– dilatación moderada de la pupila que no reacciona ante la luz
– córnea opaca
– opacidad y menor agudeza visual
– sensibilidad a la luz
– visión de halos alrededor de las luces
– náuseas y vómitos relacionados con un incremento de la presión dentro del ojo.

A menos que se trate precozmente, el glaucoma agudo de ángulo cerrado provoca ceguera en 3 a 5 días.

Se hace un diagnóstico de glaucoma:
– probando la presión en el ojo
– midiendo el campo óptico
– observando los cambios en el coeficiente taza a disco.

Para determinar si Ud. tiene glaucoma, se puede ordenar estas pruebas:
– tonometría para medir la presión en el ojo
– examen ocular
– examen para medir el ángulo dentro del ojo
– examen de visión.

Unless treated promptly, acute angle-closure glaucoma causes blindness in 3 to 5 days.

A menos que se trate precozmente, el glaucoma agudo de ángulo cerrado provoca ceguera en 3 a 5 días.

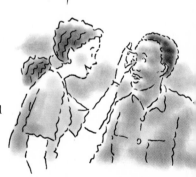

How we can treat it

Treatment of glaucoma involves the use of eye drops to reduce the production of fluid in the eye.	El tratamiento de un glaucoma requiere el uso de gotas oculares para reducir la producción de fluido en el ojo.
If you're unresponsive to drug therapy, you may require surgery.	Si Ud. no responde a la terapia de medicamentos, es posible que necesite cirugía.
Acute angle-closure glaucoma is an emergency requiring immediate treatment to reduce the pressure in the eye.	Un glaucoma con cierre de ángulo agudo es una emergencia que requiere un tratamiento inmediato para reducir la presión en el ojo.
I.V. medications to decrease pressure in the eye, pain medicine, and surgery may be needed.	Se pueden requerir medicamentos intravenosos para disminuir la presión en el ojo, analgésicos, y cirugía.
Screening for glaucoma is recommended for all persons over age 35, especially those with a family history of glaucoma.	Se recomienda hacer un examen de glaucoma a todas las personas mayores de 35 años, particularmente aquéllas con antecedentes familiars de glaucoma.

Heart failure

Heart failure is called *insuficiencia cardiaca* in Spanish. Here are some phrases to help you explain what heart failure is and its effects, diagnosis, and treatment.

What it is

In heart failure, the heart can't pump enough blood to meet the body's needs.	En la insuficiencia cardiaca, el corazón no bombea sangre suficiente para cubrir las necesidades del cuerpo.

How it happens

Heart failure can be caused by an abnormality of the heart muscle such as occurs as a result of a heart attack.	Puede causar la insuficiencia cardiaca una anormalidad en el músculo cardiaco, tal como ocurre como resultado de un ataque al corazón.
It can also be caused by mechanical problems with the heart due to arteriosclerosis, heart muscle disease, high blood pressure, kidney failure, or lung problems.	También puede ser provocado por problemas mecánicos del corazón a raíz de arterioesclerosis, enfermedad del músculo cardiaco, presión sanguínea alta, o problemas pulmonares.

How we can find it

To determine if you have heart failure, these tests may be ordered:	Para determinar si Ud. tiene insuficiencia cardiaca, voy a pedir que se le hagan unos análisis (unas pruebas), incluido(a):
– electrocardiogram	– un electrocardiograma
– chest X-ray	– una radiografía del tórax

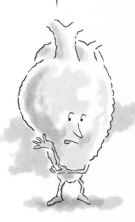

Heart failure is called *insuficiencia cardiaca* in Spanish.

– echocardiogram
– pulmonary artery monitoring
– cardiac catheterization.

– un ecocardiograma
– monitoreo de la arteria pulmonar
– un cateterismo cardiaco.

How we can treat it

The goals of treatment are to:
– identify or prevent conditions that can bring on or worsen heart failure

– reduce the heart's workload
– improve the heart's performance
– control salt intake and fluid retention.

Treatment for heart failure may include:

– physical activity or exercise
– a low-salt diet
– long-term drug therapy

– diuretics or water pills

– heart medications
    ACE inhibitors
    beta blockers.

Notify your doctor right away if you gain 3 to 5 lb (1.5 to 2.5 kg) in a week.

El objetivo del tratamiento es:
– identificar o prevenir condiciones que pueden provocar o empeorar la insuficiencia cardiaca

– reducir la carga de trabajo del corazón
– mejorar el desempeño del corazón
– controlar la ingestión de sal y la retención de líquidos.

El tratamiento para la insuficiencia cardiaca podrá incluir:

– actividad física o ejercicio
– una dieta con poca sal
– terapia de largo plazo con medicamentos

– diuréticos o píldoras contra la retención de líquidos

– medicamentos para el corazón
    inhibidores de la ECA
    bloqueadores beta.

Notifique a su médico inmediatamente si sube entre 3 a 5 libras (1.5 a 2.5 kg) en una semana.

Hepatitis

Hepatitis is called *hepatitis* in Spanish. Here are some phrases to help you explain what hepatitis is and its effects, diagnosis, and treatment.

What it is

Hepatitis is an inflammation of the liver that interferes with normal liver function.

La hepatitis es una inflamación del hígado que interfiere con el funcionamiento normal del mismo.

It can be caused by a virus.

La puede causar un virus.

There are many types of hepatitis. The most common are hepatitis A, B, and C.

Hay cinco tipos de hepatitis: hepatitis A, B, y C.

The types of hepatitis differ in their manner of transmission and severity.

Los tipos de hepatitis difieren en su forma de contagio y su gravedad.

How it happens

Some types of hepatitis are caused by transmission through blood, feces, or human secretions.

Algunos tipos de hepatitis ocurren por contagio a través de la sangre, materia fecal, o secreciones del cuerpo.

Other types can result from eating food, milk, or water contaminated by the virus.

Otros tipos pueden ocurrir a través del consumo de alimentos, leche, o agua contaminados por el virus.

What it does

The virus destroys the cells of the liver.

El virus destruye las células del hígado.

Liver cells can regrow but it takes time and lots of rest.

Las células del hígado pueden volver a crecer, pero se requiere tiempo y mucho reposo.

Older people and people with other health care problems are at increased risk for complications if they develop hepatitis.

Las personas de edad y las personas con otros problemas de salud tienen mayor riesgo de complicaciones si contraen hepatitis.

How we can find it

To determine if you have hepatitis, these tests may be ordered:

Para determinar si Ud. tiene hepatitis, voy a pedir que se le hagan unos análisis, incluido(a):

– blood tests
– liver biopsy.

– análisis de sangre
– una biopsia del hígado.

How we can treat it

There's no specific drug therapy for viral hepatitis; however, a drug called *interferon* may be used to treat hepatitis C.

No existe una terapia con medicamentos específica para la hepatitis viral; sin embargo, se puede utilizar un medicamento llamado *interferona* para el tratamiento de la hepatitis C.

It's important to rest, restrict your activities, and eat a healthy diet.

Es importante descansar, restringir sus actividades, y tener una dieta sana.

Avoid alcohol and over-the-counter drugs for at least 1 year or longer.

Evite el alcohol y los medicamentos sin receta médica durante por lo menos 1 año.

You need to have regular checkups for at least 1 year.

Necesitará chequeos periódicos durante por lo menos 1 año.

Good handwashing and personal hygiene is very important.

Es muy importante lavarse bien las manos y tener una buena higiene personal.

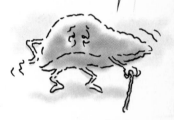

Liver cells can regrow but it takes time and lots of rest.

Las células del hígado pueden volver a crecer, pero se requiere tiempo y mucho reposo.

Herniated disk

A herniated disk is called *hernia de disco* in Spanish. Here are some phrases to help explain what a herniated disk is and its effects, diagnosis, and treatment.

What it is

A herniated disk, often called a *ruptured disk*, is a back problem.

Una hernia de disco, a menudo denominada *ruptura de disco*, es un problema de espalda.

It starts when all or part of the soft, central portion of a spinal disk, which is found between each of the bones in the back or spine, is forced through the disk's weakened or torn outer ring.

Comienza cuando toda o una parte de la porción central blanda de un disco espinal, que se encuentra entre cada uno de los huesos en la espalda o médula espinal, pasa a la fuerza por el anillo externo debilitado o desgarrado del disco.

What it does

When this happens, the protruding disk may rub against spinal nerves or the spinal cord itself, causing back, leg, or arm pain or signs of pinched nerves.

Cuando esto ocurre, el disco que sobresale puede rozar nervios espinales o la misma médula espinal, lo que provoca dolor en la espalda, la pierna o el brazo, o señales de nervios pellizcados.

The leg or arm may feel numb or tingle and feel weak.

La pierna o el brazo se pueden entumecer o cosquillear y debilitarse.

How we can find it

To determine if you have a herniated disk, these tests may be ordered:

– spinal X-ray
– CT scan
– MRI
– EMG
– myelography.

Para determinar si Ud. tiene hernia de disco, voy a pedir que se le hagan unos análisis, incluido(a):
– radiografía de la espina dorsal
– tomografía computada
– resonancia magnética
– electromiograma
– una mielografía.

How we can treat it

Treatment for a herniated disk may involve:
– bed rest
– traction
– surgery.

El tratamiento para la hernia de disco podrá comprender:
– reposo en la cama
– tracción
– cirugía.

You need to learn proper lifting techniques to prevent further injury.

Es importante aprender técnicas de levantamiento adecuadas para impedir lesiones adicionales.

You need to watch your weight carefully.

Es importante que observe su peso cuidadosamente.

> You need to watch your weight carefully.

> Es importante que observe su peso cuidadosamente.

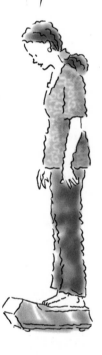

High cholesterol

High cholesterol is called *colesterol alto* in Spanish. Here are some phrases to help you explain what high cholesterol is and its effects, diagnosis, and treatment.

What it is

Cholesterol is a soft, fat-like substance found in all body cells.

El colesterol es una sustancia blanda parecida a la grasa que se encuentra en todas las células del cuerpo.

High cholesterol is the increase in fat and lipoprotein levels.

It may occur because of:
– genetics
– diet
– diabetes
– pancreatitis
– hypothyroidism
– kidney disease.

How it happens

High cholesterol comes from what you eat, family history, and what your body makes.

What it does

High cholesterol may cause:
– problems in the blood vessels in your legs
– inflamed pancreas
– nerve damage in the legs
– enlarged liver and spleen
– abdominal pain.

How we can find it

To determine if you have high cholesterol, a blood test may be ordered.

Questions about your diet and family history will be asked.

How we can treat it

The first goal of treatment is to identify and treat any underlying disorder that may be causing your high cholesterol.

Dietary management involves lowering cholesterol intake.

Weight reduction may be a priority.

Drug therapy may be needed to lower cholesterol levels.

El colesterol alto es el aumento de los niveles de grasa y lipoproteína.

Puede ocurrir debido a:
– la genética
– la dieta
– la diabetes
– pancreatitis
– hipotiroidismo
– una enfermedad renal.

El colesterol alto proviene de lo que uno come, antecedentes, y lo que produce el cuerpo.

El colesterol alto puede provocar:
– problemas en los vasos sanguíneos de las piernas
– inflamación de páncreas
– daños en los nervios de las piernas
– agrandamiento del hígado y el bazo
– dolor abdominal.

Para determinar si usted tiene colesterol alto, se puede solicitar un análisis de sangre.

Se le harán preguntas sobre su dieta y sus antecedentes familiares.

El primer objetivo del tratamiento es identificar y tratar cualquier trastorno subyacente que pueda provocar el colesterol alto.

El control dietario consiste en disminuir el consumo de fuentes de colesterol.

La reducción de peso debe ser una prioridad.

Se puede necesitar un tratamiento medicamentoso para disminuir los niveles de colesterol.

High cholesterol may occur because of diet.

El colesterol alto puede ocurrir debido a la dieta.

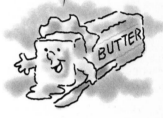

Hypertension

Hypertension is called *hipertensión* in Spanish. Here are some phrases to help you explain what hypertension is and its effects, diagnosis, and treatment.

What it is

In hypertension, also called *high blood pressure*, the blood exerts too much pressure on the walls of the arteries or blood vessels.

En los casos de hipertensión, también denominada *presión sanguínea alta*, la sangre ejerce demasiada presión sobre las paredes de las arterias o vasos sanguíneos.

What it does

When this condition persists, it eventually damages blood vessels and reduces blood flow through the vessels and tissues.

Cuando dicho problema persiste, eventualmente daña los vasos sanguíneos y reduce el flujo de sangre a través de los vasos sanguíneos y los tejidos.

This can damage the heart, kidneys, brain, and eyes.

Esto puede dañar el corazón, los riñones, el cerebro, y los ojos.

If high blood pressure damages the heart and blood vessels, it can cause a heart attack, heart failure, or a stroke.

Si la presión sanguínea alta daña el corazón y los vasos sanguíneos, puede provocar un ataque cardiaco, una insuficiencia cardiaca, o un derrame cerebral.

How we can find it

To determine if you have high blood pressure or are at risk for complications from high blood pressure, these tests may be ordered:
– frequent blood pressure measurements

– urinalysis
– chest X-ray
– echocardiogram
– electrocardiogram.

Para determinar si usted tiene presión sanguínea alta o tiene riesgo de complicaciones por presión sanguínea alta, se pueden solicitar estos análisis:
– medición frecuencia de la presión sanguínea
– un urinálisis
– una radiografía del tórax
– un ecocardiograma
– un electrocardiograma.

How we can treat it

Treatment for hypertension includes making changes in your lifestyle, including:
– losing weight
– stopping smoking
– exercising regularly
– reducing alcohol consumption
– reducing salt intake.

El tratamiento de la hipertensión incluye la realización de cambios en su estilo de vida, incluido(a):
– reducción de peso
– dejar de fumar
– ejercicio regular
– reducción del consumo de alcohol
– reducción de la ingestión de sal.

You may need to take drugs called *antihypertensives* to control your blood pressure.

Podrá necesitar tomar medicamentos llamados *antihipertensivos* para controlar la presión de su sangre.

Be sure to follow all your doctor's orders. Uncontrolled blood pressure may cause a stroke or heart attack.

Asegúrese de seguir todas las indicaciones de su médico. La presión sanguínea sin control puede provocar un ataque apopléjico o cardiaco.

Irritable bowel syndrome

Irritable bowel syndrome is called *síndrome de intestino irritable* in Spanish. Here are some phrases to help you explain what irritable bowel syndrome is and its effects, diagnosis, and treatment.

What it is

Irritable bowel syndrome is a common condition that causes:
– chronic or occasional diarrhea alternating with constipation
– straining to have a bowel movement
– stomach cramps.

El síndrome del intestino irritable es una afección común que provoca:
– diarrea crónica u ocasional que se alterna con estreñimiento
– dificultad para evacuar
– retorcijones estomacales.

How it happens

The onset of irritable bowel syndrome is associated with psychological stress or physical factors, such as:
– disease in the lower colon

– irritants (coffee, raw fruits, or vegetables)
– lactose intolerance
– abuse of laxatives.

Se asocia el síndrome de intestino irritable al estrés psicológico o factores físicos, tales como:
– una enfermedad en el colon descendiente
– sustancias irritantes (café, frutas crudas, o vegetales)
– intolerancia a la lactosa
– abuso de laxantes.

How we can find it

To determine if you have irritable bowel syndrome, these tests may be ordered:

– barium X-ray
– rectal biopsy
– stool analysis
– colonoscopy.

Para determinar si Ud. tiene el síndrome de intestino irritable, voy a pedir que se le hagan unos análisis (unas pruebas), incluido(a):
– una radiografía de bario
– una biopsia rectal
– un análisis de materia fecal
– una colonoscopia.

How we can treat it

Treatment for irritable bowel syndrome consists of reducing the symptoms by:

– reducing stress
– avoiding irritants
– avoiding certain foods
– taking sedatives
– taking drugs to reduce spasms in the bowel.

El tratamiento del síndrome de intestino irritable consiste en la reducción de los síntomas:
– disminuyendo el estrés
– evitando sustancias irritantes
– evitar determinados alimentos
– tomando sedantes
– tomando medicamentos para reducir los espasmos en el intestino.

You need to get regular checkups because irritable bowel syndrome is associated with an increased risk of colon cancer.

Necesitará chequeos periódicos, pues se asocia el síndrome de intestino irritable con un mayor riesgo de cáncer de colon.

Multiple sclerosis

Multiple sclerosis (MS) is called *esclerosis múltiple* (EM) in Spanish. Here are some phrases to help explain what MS is and its effects, diagnosis, and treatment.

What it is

Multiple sclerosis (MS) is a progressive disease of the nervous system.

La esclerosis múltiple (EM) es una enfermedad progresiva del sistema nervioso.

How it happens

It occurs when the outer coating of the nerve is damaged and nerve impulses can't be sent back and forth.

Se produce cuando la cobertura externa del nervio está dañada y los impulsos nerviosos no se pueden enviar en ninguno de los dos sentidos.

This damage to nerves happens in the brain, spinal cord, and eyes.

Este daño a los nervios se produce en el cerebro, la médula espinal y los ojos.

The exact cause is unknown, but genetic factors may play a part.

Se desconoce la causa exacta, pero es posible que los factores genéticos tengan un rol en el problema.

Emotional stress, fatigue, pregnancy, and acute respiratory infections can come before the onset of the disease.

Puede haber estrés emocional, fatiga, embarazo, e infecciones respiratorias agudas antes de la aparición de la enfermedad.

What it does

MS causes visual problems, muscle dysfunction, urinary and bowel disturbances, and fatigue. It also causes speech problems, mood swings, and memory problems.

La EM provoca problemas visuales, disfunción muscular, alteraciones urinarias e intestinales, y fatiga. También provoca problemas en el habla, cambios de ánimo, y problemas en la memoria.

How we can find it

To determine if you have MS, these tests may be ordered:

– MRI
– electroencephalogram
– psychological evaluation
– lumbar puncture.

Para determinar si Ud. tiene EM, voy a pedir que se le hagan unos análisis de diagnóstico, incluido(a):
– resonancia magnética
– un electroencefalograma
– una evaluación psicológica
– una punción lumbar.

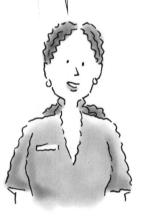

MS is a progressive disease of the nervous system.

La EM es una enfermedad progresiva del sistema nervioso.

How we can treat it

Drugs may be used to reduce the recurrence and severity of attacks.

Se pueden utilizar medicamentos para disminuir la repetición y gravedad de los ataques.

Avoid stress, fatigue, exposure to people with infections, and very hot or cold temperatures.

Evite el estrés, la fatiga, la exposición a personas con infecciones y temperaturas muy cálidas o frías.

To help maintain independence, develop new ways to perform daily activities.

Para conservar la independencia, busque nuevas maneras de realizar sus actividades diarias.

Eat a nutritious, well-balanced, high-fiber diet and drink plenty of fluids to prevent constipation.

Coma una dieta nutritiva, bien balanceada y con alto contenido de fibra y beba mucho líquido para evitar el estreñimiento.

Frequent rest periods will help reduce fatigue.

Períodos frecuentes de reposo ayudarán a reducir la fatiga.

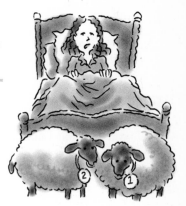

Frequent rest periods will help reduce fatigue.

Períodos frecuentes de reposo ayudarán a reducir la fatiga.

Myocardial infarction

Myocardial infarction (MI), or heart attack, is called *infarto de miocardio* (IM) or *ataque cardiaco* in Spanish. Here are some phrases to help you explain what MI is and its effects, diagnosis, and treatment.

What it is

In a heart attack, or a myocardial infarction (MI), one of the heart's arteries fails to deliver enough blood to the part of the heart muscle it serves.

En el ataque cardiaco o infarto de miocardio (IM), una de las arterias del corazón deja de suministrar suficiente sangre a la porción del músculo cardiaco que suple.

How it happens

Arteriosclerosis, or hardening of the arteries in the heart, which reduces the artery's blood flow, is the usual cause.

La causa usual es la arteriosclerosis, o el endurecimiento de las arterias del corazón, que reduce el flujo de sangre por las arterias.

Sometimes a small blood clot or a spasm of a blood vessel can cause a heart attack.

A veces un pequeño coágulo sanguíneo, o un espasmo de un vaso sanguíneo puede provocar un ataque cardiaco.

What it does

The reduced blood flow causes destruction of the localized area of the heart.

La reducción del flujo de sangre causa la destrucción de un área del corazón.

If treatment is delayed, the person can die.

Si se demora en efectuar el tratamiento, la persona puede morir.

How we can find it

To determine if you have had an MI, these tests may be ordered:

– blood tests
– cardiac catheterization
– electrocardiogram
– echocardiogram
– heart scans.

Para determinar si Ud. tuvo un IM, voy a pedir que se le hagan unos análisis, incluido(a):
– análisis de sangre
– un cateterismo cardiaco
– un electrocardiograma
– un ecocardiograma
– angiografías.

How we can treat it

You may receive drugs to:
– reduce the workload of the heart
– stabilize heart rhythm
– relieve chest pain.

Podrá recibir medicamentos para:
– reducir la carga de trabajo del corazón
– estabilizar el ritmo cardiaco
– aliviar el dolor en el pecho.

Other treatments may include:
– drugs that break up clots in the arteries
– insertion of a temporary pacemaker
– angioplasty
– open heart surgery.

Otros tratamientos pueden ser:
– medicamentos que disuelven coágulos en las arterias
– inserción de un marcapasos provisional
– angioplastía
– cirugía de corazón abierto.

Make sure you understand and follow your prescribed drug therapy and other treatments.

Asegúrese de comprender y llevar a cabo su terapia de medicamentos recetada y otros tratamientos.

Call the doctor if you have chest pain.

Llame a su médico si siente dolor en el tórax.

If you smoke cigarettes, you must stop.

Si fuma cigarrillos, debe dejar de fumar.

You may need to change your diet to cut down on salt, fat, and cholesterol.

Podrá necesitar cambiar su dieta para reducir la ingestión de sal, grasas, y colesterol.

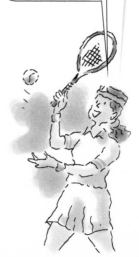

> Obesity results from consuming too many calories and lack of exercising.
>
> La obesidad surge del consumo de demasiadas calorías y la falta de ejercicio.

Obesity

Obesity is called *obesidad* in Spanish. Here are some phrases to help you explain what obesity is and its effects, diagnosis, and treatment.

What it is

Obesity is an excess of body fat, generally 20% above ideal body weight.

La obesidad es un exceso de grasa corporal, generalmente 20% mayor que el peso ideal del cuerpo.

How it happens

Obesity results from consuming too many calories and lack of exercise.

La obesidad surge del consumo de demasiadas calorías y la falta de ejercicio.

It may also be caused by:
– a problem with the hypothalamus

También puede ser provocada por:
– un problema con el hipotálamo

– genetic predisposition
– abnormal absorption of nutrients
– impaired action of certain hormones and hormone regulators such as insulin.

Socioeconomic status, environmental factors, and psychological factors also may contribute to obesity.

What it does

Obesity may lead to serious complications, such as:
– breathing difficulties
– high blood pressure
– heart disease
– diabetes
– kidney disease
– gallbladder disease
– psychosocial difficulties
– sleep apnea
– premature death.

How we can find it

To determine if you're obese, these tests may be ordered:
– observing and comparing your height and weight to a standard table
– measuring of the thickness of fat folds to determine your total body fat.

How we can treat it

Successful management of obesity involves decreasing calorie intake while increasing activity levels.

You'll be required to maintain improved eating and exercise patterns for the rest of your life.

You may be treated with hypnosis and behavior modification techniques.

Drug therapy or surgery may be indicated if your weight becomes life-threatening.

– una predisposición genética
– la absorción anormal de nutrientes
– la acción afectada de ciertas hormonas y reguladores de hormonas, como la insulina.

El status socioeconómico y los factores ambientales y psicológicos también pueden contribuir a la obesidad.

What it does

La obesidad puede conducir a complicaciones graves, tales como:
– dificultades respiratorias
– alta presión sanguínea
– enfermedad cardiaca
– diabetes
– enfermedad renal
– enfermedad de la vesícula (biliar)
– problemas psicosociales
– apnea del sueño
– muerte prematura.

How we can find it

Para determinar si Ud. está obeso, se puede prescribir estas pruebas:
– observar y comparar su altura y su peso con una tabla estándar
– medición del espesor de los pliegues de grasa para determinar el total de grasa corporal.

How we can treat it

El manejo exitoso de la obesidad implica disminuir el consumo de calorías y aumentar los niveles de actividad.

Se le solicitará que mantenga una dieta mejorada y haga ejercicios el resto de su vida.

Se le podrá tratar con hipnosis y ténicas de modificación del comportamiento.

Se puede indicar un tratamiento medicamentoso o una cirugía si su peso pone en riesgo su vida.

Parkinson's disease

Parkinson's disease is called *mal de Parkinson* in Spanish. Here are some phrases to help you explain Parkinson's disease and its effects, diagnosis, and treatment.

What it is

Parkinson's disease occurs when certain chemicals in the brain decrease slowly over time.

El mal de Parkinson se produce cuando determinados químicos en el cerebro disminuyen lentamente con el paso del tiempo.

What it does

Parkinson's disease produces progressive muscle rigidity, loss or absence of voluntary motion, and involuntary tremors due to decreased chemicals in the brain.

El mal de Parkinson produce rigidez progresiva de los músculos, pérdida o ausencia de los movimientos voluntarios, y temblores involuntarios.

Parkinson's disease also causes:
– impaired speech
– drooling
– a high-pitched, monotone voice
– difficulty swallowing
– fatigue
– muscle cramps
– shuffled gait
– tremors or shaking
– mood changes.

El mal de Parkinson produce también:
– dificultades en el habla
– el enfermo de babea
– habla con voz monótona y aguda
– dificultades para tragar
– fatiga
– calambres musculares
– caminar arrastrando los pies
– temblores o temblequeo
– cambios de humor.

How we can find it

To determine if you have Parkinson's disease, the doctor will ask what problems you are having and examine you. There is no test to diagnose this disease.

Para determinar si Ud. tiene el mal de Parkinson, el médico le preguntará qué problemas tiene y lo examinará. No existe un análisis para diagnosticar la enfermedad.

How we can treat it

Treatment aims to reduce symptoms and may include drugs, physical therapy, and surgery.

El objetivo del tratamiento es reducir los síntomas y podrá incluir medicamentos, terapia física, y cirugía.

If you have difficulty eating, eat frequent, small meals.

Si tiene dificultad para alimentarse, coma pequeñas cantidades con frecuencia.

To establish a regular bowel elimination routine, drink plenty of fluids and eat high-fiber foods.

Para establecer una rutina regular de movimiento de intestinos, tome bastante líquido y coma alimentos con alto contenido de fibra.

If you have trouble walking, consider using a walker.

Si tiene problemas para caminar, analice el uso de un andador.

If you have trouble moving from a standing to sitting position, consider installing an elevated toilet seat.

Si tiene dificultad en pasar de la posición parada a la sentada, considere la posibilidad de instalar un asiento sanitario elevado.

Take household safety measures to prevent accidents.

Tome medidas en el hogar para evitar accidentes.

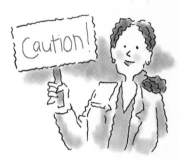

Take household safety measures to prevent accidents.

Tome medidas en el hogar para evitar accidentes.

Peptic ulcer

A peptic ulcer is called *úlcera péptica* in Spanish. Here are some phrases to help you explain peptic ulcer and its effects, diagnosis, and treatment.

What it is

Peptic ulcers are sores that develop in the mucous lining of the lower esophagus, stomach, and upper sections of the intestine.

Las úlceras pépticas son llagas que se desarrollan en el revestimiento mucoso del esófago inferior, el estómago, y las secciones superiores del intestino.

How it happens

Peptic ulcers may be caused by:

– infection with an organism called *Helicobacter pylori*
– too much acid in the stomach
– use of anti-inflammatory drugs such as aspirin.

Las causas de la úlcera péptica pueden ser:

– infección con un organismo llamado *Helicobacter pylori*
– demasiada acidez en el estómago
– uso de drogas antinflamatorias, como la aspirina.

What it does

Symptoms vary with the type of ulcer but may include:
– pain that is gnawing, burning, or cramplike
– pain that worsens with eating
– pain that is relieved by eating
– nausea
– loss of appetite
– pain that's relieved by antacids but usually recurs several hours later.

Los síntomas varían de acuerdo con el tipo de úlcera pero podrán incluir:
– dolor que es lacerante, quema, o se expresa en forma de calambres
– dolor que se agrava al comer
– dolor que se calma al comer
– náusea
– pérdida de apetito
– dolor que se calma con antiácidos pero generalmente vuelve a producirse varias horas más tarde.

If a peptic ulcer is not treated, bleeding in the intestines may occur and cause bloody vomit or bloody bowel movements.

Si no se trata una úlcera péptica, se puede producir sangrado en los intestinos, lo que puede provocar vómitos o materia fecal con sangre.

How we can find it

To determine if you have a peptic ulcer, these tests may be ordered:
– upper GI series
– endoscopy

Para determinar si usted tiene una úlcera péptica, su médico ha solicitado:
– una serie gastrointestinal superior
– una endoscopia

– blood or breath test for *H. pylori*

– un análisis de *H. Pylori* en la sangre o en el aliento

– blood testing of stools.

– control de sangre en las deposiciones.

How we can treat it

Treatment of peptic ulcer may include combination drug therapy.

El tratamiento de la úlcera péptica podrá incluir la terapia de combinación de medicamentos.

You may need to undergo surgery.

Podrá necesitar cirugía.

Get plenty of rest.

Haga mucho reposo.

Don't smoke; it stimulates gastric acid.

No fume, ya que estimula el ácido gástrico.

Cut down on alcohol and coffee.

Reduzca la ingestión de alcohol y café.

Avoid spicy food.

Evite las comidas picantes.

Pneumonia

Pneumonia is called *neumonía* or *pulmonía* in Spanish. Here are some phrases to help you explain what pneumonia is and its effects, diagnosis, and treatment.

What it is

Pneumonia is an inflammation of the lungs that prevents adequate exchange of oxygen.

La neumonía es una inflamación de los pulmones que impide un intercambio adecuado de oxígeno.

How it happens

It's caused most commonly by a virus or bacteria that infect the lungs; however, you can also get pneumonia from breathing in chemicals.

Generalmente es provocada por un virus o bacterias que infectan los pulmones; sin embargo, también se puede contraer neumonía por inspirar químicos.

Symptoms include:
– coughing
– sputum production
– chest pain when taking deep breaths

– shaking chills and fever
– shortness of breath.

Los síntomas incluyen:
– tos
– producción de esputo
– dolor en el pecho al inhalar profundamente
– escalofríos y fiebre
– falta de aliento.

How we can find it

To determine if you have pneumonia, these tests may be ordered:

Para determinar si Ud. tiene neumonía, voy a pedir que se le hagan unos análisis, incluido(a):

– chest X-ray
– blood tests
– bronchoscopy
– sputum culture.

– una radiografía del tórax
– un análisis de sangre
– una broncoscopia
– un cultivo de esputo.

How we can treat it

Treatment involves antibiotic therapy, which varies depending upon the cause of the pneumonia.

El tratamiento consiste en un tratamiento con antibióticos que varía según la causa de la neumonía.

Other measures include:
– oxygen
– bed rest
– a high-calorie diet
– adequate fluid intake
– drugs to relieve pain.

Otras medidas incluyen:
– oxígeno
– reposo en la cama
– dieta con alto contenido calórico
– ingestión adecuada de líquidos
– medicamentos para aliviar el dolor.

Sneeze and cough into a disposable tissue to avoid giving others your infection.

Estornude y tosa en un pañuelo de papel para evitar contagiar a los demás con su infección.

Get yearly flu shots and a vaccine against pneumonia (Pneumovax) if you have chronic obstructive pulmonary disease, heart disease, sickle cell disease, or are over 50 years old.

Lo recomendable es darse vacunas anuales contra la gripe y una vacuna contra la neumonía (Pneumovax) si tiene enfermedad crónica obstructiva del pulmón, enfermedad cardiaca, anemia falciforme, o tiene más de 50 años.

Renal failure

Renal failure is called *insuficiencia renal* in Spanish. Here are some phrases to help you explain what renal failure is and its effects, diagnosis, and treatment.

What it is

Renal failure is a sudden or gradual loss of kidney function.

La insuficiencia renal es la pérdida repentina o gradual del funcionamiento de los riñones.

How it happens

Acute (sudden) renal failure can be caused by:
– any condition that reduces blood flow to the kidneys, such as:

    infection
    shock
    blood loss
    burns
    heart disorders.
– damage to the kidneys.

La insuficiencia renal aguda (repentina) puede tener como causa:
– cualquier problema de salud que reduzca el flujo de la sangre a los riñones, tal como:

    infección
    shock
    pérdida de sangre
    quemaduras
    trastornos cardiacos.
– daño a los riñones.

Chronic (gradual) renal failure may result from:
– complications of diabetes, hypertension, lupus, or other disorders.
– long-term treatment with certain drugs.

La insuficiencia renal crónica (gradual) puede tener como causa:
– complicaciones de diabetes, hipertensión, lupus, u otros trastornos.
– tratamiento a largo plazo con drogas determinadas.

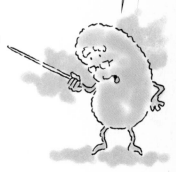

Renal failure is a sudden or gradual loss of kidney function.

La insuficiencia renal es la pérdida repentina o gradual del funcionamiento de los riñones.

What it does

Renal failure can cause:
– decreased urination
– nausea
– vomiting
– constipation
– dry mucous membranes
– itchy skin
– headache
– drowsiness
– irritability
– confusion
– high blood pressure
– irregular heartbeat
– fluid buildup.

La insuficiencia renal puede provocar:
– reducción de micción
– náuseas
– vómitos
– estreñimiento
– membranas mucosas secas
– picazón en la piel
– dolor de cabeza
– somnolencia
– irritabilidad
– confusión
– presión sanguínea alta
– ritmo cardiaco irregular
– acumulación de fluidos.

How we can find it

To determine if you have renal failure, these tests may be ordered:
– blood test
– urine test
– ultrasound
– X-ray of the:
    kidneys
    ureter
    bladder.

Para determinar si usted tiene insuficiencia renal, su médico ha solicitado:
– un análisis de sangre
– un análisis de orina
– un ultrasonido
– una radiografía de:
    los riñones
    la uretra
    la vejiga.

How we can treat it

You may receive drugs to improve blood flow to your kidneys or to stimulate urine production.

Podrá recibir medicamentos para mejorar el flujo de sangre a los pulmones o para estimular la producción de orina.

You may need:
– dialysis
– kidney transplant.

Puede necesitar:
– diálisis
– un transplante de riñón.

You'll need to restrict your diet and fluid intake.

Tendrá que restringir su dieta y la ingestión de líquidos.

SARS

Severe acute respiratory syndrome (SARS) is called *síndrome respiratorio agudo grave (SARS)* in Spanish. Here are some phrases to help you explain what SARS is and its effects, diagnosis, and treatment.

What it is

SARS is a lung illness that has recently been discovered.

El SARS es una enfermedad pulmonar descubierta recientemente.

Reports of SARS have come from Asia, North America, and Europe.

Hay informes de SARS de Asia, América del Norte, y Europa.

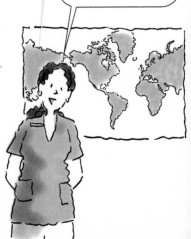

Reports of SARS have come from Asia, North America, and Europe.

Hay informes de SARS de Asia, América del Norte, y Europa.

How it happens

SARS is caused by a coronavirus believed to spread by close person-to-person contact.

SARS also may spread through the air or by other ways that are currently unknown.

El SARS es provocado por un coronavirus que se cree que se transmite por contacto cercano de persona a persona.

SARS también se puede propagar por el aire o de otras formas que se desconocen actualmente.

What it does

SARS begins with a fever greater than 100.4° F (38° C).

Other symptoms may include:
– headache
– body aches
– mild respiratory symptoms
– chills.

If you have SARS, you may develop a dry cough and breathing difficulties after 2 to 7 days.

In some cases, rapid decline has led to acute breathing problems requiring intensive care and the use of a ventilator.

SARS comienza con una fiebre mayor a 100.4° F (38° C).

Otros síntomas pueden incluir:
– dolor de cabeza
– dolores de cuerpo
– síntomas respiratorios moderados
– escalofríos.

Si tiene SARS, Ud. puede tener una tos seca y dificultades respiratorias después de 2 a 7 días.

En algunos casos, un desmejoramiento rápido ha provocado problemas respiratorios agudos que requieren cuidados intensivos y el uso de un respirador artificial.

How we can find it

To help determine if you have SARS, these tests may be ordered:
– chest X-ray
– pulse oximetry
– blood tests
– tests of urine and sputum specimens.

Para ayudar a determinar si Ud. tiene SARS, se puede prescribir estas pruebas:
– radiografía del tórax
– oximetría del pulso
– análisis de sangre
– análisis de orina y especimenes de esputo.

How we can treat it

SARS is treated the same way as another atypical pneumonia of unknown cause:

– by using antibiotics.

Patients with SARS are isolated until they're no longer contagious.

To help avoid contracting SARS, consider postponing nonessential travel to areas where there have been outbreaks of the disease.

El SARS se trata del mismo modo que otras neumonías atípicas con causas desconocidas:
– usando antibióticos.

Los pacientes con SARS son aislados hasta que ya no son contagiosos.

Para evitar contraer SARS, considere postergar viajes no esenciales a áreas donde ha habido brotes de la enfermedad.

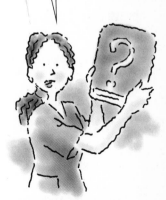

To determine if you have SARS, a chest X-ray may be ordered.

Para determinar si Ud. tiene SARS, se puede prescribir una radiografía del tórax.

If you must travel, wash your hands frequently and avoid close contact with
large numbers of people.

Si debe viajar, lávese las manos frecuentemente y evite el contacto cercano
con grandes cantidades de personas.

Seizure disorders

Seizure disorder, or epilepsy, is called *ataque epiléptico* or *epilepsia* in Spanish. Here
are some phrases to help you explain seizure disorder and its effects, diagnosis, and
treatment.

What it is

Seizure disorder (also known as *epilepsy*) is a brain condition that is caused by
abnormal electrical discharges of nerve
cells.

El trastorno convulsivo (también cono-
cido como *epilepsia*) es una afección
cerebral provocada por descargas eléc-
tricas anormales de células nerviosas.

> Epilepsy is a
> brain condition.

> La epilepsia es
> una afección
> cerebral.

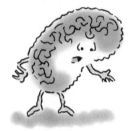

How it happens

Seizure disorders can be caused by:

– birth trauma
– lack of oxygen
– infections
– brain tumors
– ingestion of poisons
– inherited disorders
– strokes
– high fever
– low blood sugar
– drug overdose.

Las convulsiones pueden tener como
causa:

– trauma en el parto
– falta de oxígeno
– infecciones
– tumores cerebrales
– ingestión de venenos
– trastornos hereditarios
– apoplejía
– fiebre alta
– nivel bajo de azúcar en sangre
– sobredosis de drogas.

What it does

Several types exist, and symptoms may
include:
– stiffening or jerking of one extremity

– loss of consciousness
– dizziness
– flashing lights
– body stiffness
– tongue biting
– loss of bowel and bladder control

– labored breathing
– periods of not breathing.

Los síntomas podrán incluir:

– endurecimiento o espasmos musculares en una extremidad
– pérdida de conocimiento
– mareos
– destellos
– endurecimiento del cuerpo
– mordedura de la lengua
– pérdida de control del intestino y la
  vejiga
– respiración trabajosa
– períodos sin respirar.

How we can find it

To determine if you have seizure disorders, these tests may be ordered:

– electroencephalogram

Para determinar si usted tiene ataques
epilépticos (convulsiones) su médico ha
solicitado:
– un electroencefalograma

– CT scan	– tomografía computada
– MRI	– resonancia magnética
– skull X-rays	– radiografías de cráneo
– brain scan	– un ultrasonido cerebral
– lumbar puncture.	– una punción lumbar.

How we can treat it

Seizure disorders are treated with drugs.	Las convulsiones se tratan con medicamentos.
The treatment is specific to the type of seizure and is intended to reduce frequency or prevent occurrence.	El tratamiento es específico para el tipo de ataque y tiene previsto reducir frecuencia o impedir ocurrencia.
The doctor may prescribed:	El médico puede recetar:
– phenytoin.	– fenitoína.
– carbamazepine.	– carbamecepina.
– valproic acid.	– acido valproico.
– clonazepam.	– clonacepam.
– ethosuximide.	– etosuximida.
Sometimes surgery is needed to treat the cause.	A veces se necesita realizar una cirugía para tratar la causa.

Smallpox

Smallpox is called *viruela* in Spanish. Here are some phrases to help you explain what smallpox is and its effects, diagnosis, and treatment.

What it is

Smallpox is a highly contagious infectious disease caused by the poxvirus variola.	La viruela es una enfermedad muy contagiosa causada por el poxvirus variolae.
Smallpox may now be used in biochemical warfare.	Actualmente se puede usar la viruela en guerras bioquímicas.

How it happens

Smallpox is transmitted directly by respiratory droplets or dried scales of virus-containing lesions or indirectly through contact with contaminated clothes or other objects.	La viruela se transmite directamente por gotitas respiratorias o escamas secas de lesiones que contienen el virus, or indirectamente por contacto con ropas contaminadas u ortos objetos.

What it does

After 10 to 14 days, smallpox causes chills, fever, backache, malaise, and vomiting.	Después de 10 a 14 días, la viruela causa escalofríos, fiebre, dolor de espalda, malestar, y vómitos.
Occasionally, violent delirium, stupor, or coma also occurs.	Ocasionalmente, también se produce un delirio violento, estupor, o coma.

You may develop a sore throat, cough, and lesions on the mucous membranes of the mouth, throat, and respiratory tract.

Ud. podrá tener dolor de garganta, tos y lesiones en las membranas mucosas de la boca, garganta, y mías respiratories.

Skin lesions appear and commonly leave permanent scars.

Aparecen lesiones en la piel que comúnmente dejan cicatrices permanentes.

Smallpox may cause death.

La viruela puede provocar la muerte.

How we can find it

To determine if you have smallpox, cultures of the skin lesions may be ordered.

Para determinar Ud. tiene viruela, se pueden solicitar cultivos de las lesiones en la piel.

How we can treat it

Treatment includes:
– isolation
– antibiotics
– pain medication.

El tratamiento incluye:
– aislamiento
– antibióticos
– analgésicos.

> To determine if you have smallpox, cultures of the skin lesions may be ordered.

> Para determinar si Ud. tiene viruela, se pueden solicitar cultivos de las lesiones en la piel.

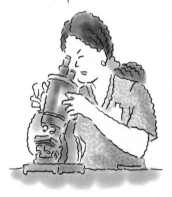

Stroke

A stroke is called *accidente cerebrovascular* or *un ataque apopléjico* in Spanish. Here are some phrases to help you explain what a stroke is and its effects, diagnosis, and treatment.

What it is

A stroke is a sudden circulation problem in one or more of the blood vessels supplying the brain.

Un derrame cerebral es un problema repentino de circulación en uno o más de los vasos sanguíneos que alimentan el cerebro.

It affects oxygen supply, causing serious damage to the brain.

Afecta el suministro de oxígeno, lo que provoca un daño severo al cerebro.

How it happens

Major causes of a stroke include:

– a clot in a blood vessel
– bleeding from an aneurysm
– high blood pressure.

Las causas principales de la apoplejía incluyen:
– un coágulo en un vaso sanguíneo
– hemorragia de un aneurisma
– presión alta.

What it does

The symptoms vary according to the amount of the damage and the part of the brain involved.

Los síntomas varían según el grado de daño y la parte del cerebro afectada.

Generalized symptoms include:
– sudden headache
– sudden confusion

Los síntomas generales incluyen:
– dolor de cabeza repentino
– confusión repentina

– seizures
– trouble talking
– vision problems
– sudden weakness on one side of the body
– loss of consciousness.

– convulsiones
– problemas para hablar
– problemas en la visión
– debilitamiento repentino en un lado del cuerpo
– pérdida del conocimiento.

How we can find it

To determine if you have had a stroke, these tests may be ordered:

– evaluation of your symptoms
– physical examination
– CT scan
– MRI
– brain scan
– angiography
– ultrasound
– blood flow studies of the brain

– electroencephalogram.

Para determinar si usted tuvo un derrame cerebral, se pueden solicitar los siguientes estudios:

– evaluación de los síntomas
– un examen físico
– tomografía computada
– resonancia magnética
– encefalograma
– angiografía
– ecografía
– exámenes del flujo sanguíneo en el cerebro
– electroencefalograma.

How we can treat it

Treatment includes:
– antiseizure drugs
– drugs to thin your blood
– drugs to dissolve clots
– surgery to remove atherosclerotic plaque
– surgery to bypass a blocked artery or repair a blood vessel.

El tratamiento incluye:
– medicamentos anticonvulsivos
– medicamentos para diluir la sangre
– medicamentos para disolver coágulos
– cirugía para la remoción de la placa arterosclerótica
– cirugía para realizar un bypass de una arteria bloqueada o reparar un vaso sanguíneo.

Tuberculosis

Tuberculosis is called *tuberculosis* in Spanish. Here are some phrases to help you explain tuberculosis and its effects, diagnosis, and treatment.

What it is

Tuberculosis is an infection of the lungs caused by airborne bacteria.

La tuberculosis es una infección de los pulmones provocada por bacterias transportadas en la sangre.

In this disease, abnormal cavities and masses develop in the lungs that make breathing difficult.

En dicha enfermedad, se desarrollan cavidades y masas anormales en los pulmones que dificultan la respiración.

How it happens

Tuberculosis is caused by bacteria and can be easily spread to other people.

La tuberculosis es provocada por bacterias y puede contagiarse con facilidad a otras personas.

It may not cause any obvious symptoms but may cause vague symptoms, including:
– fatigue
– weakness
– loss of appetite
– weight loss
– night sweats
– low-grade fever.

Puede no provocar síntomas evidentes, pero puede provocar síntomas imprecisos, entre ellos:
– fatiga
– debilidad
– pérdida del apetito
– pérdida de peso
– sudores nocturnos
– fiebre baja.

How we can find it

To determine if you have tuberculosis, these tests may be ordered:

– chest X-ray
– sputum culture
– TB test.

Para determinar si Ud. tiene tuberculosis, voy a pedir que se le hagan unos análisis, incluido(a):
– una radiografía del tórax
– un cultivo de esputo
– examen de tuberculosis.

How we can treat it

You may need to be isolated from other people while you are contagious.

Es posible que deba estar aislado de otras personas mientras pueda contagiar.

After 2 to 4 weeks, you should no longer be contagious.

Después de dos a cuatro semanas, ya no contagiará a los demás.

You'll need to have long-term drug treatment.

Deberá someterse a un tratamiento medicamentoso prolongado.

The drugs you're taking can cause many side effects.

Las drogas que usted toma pueden provocar diversos efectos secundarios.

Report any side effects immediately.

Informe inmediatamente cualquier efecto secundario.

Be sure to get regular follow-up examinations.

Asegúrese de obtener exámenes de acompañamiento regulares.

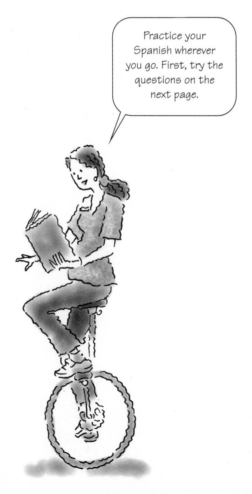

Practice your Spanish wherever you go. First, try the questions on the next page.

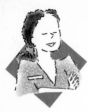

Practice makes perfecto

1. Help Joy ask her patient if she has ever had chest pain.

_____

_____

_____

_____

> ¿Alguna vez ha sentido
>
> _____?

> Tendrá que realizarse
>
> _____.

2. Help Joy explain to her patient that he's going to need a chest X-ray.

_____

_____

_____

_____

> La diabetes es una enfermedad en la que el cuerpo no produce
>
> _____.

3. Help Joy teach her patient that diabetes is a disease in which the body doesn't produce enough insulin.

_____

_____

_____

_____

Answer key

1. Do you ever have chest pain?
   ¿Alguna vez ha sentido <u>dolor en el tórax</u>?

2. You're going to need a chest X-ray.
   Tendrá que realizarse <u>una radiografía del tórax.</u>

3. Diabetes is a disease in which the body doesn't produce enough insulin.
   La diabetes es una enfermedad en la que el cuerpo no produce <u>suficiente insulina.</u>

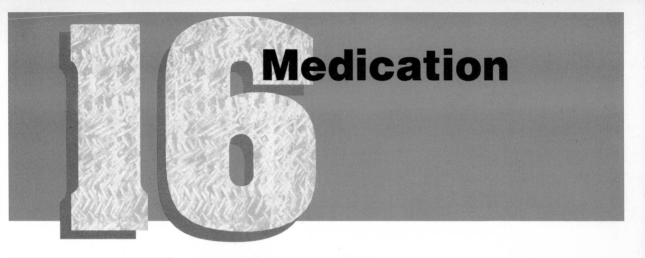

Medication

16

Fast fact

Key terms related to the administration of medication include:

- *de receta (prescription)*
- *de venta libre (over the counter)*
- *efectos adversos (adverse effects)*
- *una reacción alérgica (allergic reaction)*
- *dosis (dose)*

Taking the history

You need to find out if your patient takes medications routinely at home.

The program already in progress

Do you take any medications?
– Prescription?
– Over the counter?
–Herbal drugs?
–Vitamins?
– Other?

Which prescription drugs do you take routinely?
– How often do you take them?
    Once daily?
    Twice daily?
    Three times daily?
    Four times daily?
    More often?
    As needed?
(See *OTC medication use among elderly Latinos.*)

¿Toma Ud. medicamentos?
– ¿Con receta?
– ¿De venta libre?
–¿Homeopáticos?
–¿Vitaminas?
– ¿Otros?

¿Qué medicamentos de receta toma Ud. habitualmente?
– ¿Con qué frecuencia los toma Ud.?
    ¿Una vez al día?
    ¿Dos veces al día?
    ¿Tres veces al día?
    ¿Cuatro veces al día?
    ¿Con más frecuencia?
    ¿Sies necesario?

La cultura

OTC medication use among elderly Latinos

According to a study published in the *Journal of the American Geriatric Society*, elderly Latino people tend to use fewer over-the-counter medications than do their peers in other ethnic groups. Possible explanations for this underuse include lack of access to health care in the Latino population (due in part to lack of coverage—both private insurance and Medicare) and cultural preferences that reject medication use in treatment.

Which over-the-counter medications do you take?	¿Qué medicamentos de venta libre toma?
What do you take them for?	¿Para qué los toma?
– How often do you take them?	– ¿Con qué frecuencia los toma?
Did you bring them with you?	¿Los trajo Ud. consigo?
Do you have a list of your medications?	¿Tiene Ud. una lista de sus medicamentos?
– How often do you take them?	– ¿Con qué frecuencia los toma?
Once daily?	¿Una vez al día?
Twice daily?	¿Dos veces al día?
Three times daily?	¿Tres veces al día?
Four times daily?	¿Cuatro veces al día?
More often?	¿Con más frecuencia?
What herbal drugs do you take?	¿Qué medicamentos homeopáticos toma Ud.?
–What for?	–¿Para qué?
–How often?	–¿Con qué frecuencia?
What vitamins do you take?	¿Qué vitaminas toma Ud.?
–How often?	–¿Con qué frecuencia?
What illicit drugs to you use?	¿Qué drogas ilícitas usa?
What's the dosage for each medication?	¿Qué dosis toma de cada medicamento?
How does each medication make you feel?	¿Cómo le hace sentirse cada uno de estos medicamentos?
Are you allergic to any medications?	¿Es Ud. alérgico(a) a algún medicamento?
– Which medications?	– ¿A qué medicamentos?
– What happens when you have an allergic reaction?	– ¿Qué pasa cuando Ud. tiene una reacción alérgica?

(See *Therapeutic drug classifications.*)

Teaching about medication

After you have established your patient's medication history, you may have to teach him about medication the doctor has prescribed. (See *Teaching your patient about his medication*, pages 228 and 229.)

Laying the groundwork

I need to give you:	Necesito darle:
– an injection.	– una inyección.
– an I.V. medication.	– un medicamento por vía intravenosa.
– a liquid medication.	– un medicamento en forma líquida.
– a medicated cream or powder.	– un medicamento en pomada o polvo.
– a medication through your epidural catheter.	– un medicamento por el catéter epidural.
– a medication through your rectum.	– un medicamento por el recto.
– a medication through your _____ tube.	– un medicamento por su tubo _____.

Therapeutic drug classifications

Here are Spanish translations for major drug classifications.

Analgesic	Analgésico	Antituberculosis agent	Agente antituberculoso
Anesthetic	Anestético	Antitussive agent	Agente antitusivo
Antacid	Antiácido	Antiviral agent	Agente antiviral
Antiamebic agent	Agente antiamebiano	Appetite stimulant	Estimulante para el apetito
Antianginal agent	Agente antianginal	Appetite suppressant	Supresor de apetito
Antianxiety agent	Agente ansiolítico	Bronchodilator	Broncodilatador
Antiarrhythmic agent	Agente antiarrítmico	Cardiac glycoside	Digital glucósido
Antibiotic	Antibiótico	Decongestant	Descongestivo
Anticancer agent	Agente anticarcinógeno	Digestant	Digestivo (agente que estimula la digestión)
Anticoagulant	Anticoagulante		
Anticonvulsant	Anticonvulsivo	Disinfectant	Desinfectante
Antidepressant	Antidepresivo	Diuretic	Diurético
Antidiarrheal	Antidiarréico	Emetic	Emético
Antiemetic	Antiemético	Fertility agent	Agente para la fertilidad
Antifungal agent	Agente antifúngico	Hypnotic	Hipnótico
Antigout agent	Agente antigota	Insulin	Insulina
Antihelmintic	Antihelmíntico	Laxative	Laxante
Antihemorrhagic agent	Agente antihemorrágico	Muscle relaxant	Relajante muscular
Antihistamine	Antihistamínico	Oral contraceptive	Anticonceptivo oral
Antihyperlipidemic agent	Agente hiperlipémico	Oral hypoglycemic agent	Agente hipoglicémico oral
Antihypertensive agent	Agente antihipertenso	Oxytocic	Oxitócico
Anti-inflammatory agent	Agente antiinflamatorio	Sedative	Sedante
Antimalarial agent	Agente antimalárico	Steroid	Esteroide
Antiparkinsonian agent	Agente antiparkinsoniano	Thyroid hormone	Hormona de la glándula tiroides
Antipsychotic agent	Agente antipsicótico		
Antipyretic	Antipirético	Tranquilizer	Tranquilizante
Antiseptic	Antiséptico	Vaccine	Vacuna
Antispasmodic	Antiespasmódico	Vasodilator	Vasodilatador
Antithyroid agent	Agente antitiroideo	Vitamin	Vitamina

– a medication under your tongue.	– un medicamento debajo de la lengua.
– some pills.	– unas píldoras.
– a suppository.	– un supositorio.
This is how you take this medication.	Así se toma este medicamento.

A spoonful of sugar

If you can't swallow this pill, I can crush it and mix it in some food or liquid such as:	Si Ud. no se puede tragar esta píldora, yo puedo molerla y mezclarla en un alimento o líquido, tal como:
– applesauce.	– puré de manzana.
– pudding.	– pudín.
– yogurt.	– yogur.
– juice.	– jugo.

Teaching your patient about his medication

When you teach your patient about his medication, use these phrases to explain how his medication will work and how it will help him.

What's gonna happen

This medication will:
– increase your blood pressure.
– improve circulation to your _____.
– lower your blood pressure.
– lower your blood sugar.
– make your heart rhythm more even.
– raise your blood sugar.
– reduce or prevent the formation of blood clots.
– remove fluid from your body.
– remove fluid from your feet, ankles, or legs.
– remove fluid from your lungs so that they work better.

Este medicamento hará que:
– su presión sanguínea suba.
– la circulación por mejore _____.
– su presión sanguínea baje.
– el nivel de azúcar en la sangre baje.
– el ritmo del corazón sea más uniforme.
– el nivel de azúcar en la sangre suba.
– se reduzca o evite la formación de coágulos de sangre.
– su cuerpo elimine los fluidos.
– su cuerpo elimine el fluido de los pies, tobillos o piernas.
– su cuerpo elimine el fluido de los pulmones para que funcionen mejor.

Benefits for your body

This medication will help your body to:
– kill the bacteria in your _____.
– slow down your heart rate.
– soften your bowel movements.
– speed up your heart rate.
– use insulin more efficiently.

Este medicamento ayudará a su cuerpo a:
– destruir la bacteria de _____.
– reducir el latido del corazón.
– ablandar sus evacuaciones.
– acelerar el latido del corazón.
– usar la insulina más eficazmente.

Do what you wanna do

This medication will help you to:
– breathe better.
– fight infections.
– relax.
– sleep.
– think more clearly.

Este medicamento le ayudará a:
– respirar con mayor facilidad.
– luchar contra infecciones.
– relajarse.
– dormir.
– pensar con mayor claridad.

Ah, relief

This medication will relieve or reduce:
– the acid production in your stomach.
– anxiety.
– bladder spasms.
– burning in your stomach or chest.
– burning when you urinate.
– diarrhea.
– constipation.
– muscle cramps.
– nausea.
– pain in your _____.

Este medicamento le aliviará o disminuirá:
– la producción de ácido en el estómago.
– la ansiedad.
– los espasmos en la vejiga.
– la sensación de ardor en el estómago o tórax.
– la sensación de ardor al orinar.
– la diarrea.
– la estreñimiento.
– los espasmos musculares.
– la náusea.
– el dolor en la (el) _____.

Teaching your patient about his medication *(continued)*

More or less

This medication will help your body to produce more or less:

– antibodies.
– clotting factors.
– insulin.
– platelets.
– red blood cells.
– white blood cells.

Este medicamento ayudará a su cuerpo a producir más o menos:

– anticuerpos.
– factores o agentes coagulantes.
– insulina.
– plaquetas.
– glóbulos rojos.
– glóbulos blancos.

Gone, gone, gone

This medication or treatment will destroy:

– antibodies.
– bacteria.
– cancer cells.
– clotting factors.
– platelets.
– red blood cells.
– white blood cells.

Este medicamento o tratamiento destruirá:

– anticuerpos.
– bacteria.
– células cancerosas.
– factores o agentes coagulantes.
– plaquetas.
– glóbulos rojos.
– glóbulos blancos.

If you can't swallow this pill, I can get it in another form.

Si Ud. no puede tragarse esta píldora, puedo obtenerla en otra forma.

I need to mix this medication in juice or water.

Tengo que mezclar este medicamento en jugo (zumo) o agua.

Hold still

I need to give you this injection in your:
– abdomen.
– buttocks.
– hip.
– outer arm.
– thigh.

Tengo que ponerle esta inyección:
– en el abdomen.
– en las nalgas.
– en la cadera.
– en el brazo.
– en el muslo.

I need to give you this medication I.V.

Tengo que darle este medicamento por vía intravenosa.

Tied to the tongue

This medication must be placed under your tongue to dissolve.
– You should feel some burning or tingling when it's under your tongue. This indicates that it's working.

Este medicamento debe ser colocado debajo de la lengua para disolverlo.
– Ud. debiera sentir un poco de ardor cuando se lo pone debajo de la lengua. Esto indica que está haciendo efecto.

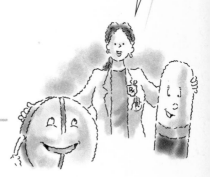

If you can't swallow this pill, I can get it in another form.

Si Ud. no puede tragarse esta píldora, puedo obtenerla en otra forma.

Note the coat

Some medications are coated to protect your stomach from getting upset.

– Don't chew:
    enteric-coated pills.

    long-acting pills.
    capsules.
    sublingual medication.

Algunos medicamentos están recubiertos para evitar posibles malestares estomacales.

– No masque Ud.:
    píldoras con recubrimiento entérico.
    píldoras de efecto prolongado.
    cápsulas.
    medicamentos sublinguales.

Speak up

Ask your doctor or pharmacist if you can:
– mix your medication with food or fluids.
– take your medication with or without food.

Pregúntele Ud. a su doctor o farmacéutico si debiera:
– mezclar su medicamento con un alimento o con líquidos.
– tomar su medicamento con o sin alimento.

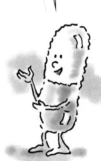

Don't take an extra dose.

No se tome una dosis extra.

Meal plan

You need to take your medication:
– on an empty stomach.
– before meals.
– after meals.
– with meals or food.

Ud. tiene que tomarse el medicamento:
– con el estómago vacío.
– antes de las comidas.
– después de las comidas.
– con las comidas o con un alimento.

Skipping doses

If you skip or miss a dose:
– take it as soon as you remember it.
– wait until the next dose.
– call the doctor if you aren't sure.

– don't take an extra dose.

Si Ud. omite o se salta una dosis:
– tómesela en cuanto se acuerde.
– espérese hasta la siguiente dosis.
– llame al doctor si Ud. no está seguro(a).
– no se tome una dosis extra.

Adverse effects

Some common adverse effects of _____ are:

– constipation
– diarrhea
– difficulty sleeping
– dry mouth
– fatigue
– headache
– itching

Algunos efectos adversos comunes de _____ son:

– estreñimiento
– diarrea
– dificultad en dormir
– boca seca
– cansancio
– dolor de cabeza
– picazón

– light-headedness
– nausea
– poor appetite
– rash
– upset stomach
– weight loss or gain
– frequent urination.

– mareo
– náusea
– poco apetito
– erupción
– trastorno estomacal
– pérdida o aumento de peso
– orinar con frecuencia.

Coping

These side effects:
– will go away after your body gets used to the medication.
– may continue as long as you take the medication.

Estos efectos secundarios:
– desaparecerán una vez que su cuerpo se acostumbre al medicamento.
– pueden continuar todo el tiempo que usted tome el medicamento.

If they bother you, speak to your doctor about changing your medication.

Si le molestan, hable con su doctor acerca de un posible cambio de medicamento.

If you have a side effect to your medication, call your doctor right away. Especially if you have:
– a rash
– itching.

Si sufre un efecto secundario a su medicamento, llame a su médico inmediatamente, especialmente si tiene:
– un sarpullido
– picazón.

Go to the emergency room right away if you have trouble breathing.

Vaya inmediatamente a emergencias si tiene problemas para respirar.

Other concerns

Tell your doctor if you're pregnant or breast-feeding.

Dígale a su doctor si Ud. está embarazada o si está amamantando.

While you're taking this medication, ask your doctor if:
– you can safely take other over-the-counter medications.
– you can drink alcoholic beverages.
– your medications interact with one another.

Mientras Ud. tome este medicamento, pida a su doctor si:
– puede tomar medicamentos de venta libre.
– puede tomar bebidas alcohólicas.
– sus medicamentos interactúan uno con el otro.

Ask your doctor if you can drink alcoholic beverages.

Pida a su doctor si puede tomar bebidas alcohólicas.

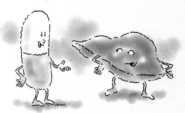

Storing medication

You should keep your medication:
– in a cool, dry place.
– in the refrigerator.

Ud. debiera guardar sus medicamentos:
– en un lugar fresco y seco.
– en el refrigerador.

Don't keep your medication:
– in a warm place or near heat.

– in the sun.
– in your pocket.

No guarde Ud. su medicamento:
– en un lugar caliente ni cerca de la calefacción.
– bajo el sol.
– en su bolsillo.

– in the bathroom medicine cabinet.

– en el botiquín del baño.

Keep your medications away from children.

Mantenga sus medicamentos alejados de los niños.

Teaching related procedures

You'll need to teach your patient how to perform medication-related procedures. (See *What, how, when, and where.*)

Always something new to learn

Your doctor wants you to learn how to:
– draw up and mix your insulin.
– give yourself an injection.
– check your blood sugar level.

Su doctor quiere que Ud. sepa cómo:
– extraer y mezclar su insulina.
– inyectarse.
– controle su nivel de azúcar en sangre.

What, how, when, and where

When you teach your patient about his medication, use these phrases to tell him the route of the medication, how it's prepared, the frequency of the administration, and how to store it.

Routes

Intradermal	Intradérmica
I.M.	Intramuscular
I.V.	Intravenosa
Oral	Oral
Rectal	Rectal
Subcutaneous	Subcutánea
Topical	Tópica
Vaginal	Vaginal

Preparations

Capsule	Cápsula
Cream	Pomada
Drops	Gotas
Elixir	Elixir
Injection	Inyección
Inhaler	Inhalador
Lotion	Loción
Lozenge	Pastilla
Powder	Polvo
Spray	Atomizador
Suppository	Supositorio
Suspension	Suspensión
Syrup	Jarabe
Tablet	Tableta

Frequency

Once daily	Una vez al día
Twice daily	Dos veces al día
Three times daily	Tres veces al día
Four times daily	Cuatro veces al día
In the morning	Por la mañana
In the evening	A la noche
With meals	Con las comidas
Before meals	Antes de las comidas
After meals	Después de las comidas
Before bedtime	Antes de acostarse
When you have _____	Cuando Ud. tome _____
Only when you need it	Sólo cuando lo necesite
Every 4 hours	Cada 4 horas
Every 6 hours	Cada 6 horas
Every 8 hours	Cada 8 horas

Storage

At room temperature	A temperatura ambiente
In the refrigerator	En el refrigerador
Out of direct sunlight	Fuera de la luz del sol
In a dry place	En un lugar seco
Away from heat	Lejos de la calefacción
Away from children	Lejos del alcance de los niños

Working together

Let me show you how to do it.	Permítame enseñarle cómo hacerlo.
Let's practice together.	Vamos a ensayar juntos(as).
I want you to do it yourself.	Quiero que Ud. lo haga por sí solo(a).
I'll watch to make sure you can do it correctly.	Le observaré para estar seguro(a) que Ud. lo puede hacer por sí solo(a).
Let me know if you have trouble:	Dígame si Ud. tiene dificultad en:
– handling the equipment.	– manejar el aparato.
– seeing the directions.	– ver las instrucciones.
– understanding the directions.	– comprender las instrucciones.
– reading the directions.	– leer las instrucciones.

Inject yourself

To give yourself an injection, follow these steps:	Para inyectarse a sí mismo(a), siga estas instrucciones:
– Draw up the medication.	– Extraiga el medicamento.
– Replace the cap carefully.	– Coloque de nuevo la tapa con cuidado.
– Decide where you're going to give the injection.	– Decida Ud. dónde va a ponerse la inyección.
– Clean the skin area with alcohol.	– Limpie el área de la piel con alcohol.
– Gently pinch up a little skin over the area.	– Suavemente pellizque un poco de piel sobre el área.
– Using a dartlike motion, stab the needle into your skin.	– Con un movimiento rápido, penetre la aguja en su piel.
– Gently pull back on the plunger to see if there's any blood in the syringe.	– Con cuidado retire el émbolo para ver si hay sangre en la jeringa.
– Steadily push the medication into your skin.	– Empuje el medicamento dentro de su piel.
– Pull the needle out.	– Saque la aguja.
– Apply gentle pressure with the alcohol pad.	– Ejerza presión suavemente con un algodón mojado en alcohol.
– Dispose of the needle in a proper container.	– Descartar la aguja en el recipiente apropiado.

Insights into insulin

The doctor has ordered insulin for you.

To draw up insulin, follow these steps:

– Wipe the rubber top of the insulin bottle with alcohol.
– Remove the needle cap.
– Pull back the plunger until the end of the plunger in the barrel aligns with the number of units of insulin that you need.
– Push the needle through the rubber top of the insulin bottle.

– Inject the air into the bottle.
– Without removing the needle from the bottle, turn it upside down.
– Withdraw the plunger until the end of the plunger aligns with the number of units you need.
– Gently pull the needle out of the bottle.

El doctor ha recetado insulina para Ud.

Para extraer la insulina siga los siguientes pasos:
– Limpie la tapa de la botella de insulina con alcohol.
– Quítele el capuchón a la aguja.
– Retraiga el émbolo hasta que el extremo del émbolo en el tubo quede alineado con el número de unidades de insulina que Ud. necesita.
– Coloque la aguja en la insulina turbia sin inyectar ningún medicamento en la botella.
– Inyecte el aire dentro de la botella.
– Sin sacar la aguja de la botella, póngala al revés.
– Retire el émbolo hasta que llegue la insulina al número de unidades que Ud. necesita.
– Retire Ud. la aguja de la botella con cuidado.

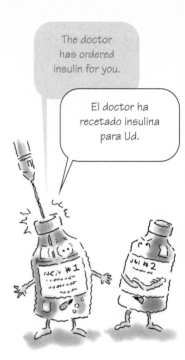

The doctor has ordered insulin for you.

El doctor ha recetado insulina para Ud.

Mixing it up

When mixing insulins, always draw up clear insulin first, then cloudy.

To mix insulin, follow these steps:

– Gently roll the cloudy insulin between your palms.
– Wipe the rubber tops of the insulin bottles with alcohol.
– Remove the needle cap.
– Pull back the plunger until the end of the plunger in the barrel aligns with the number of units of cloudy insulin that you need.

– Push the needle through the rubber top of the cloudy insulin bottle.
– Inject the air into the bottle.
– Remove the needle from the bottle.
– Pull back the plunger until the end of the plunger in the barrel aligns with the number of units of clear regular insulin that you need.

Cuando mezcle insulinas, siempre extraiga primero la insulina límpida y luego la turbia.

Para mezclar la insulina siga los siguientes pasos:
– Suavemente mueva la insulina turbia entre las palmas de la mano.
– Limpie la tapa de las botellas de insulina con alcohol.
– Retire el capuchón de la aguja.
– Retraiga el émbolo hasta que el extremo del émbolo en el tubo quede alineado con el número de unidades de insulina regular cristalina que Ud. necesita.
– Empuje la aguja por la tapa de la botella de insulina turbia.
– Inyecte el aire dentro de la botella.
– Retire la aguja de la botella.
– Retraiga el émbolo hasta que el extremo del émbolo en el tubo quede alineado con el número de unidades de insulina regular cristalina que Ud. necesita.

– Push the needle through the rubber top of the clear insulin bottle.

– Inject the air into the bottle.

– Without removing the needle, turn the bottle upside down.

– Withdraw the plunger until it aligns with the number of units of clear regular insulin that you need.

– Gently pull the needle out of the bottle.

– Push the needle into the cloudy insulin without injecting any medication into the bottle.

– Withdraw the plunger until you reach your total dosage of insulin in units (clear combined with cloudy).

– We'll practice again.

– Empuje Ud. la aguja por la tapa de goma de la botella de insulina clara.

– Inyecte el aire dentro de la botella.

– Sin sacar la aguja, voltee la botella al revés.

– Retire el émbolo hasta que llegue a la dosis de insulina (regular) clara (número de unidades) que Ud. necesita.

– Suavemente saque Ud. la aguja de la botella.

– Coloque la aguja en la insulina turbia sin inyectar ningún medicamento en la botella.

– Retire el émbolo hasta que llegue a su dosis total de insulina en unidades (regular y combinadas).

– Practicaremos juntos(as) otra vez.

Minding the monitor

The doctor wants you to check your blood sugar level at home.

This is done by using a special machine called a *blood sugar monitor*.

To work the blood sugar monitor, follow these steps:
– Turn the machine on.
– Wash your hands with soap and water.
– Prick your finger with the lancet.
– Place a drop of blood onto the strip on the designated area on the strip.
– Insert the strip into the monitor.

El médico quiere que usted controle su nivel de azúcar en sangre en su casa.

Esto se hace por medio de un aparato especial que se llama *monitor de azúcar en la sangre*.

Para hacer funcionar el monitor de azúcar en sangre, siga estos pasos:
– Conecte Ud. el aparato.
– Lávese las manos con agua y jabón.
– Pínchese el dedo con la lanceta.
– Ponga una gota de sangre en la banda en el lugar que se indica.
– Inserte la tira en el monitor.

– The machine will count for _____ seconds.
– You can read your blood sugar number here.
– If the number is high:
    call your doctor.
    follow his directions.
– If it's low:
    drink some orange juice.
    eat a candy bar.
    suck on hard candy.
    call your doctor.

– El aparato contará por _____ segundos.
– Aquí puede Ud. leer el número de azúcar en la sangre.
– Si indica un número alto:
    llame Ud. a su doctor.
    siga sus instrucciones.
– Si indica uno bajo:
    tome jugo (zumo) de naranja.
    coma un caramelo.
    chupar dulces duro.
    llame a su doctor.

It happens to be hypoglycemia

Signs and symptoms of hypoglycemia (low blood sugar) are:
– shakiness
– nervousness
– hunger
– nausea
– light-headedness
– confusion.

Los síntomas de hipoglicemia son:

– inestabilidad
– nerviosismo
– hambre
– náusea
– mareo
– desorientación.

If you have signs or symptoms of hypoglycemia:
– Check your blood sugar level.

– Drink some orange juice.

– Call your doctor. He may want to adjust your medication dosage.

Si Ud. tiene síntomas de hipoglicemia:

– Confirme el nivel de azúcar en la sangre.
– Beba un poco de jugo (zumo) de naranja.
– Llame a su doctor. Es posible que él quiera modificar su dosis de medicamento.

It happens to be hypERglycemia

Signs and symptoms of hyperglycemia (high blood sugar) are:
– thirst
– sleepiness
– frequent urination
– fruity smell to breath.

Síntomas de hiperglucemia (aumento excesivo de azúcar en su sangre) son:
– sed
– somnolencia
– orinar con frecuencia
– un olor de fruta en el aliento.

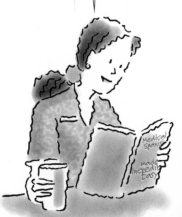

Drink some orange juice.

Beba un poco de jugo de naranja.

If you have signs or symptoms of high blood sugar:

– check your blood sugar level.

– call your doctor.

Si Ud. tiene síntomas de hiperglucemia o aumento excesivo de azúcar en su sangre:

– confirme el nivel de azúcar en la sangre.

– llame a su doctor.

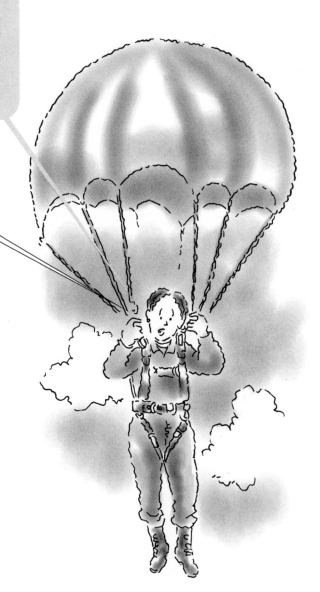

Make sure you aren't jumping without a parachute by guessing at the correct Spanish word. Use the practice questions on the next page to help you get it right!

Asegúrese de no saltar sin paracaídas al adivinar la palabra correcta en Español. ¡Use las preguntas de práctica de la próxima página como ayuda para encontrar la opción correcta!

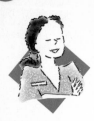

Practice makes perfecto

1. Help Joy ask her patient if he takes any medications.

_____

_____

_____

_____

> ¿Toma Ud.
> _____?

2. Help Joy teach her diabetic patient how to push the needle through the top of the insulin bottle.

_____

_____

_____

_____

> Empuje la aguja
> por la tapa de
> _____.

3. Joy wants to explain to her patient that the doctor wants her to check her blood sugar level at home. _Hint:_ The Spanish word for blood is _sangre._

_____

_____

_____

_____

> El médico quiere
> que usted
> _____.

Answer key

1. Do you take any medications?
¿Toma Ud. <u>medicamentos</u>?

2. Push the needle through the top of the insulin bottle.
Empuje la aguja por la tapa de <u>la botella de insulina</u>.

3. The doctor wants you to check your blood sugar level at home.
El médico quiere que usted <u>controle su nivel de azúcar en sangre en su casa</u>.

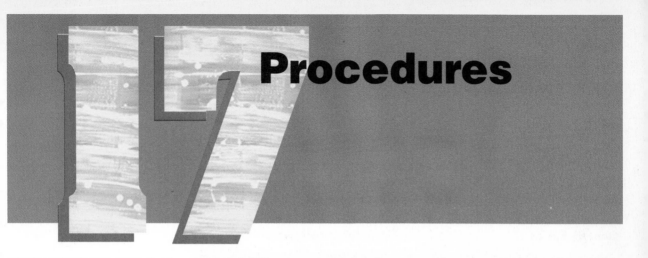

17 Procedures

Fast fact

Key terms related to medical procedures include:
- *percusión del tórax* (chest percussion)
- *ejercicios fortificantes* (strengthening exercises)
- *diálisis* (dialysis)
- *cateterismo urinario* (urinary catheterization)
- *transfusión de sangre* (blood transfusion).

Cardiovascular procedures

Cardiovascular procedures that you may need to discuss with your patient include antiembolism stockings, synchronized cardioversion, intermittent pneumatic compression, pericardiocentesis, and Valsalva's maneuver.

Antiembolism stockings

These stockings help decrease the risk of blood clots that may form in your legs.	Estas medias ayudan a disminuir el riesgo de coágulos de sangre que se pueden formar en las piernas.
These stockings may be used before and after surgery.	Estas medias pueden usarse antes y después de la cirugía.

Keep 'em on

The stockings are worn continuously, while in bed and while walking.	Estas medias se llevan puestas continuamente en la cama y mientras camina.
I need to measure your legs so that the stockings fit properly.	Necesito medirle las piernas para que las medias le queden bien.
Powder may be applied to your legs before you put on the stockings.	Es posible que se le aplique talco a sus piernas antes de ponerle las medias.
They may feel a little tight.	Pueden ser un poco ajustadas.
They may feel a little uncomfortable.	Pueden ser un poco incómodas.
The stockings are removed every shift to check your skin.	Se le sacan las medias cada turno para ver cómo está su piel.

Synchronized cardioversion

Cardioversion is the delivery of an electric shock to your heart.	Una cardioversión es la aplicación de una descarga eléctrica directa al corazón.
It's used to stop an abnormal heart rhythm.	Se utiliza para detener el ritmo cardiaco anormal.

You need to sign this consent form.

Necesita firmar este papel para dar su autorización.

Before

You'll have an electrocardiogram (ECG) done before the procedure.

Le harán un electrocardiograma (ECG) antes de los procedimientos.

Your heart will be monitored during the procedure.

Se monitorizará su corazón durante el procedimiento.

Your blood pressure will be monitored during the procedure.

Se monitorizará su presión sanguínea durante el procedimiento.

This probe on your finger will monitor your oxygen level.

Esta sonda en su dedo controlará su nivel de oxígeno.

An I.V. line will be started.

Se le pondrá una línea intravenosa.

You'll be given a sedative.

Se le dará un sedante.

You'll receive oxygen during the procedure.

Ud. recibirá oxígeno durante el procedimiento.

Your heart will receive a low-energy shock.

Su corazón recibirá un pequeño choque eléctrico.

After

You won't remember the procedure.

Ud. no recordará el procedimiento.

You'll have an ECG done after the procedure.

Le harán un ECG después del procedimiento.

You'll be checked for at least 2 hours after the procedure.

Se le controlará por lo menos durante 2 horas después del procedimiento.

> Common cardiac procedures include intermittent pneumatic compression and Valsalva's maneuver.

> Los procedimientos cardiacos usuales incluyen la compresión intermitente neumática y la maniobra de Valsalva.

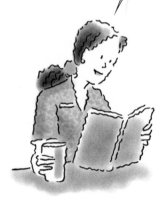

Intermittent pneumatic compression

This machine is called an *SCD machine.*

Esta máquina se llama *máquina de SCD.*

It involves wrapping cuffs around your legs to prevent blood clots.

Se requiere envolver las piernas con bandas para evitar que se formen coágulos de sangre.

The cuffs are connected to a pump.

Las bandas están conectadas a una bomba.

The cuffs inflate and deflate, gently compressing the legs.

Los manguitos se inflan y desinflan, comprimiendo suavemente las piernas.

Imitation of the heart

This inflation and deflation mimics the normal pumping action of the heart.

Este inflado y desinflado imita la acción normal del latir del corazón.

It helps blood return to the heart.

Esto incrementa el regreso de la sangre al corazón.

The cuffs will stay in place until you're no longer at risk for developing blood clots.

Las bandas permanecerán puestas hasta que Ud. no esté en peligro de desarrollar coágulos de sangre.

Walk on

If you walk around in your room or in the hallway, the cuffs should be removed.

Si camina por su cuarto o en el pasillo, se deben quitar las bandas.

The cuffs will be removed every shift so that we can check your skin.

Se le retirarán los manguitos cada turno para ver cómo está su piel.

Pericardiocentesis

This procedure is called *pericardiocentesis*.

Este procedimiento se llama *pericardiocentesis*.

Pericardiocentesis involves the removal of fluid from the sac that surrounds the heart.

La pericardiocentesis supone la extracción de líquido del saco que rodea el corazón.

Pericardiocentesis removes fluid from the sac around the heart. It can be done at the bedside.

Pericardiocentesis es la extracción de líquido del saco que rodea el corazón. Se puede hacer en la cama.

Pump it up

Your heart will be able to pump easier when we remove the fluid around your heart.

La extracción del el líquido que se ha acumulado alrededor del corazón lo ayudará a latir mejor.

This procedure may be done at the bedside.

Este procedimiento se puede hacer en la cama.

You'll receive tranquilizers or sedatives.

A Ud. se le dará un sedante.

An I.V. catheter will be inserted for administration of medicine.

Se le insertará un catéter intravenoso para administrar la medicina.

Your chest may be shaved and will be cleaned with an antiseptic solution.

Se le limpiará el área con una solución antiséptica y si es necesario se le rasurará el pecho.

Your heart will be monitored during the procedure.

Se le chequeará el corazón durante el el procedimiento.

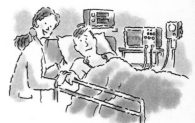

Through the needle

The doctor will numb an area on your chest and then insert a needle to remove the fluid.

El médico adormecerá un área en su pecho y luego le insertará una aguja para extraer el líquido.

After the fluid has been removed, a bandage will be placed over the site.

Después de haberle extraído el líquido, se le colocará una venda en el lugar.

Your heart will be monitored during and after the procedure.

Su corazón estará bajo observación continuamente durante y después del procedimiento.

Your vital signs will be monitored every 15 minutes after the procedure.

Sus signos vitales se observarán cada 15 minutos después de este procedimiento.

Valsalva's maneuver

Valsalva's maneuver is a procedure in which you hold your breath and bear down.

La maniobra de Valsalva es un procedimiento en el que Ud. retiene la respiración y a la vez puja.

It's like trying to breathe out while holding your breath.

Es como tratar de soltar el aire mientras sostiene la respiración.

Back on the beat

This maneuver may correct certain abnormal heart rhythms.

Esta maniobra puede corregir ciertos ritmos cardiacos anormales.

You'll be placed on a heart monitor.

Le pondremos a Ud. un monitor cardiaco.

An I.V. catheter will be inserted to give medicine if needed.

Se le insertará un catéter intravenoso para darle medicamentos, si fuera necesario.

You'll lie on your back, breathe in deeply, hold your breath, and bear down as if you're trying to have a bowel movement.

Se acostará sobre la espalda, respirará profundamente, sostendrá su respiración y hará fuerza como si estuviera tratando de evacuar.

I feel dizzy

You may feel faint or dizzy during the procedure.

Ud. puede sentirse mareado(a) durante el procedimiento.

You'll hold your breath and bear down for 10 seconds.

Ud. contendrá la respiración y pujará por 10 segundos.

Then you'll breathe normally.

Luego respirará normalmente.

If the procedure works, your heart rate will begin to slow down before you exhale.

Si el procedimiento funciona, su ritmo cardiaco comenzará a desacelerarse antes de que Ud. exhale.

Respiratory procedures

Respiratory procedures you may need to discuss with your patient include chest drainage, chest physical therapy, incentive spirometry, mechanical ventilation, nebulizer treatments, oxygen therapy, and thoracentesis.

Chest drainage

A chest tube is inserted to remove air, blood, or pus from the lung.

Se inserta un tubo en el pecho para extraer aire, sangre, o pus del pulmón.

It allows your lung to reinflate.

Permitirá que el pulmón se vuelva a inflar.

You'll receive a sedative.

Se le dará a Ud. un sedante.

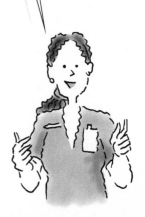

Important respiratory procedures include nebulizer treatments, mechanical ventilation, and thoracentesis.

Los procedimientos respiratorios importantes incluyen tratamientos de nebulizadoc, ventilación mecánica, y toracentesis.

How it's done

The doctor inserts a tube into your chest.	El médico le introducirá un tubo en el pecho.
The chest tube is sutured into place.	Se sutura el tubo torácico en su lugar.
It's attached to a collection container.	El tubo se conecta a una cámara colectora.
The doctor will put a dressing over the site.	El médico pondrá un vendaje sobre el lugar.
You'll have a chest X-ray to make sure the tube is in the right place.	Se le hará una radiografía de tórax para asegurar que el tubo esté en el lugar correcto.

Afterward

Your dressing will be checked and your vital signs will be monitored.	Se le examinará el vendaje y se observarán sus signos vitales.
A nurse will check the drainage every few hours.	Un(a) enfermero(a) verificará el drenaje con intervalos de algunas horas.

Chest physical therapy

Chest physical therapy includes: – coughing and deep-breathing exercises – positioning to encourage drainage – tapping on your back.	La terapia física del tórax incluye: – ejercicios de toser y respirar profundamente – posicionamiento para incentivar el drenaje – golpes en la espalda.
It's performed to loosen mucus in the lungs.	Se realiza para aflojar la mucosidad en los pulmones.

What happens

You'll be told to cough while performing deep-breathing exercises.	Se le dirá que tosa al hacer ejercicios de respiración profunda.
Coughing helps move mucus from the lungs.	Toser ayuda a eliminar más mucosidad de los pulmones.
Deep breathing increases the amount of air in the lungs.	El respirar profundamente aumenta la cantidad de aire en los pulmones.
You'll lie in a position that results in the best drainage for each part of the lung.	Se acostará en una posición que permita el mejor drenaje para cada parte del pulmón.

Percussion and vibration

Percussion is performed by tapping the back with cupped hands or with a special device.	La percusión se realiza golpeando la espalda con las manos ahuecadas o con un dispositivo especial.

This action helps loosen mucus in the lungs.

Esta acción ayuda a aflojar la mucosidad en los pulmones.

You can then cough up and spit out the mucus, or we can use suctioning.

Luego, puede toser y escupir la mucosidad, o podemos succionar.

Incentive spirometry

Incentive spirometry is used to encourage you to take deep breaths.

El estímulo de espirometría se usa para tomar respiraciones a fondo.

It's used to prevent problems with your lungs.

Se usa para evitar problemas con sus pulmones.

Deep breathing

Sit up as straight as you can. Hold the mouthpiece with one hand and the meter with the other.

Siéntese lo más desecho(a) que pueda. Sujete la boquilla con una mano y el medidor con la otra.

Take a deep breath in and watch the balls in the meter rise.

Inspire profundamente y mire cómo suben las esferas en el medidor.

The deeper you breathe, the higher the balls will rise.

Cuanto más profundamente respire, más alto subirán las esferas.

Mechanical ventilation

A ventilator is a machine that helps you breathe.

Un respirador es una máquina que le ayuda a respirar.

It supplies oxygen and can help you breathe easier.

Puede suplir oxígeno y le ayuda a respirar más fácilmente.

Breath savers

Mechanical ventilation is only temporary.

La ventilación mecánica es solo temporal.

You'll need a breathing tube inserted that connects to the ventilator.

Ud. necesitará que se le inserte un tubo que se conecta al respirador.

You won't feel a thing

You'll be given some sedation so that you won't feel the tube going in.

Se le dará algún sedante para que Ud. no sienta el ingreso del tubo.

After the breathing tube is in place, you'll have a chest X-ray.

Una vez que el tubo endotraqueal esté dentro se le tomará una radiografía.

Don't pull out the breathing tube.

No tire del tubo de respiración.

Finding an alternative

You won't be able to talk or eat while the breathing tube is in.

Ud. no podrá hablar o comer mientras tenga el tubo de respiración insertado.

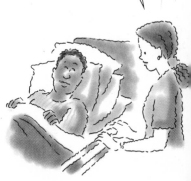

Mechanical ventilation can help you breathe.

La ventilación mecánica le puede ayudar a respirar.

Nebulizer treatments

Nebulizer treatments are a way to administer medication directly into your lungs.

Los tratamientos de nebulizador son una manera de administrar medicamentos directamente a los pulmones.

The lung and short of it

The nurse or a respiratory therapist will listen to your lungs with a stethoscope.

La enfermera o una terapeuta de la respiración escuchará sus pulmones con un estetoscopio.

Liquid medication will be placed into the nebulizer cup.

Luego pondrá medicamento líquido en la tasa del nebulizador.

The cup is then attached to a compressed air machine.

Luego se sujeta la tasa a un aparato de compresión de aire.

As the air passes through the cup, it creates a mist of medication that you breathe into your lungs.

El aire al pasar por la tasa produce una neblina de medicamento que Ud. respira adentro de los pulmones.

You should take slow, deep breaths during the treatment.

Ud. debe respirar despacio pero a fondo durante este tratamiento.

Afterward

After the treatment, the respiratory therapist or nurse will listen to your lungs again.

Después de este tratamiento la terapeuta de la respiración o la enfermera le volverá a escuchar los pulmones.

Oxygen therapy

Oxygen therapy helps maintain the oxygen level in your blood.

La terapia de oxígeno sirve para mantener un nivel de oxígeno en la corriente sanguínea.

The curved prongs of the nasal tube go into your nose.

Las puntas curvas del tubo nasal van en la nariz.

The tubing hooks behind your ears and under your chin.

Los tubos se enganchan detrás de las orejas y debajo de la barbilla (el mentón).

Mask maneuvers

This mask goes on your face, over your nose and mouth.

La máscara va en la cara sobre la nariz y la boca.

Oxygen flows through the mask.

El oxígeno fluye a través de la máscara.

Keep the mask on your face.

Mantenga la máscara sobre el rostro.

Thoracentesis

Thoracentesis removes fluid or air from the lungs with a needle or catheter.

La toracentesis extrae el líquido o aire de los pulmones con una aguja o catéter.

The needle or catheter is inserted through the chest wall.

La aguja o catéter se introduce por la pared del tórax.

It will help relieve pressure on the lungs.

Ayuda a disminuir la presión en los pulmones.

It can also be used to put medication around the lungs.

También se puede usar para poner medicamento alrededor de los pulmones.

You'll receive sedation before the procedure is performed.

Ud. recibirá un sedante antes que se le practique el procedimiento.

Strike a pose

Lean on the bedside table.

Apóyese en la mesita de luz.

Sit up in bed with your arms over your head.

Siéntese en la cama con los brazos sobre la cabeza.

A little sting

You may feel a stinging sensation when the doctor injects the local anesthetic.

Es posible que sienta una sensación de ardor cuando el médico inyecte el anestésico local.

You may feel some pressure during the needle insertion and when the fluid is removed.

Es posible que Ud. sienta algo de presión al introducir la aguja y cuando se extrae el líquido.

It's important to remain still during the procedure.

Es importante estar quieto(a) durante el procedimento.

A chest X-ray or an ultrasound may be done to find the exact location of the fluid.

Se le hará una radiografía del tórax o un ultrasonido para encontrar el lugar exacto del líquido.

Gastrointestinal procedures

GI procedures that you may need to discuss with your patient include enemas, nasogastric decompression, and tube feedings.

Enema administration

Enemas involve putting a solution into the rectum and colon.

En la enema, se coloca una solución dentro del recto y el colon.

You need an enema:
– to clean the lower bowel.

Ud. necesita una enema:
– para limpiar la parte inferior del intestino.

– to relieve constipation and gas.

– aliviar el estreñimiento y el gas.

> Common gastrointestinal procedures include enemas, nasogastric decompression, and tube feedings.

> Los procedimientos gastrointestinales comunes incluyen enemas (lavativas), decompresión nasogástrica, y la alimentación por tubo.

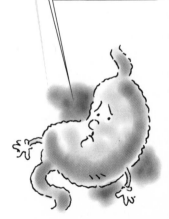

Lie on your left side with your right knee bent.	Acuéstese sobre su lado izquierdo con la rodilla derecha flexionada.
This position helps the flow of enema solution.	Esta posición facilita el fluir de la solución.
The tip of the enema tube is lubricated.	La punta del tubo de la enema se lubrica.
I'm going to gently insert the tube into your rectum.	Le voy a insertar el tubo en el recto suavemente.

Breathe easy

Take slow, easy breaths through your mouth.	Respirar despacio por la boca.
Retain the fluid for 5 to 15 minutes, if possible, before emptying your bowels.	Retenga el líquido por 5 a 15 minutos, si posible, antes de evacuar el intestino.
Retain the fluid for 30 minutes if possible.	Retenga el líquido por 30 minutos, si posible.
You may sit on a bedpan while lying in bed.	Ud. se puede sentar en una cuña mientras está acostado en la cama.
You'll be helped to the bathroom or a commode.	Se le ayudará a ir al baño o a una silla-retrete.

Nasogastric decompression

A tube is needed to remove stomach contents to prevent nausea and vomiting.	Se necesita un tubo para extraer el contenido del estómago para evitar náuseas y vómitos.

Nasal appraisal

Please sit up while the tube is inserted into your nose.	Siéntese mientras se le introduce el tubo en la nariz.
You may feel mild discomfort as the tube is inserted.	Es posible que Ud. sienta algo de molestia al introducir el tubo.
Please swallow as the tube is advanced.	Por favor trague para que el tubo pueda entrar en el estómago.
The tube is connected to suction.	Luego el tubo se conecta a una succión.
The tube must be taped to your nose.	Se debe adherir el tubo a su nariz con cinta adhesiva.

Drain stains?

The drainage will be checked every few hours.	Se verificará el drenaje con intervalos de algunas horas.
The tube may be flushed with saline to keep it from clogging.	Se puede lavar el tubo con solución salina para evitar que se tape.

Your abdomen will be checked for the return of bowel sounds.

Se verificará el regreso de sonidos de los intestinos en su abdomen.

You won't be able to eat or drink while the tube is in place.

Usted no podrá comer ni beber mientras el tubo esté insertado.

Tube feeding

A tube feeding delivers pureed foods or liquid formula directly into the stomach.

En la alimentación por tubo se administran alimentos en puré o líquidos.

A tube is inserted into the stomach through the nose.

Se inserta un tubo en el estómago a través de la nariz.

Food fortification

Tube feedings provide nutrition when you can't eat.

La alimentación por tubo provee nutrición cuando Ud. no puede comer.

Location, location, location

The feeding will be given through the tube.

Se lo(a) alimentará a través del tubo.

You'll be weighed daily to check how you're doing.

Se lo(a) pesará todos los días para ver cómo anda.

Tube feedings are given to provide necessary nutrition when you can't eat.

La alimentación por tubo es dada para proveer la nutrición necesaria cuando Ud. no puede comer.

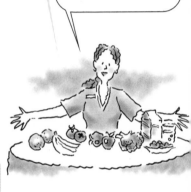

Musculoskeletal procedures

Musculoskeletal procedures that you may need to discuss with your patient include hydrotherapy, range-of-motion (ROM) exercises, strengthening exercises, and traction.

Hydrotherapy

Hydrotherapy is the external use of water to promote relaxation and increase circulation.

La hidroterapia es el uso externo de agua para fomentar la relajación y aumentar la circulación.

It can be used to alter body temperature.

Se puede usar para alterar la temperatura del cuerpo.

It can strengthen muscles and improve movement.

Puede fortalecer los músculos y mejorar el movimiento.

It can help the cleaning of wounds.

Puede ayudar a limpiar las heridas.

Water, water everywhere

Hydrotherapy can be performed in a whirlpool, tank, or swimming pool.

La hidroterapia puede realizarse en una bañera de hidromasaje, tanque, o piscina.

Most whirlpool treatments are performed with warm water.

La mayoría de los tratamientos en hidromasajes se hacen con agua tibia.

If the treatment involves covering the whole body, your body will be lowered into the tank by a hoist.

Si el tratamiento incluye cubrir el cuerpo entero, su cuerpo será izado hacia dentro del tanque.

You're positioned so that a headrest supports your head.

Se le colocará un apoyo para la cabeza.

Smaller tanks may be used if only one body part, such as an arm or a leg, requires therapy.

Se usarán tanques más pequeños si sólo una parte del cuerpo, tal como un brazo o una pierna, requiere terapia.

Underwater maneuvers

Other treatments, such as removing dead tissue from wounds, may be performed.

Es posible que se realicen otros tratamientos como extraer el tejido muerto de heridas.

Exercises may be done in water.

Es posible que se realicen ejercicios en el agua.

Hydrotherapy usually lasts 20 minutes.

La hidroterapia normalmente dura veinte minutos.

After the treatment, you'll be slowly removed from the tank, dried, and covered with a warm sheet or blanket.

Después del tratamiento, se le sacará despacio del tanque, se le secará, y se le cubrirá con una sábana o manta caliente.

Range-of-motion exercises

ROM exercises are exercises that contract and shorten muscles.

La escala de movimiento de ejercicios son aquellos que contraen y acortan los músculos.

They move the joints through full range of motion.

Están diseñados para mover lo más posible las articulaciones.

Each joint of the body has a normal range of motion.

Cada articulación del cuerpo tiene una escala normal de movimiento.

The joint is jumpin'

ROM exercises help improve movement.

Los ejercicios ROM ayudan a mejorar el movimiento.

ROM exercises improve circulation.

Los ejercicios ROM mejoran la circulación.

They also enhance muscle tone and prevent contractures.

También mejoran el tono muscular y previenen contracturas.

The exercises should be done at least twice per day.

Se debe hacer los ejercicios por lo menos dos veces al día.

You shouldn't overdo it.

No exagere.

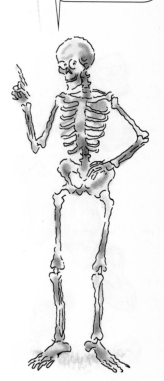

Each joint of the body has a normal range of motion.

Cada articulación del cuerpo tiene una escala normal de movimiento.

Flex appeal

ROM therapy will include:
– bending your limb forward and backward.
– moving your limb away from your body and then back toward your body.

Someone will help you move your limbs through the exercises.

La terapia de ROM incluirá:
– doblando su extremidad hacia delante y hacia atrás.
– alejando su extremidad de su cuerpo y luego moviéndola nuevamente hacia su cuerpo.

Alguien le ayudará a mover las extremidades durante los ejercicios.

Best supporting actor

If the joint is painful, it will be supported as much as possible without causing pain.

Only one limb at a time will be exercised.

If you're doing the exercises yourself, you must move the joints slowly and smoothly through their range of motion.

You'll do these exercises about three to four times per day.

You'll receive pain medication if pain develops.

Si la articulación le duele, se le sostendrá tanto como sea posible sin causarle dolor.

Solo se ejercitará una extremidad a la vez.

Si está haciendo los ejercicios solo(a), debe mover las articulaciones lentamente y suavemente a través de su rango de movimiento.

Ud. hará estos ejercicios alrededor de tres o cuatro veces.

Ud. recibirá un analgésico si tiene dolor.

Strengthening exercises

Strengthening exercises are done to increase muscle strength.

They improve your ability to do things.

The exercise program will be set up for your specific needs.

Los ejercicios fortificantes se hacen para aumentar la fuerza de los músculos.

También se pueden hacen para mejorar su capacidad para hacer actividades.

El programa de ejercicios será establecido para sus necesidades específicas.

Bulking up

You may exercise with weights, including barbells, pulleys, and ankle or wrist cuff weights.

You may use equipment that supplies resistance.

You'll be asked to contract the muscle, hold for 6 seconds, and then relax and repeat.

Ud. puede hacer ejercicio con pesas, incluidas barras con pesas, poleas, y pesas con bandas.

Ud. puede usar un equipo que incluya resistencia.

Se le pedirá que Ud. contraiga el músculo, manteniéndolo así por 6 segundos, luego lo afloja y vuelve a repetirlo.

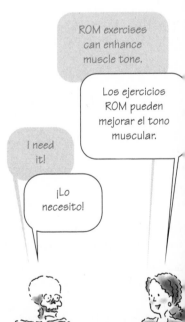

ROM exercises can enhance muscle tone.

Los ejercicios ROM pueden mejorar el tono muscular.

I need it!

¡Lo necesito!

Traction

Mechanical traction exerts a pulling force on a part of the body.

La tracción mecánica ejerce una fuerza que tira de una parte del cuerpo.

Skin traction is applied directly to the skin.

La tracción a la piel se aplica directamente a la piel.

In skeletal traction, a pin or wire is surgically placed through the bone and attaches the traction equipment to the pin or wire.

En la tracción esqueletal, un alfiler o alambre se coloca quirúrgicamente a través de un hueso y luego se conecta el equipo de tracción al alfiler o al alambre.

Traction exerts a direct pulling force on the bones to help move them into proper position for healing.

La tracción ejerce una fuerza directa a los huesos para ayudar a que vuelvan a su posición correcta para que sanen.

The overhead trapeze helps you move around.

El trapecio elevado le ayuda a moverse de un lado a otro.

The amount of weight most often used is 5 pounds (2.5 kg).

La cantidad de peso para su tracción es 2.5 kg (5 libras).

Kidney and urinary tract procedures

Kidney and urinary tract procedures that you may need to discuss with your patient include hemodialysis, peritoneal dialysis, and urinary catheterization.

Hemodialysis

Hemodialysis removes wastes and other impurities from the blood.

La hemodiálisis elimina desechos y otras impurezas de la sangre.

This procedure removes blood from the body, circulates it through a filter, and then returns it to the body.

Este procedimiento extrae sangre del cuerpo, la circula a través de un filtro, y luego la regresa al cuerpo.

Blood filter

You need to have this procedure performed because your kidneys aren't working properly.

Ud. necesita que se le haga este procedimiento porque sus riñones no funcionan debidamente.

The doctor inserts a device in your shoulder, groin, or arm to connect to the machine.

El médico inserta un dispositivo en su hombro, ingle, o brazo para conectar a la máquina.

You will be weighed before and after dialysis.

Se lo(a) pesará antes y después de la diálisis.

Common kidney and urinary tract procedures include hemodialysis, peritoneal dialysis, and urinary catheterization.

Los procedimientos normales para el riñon y el tracto urinario incluyen hemodiálisis, diálisis peritoneal, y cateterismo urinario.

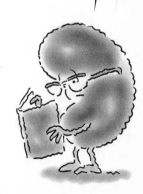

Free samples

We'll take blood samples from the site.	Se le tomará una muestra de sangre de esa área.
You'll then be connected to a dialysis unit.	Luego se le conectará a una unidad de diálisis.
The procedure usually lasts 3 to 6 hours.	El procedimiento normalmente dura de 3 a 6 horas.
At the end of dialysis, more blood samples will be drawn.	Al final de la diálisis, se le extraerán más muestras de sangre.
You'll probably have dialysis three times per week.	Probablemente, tendrá diálisis tres veces por semana.

Peritoneal dialysis

In peritoneal dialysis, a solution is put into the abdomen to remove toxins from the body.	En la diálisis peritoneal, se coloca una solución en el abdomen para eliminar toxinas del cuerpo.

Waste removal

You need to have this procedure performed because your kidneys aren't working properly.	Ud. necesita que se le haga este procedimiento porque sus riñones no funcionan debidamente.
The doctor will insert a dialysis catheter into your abdomen.	El médico le insertará un catéter de diálisis en el abdomen.
The catheter is attached to a bag that contains the dialysis solution.	El catéter está sujeto a una bolsa que contiene la solución de diálisis.

Pollution solution

The dialysis solution is then allowed to run into your abdomen by gravity.	Luego, se deja que la solución de diálisis entre en su abdomen por efecto de la gravedad.
The solution will stay in your abdomen for a prescribed amount of time.	La solución permanecerá en el abdomen por un tiempo designado.
You may feel cramping, shoulder aching, and a fullness in the abdomen or rectum.	Ud. puede sentir calambres, dolor de hombro, plenitud en el abdomen o en el recto.
When the prescribed time has passed, the solution from the abdomen will drain by gravity into a drainage bag.	Cuando el tiempo prescrito haya pasado, la solución del abdomen drenará por efecto de la gravedad hacia dentro de una bolsa de drenaje.

In peritoneal dialysis, a solution is put into the abdomen to remove toxins from the body.

En la diálisis peritoneal, se coloca una solución en el abdomen para eliminar toxinas del cuerpo.

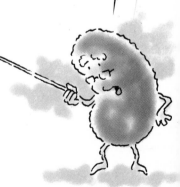

Repetition all over again

This process may take 6 to 8 hours.

Este procedimiento toma de 6 a 8 horas.

It may be repeated five or six times per week.

Se puede repetir cinco o seis veces por semana.

You have a type of dialysis that allows you to walk around during the procedure.

Ud. tiene un tipo de diálisis que le permite moverse durante el procedimiento.

This type of dialysis is performed 24 hours per day 7 days per week.

Este tipo de diálisis se realiza 24 horas por día, los 7 días de la semana.

Urinary catheterization

Urinary catheterization is the insertion of a drainage tube into the bladder.

El cateterismo urinario es la introducción de un tubo de drenaje en la vejiga.

One-time catheterization drains urine that remains in the bladder after urination or if you can't urinate naturally.

Una cateterización que se hace una vez sola drena la orina que queda en la vejiga después de orinar o si Ud. no puede orinar naturalmente.

The tube is left in place only long enough to empty the bladder.

El tubo se deja colocado solo el tiempo necesario para vaciar la vejiga.

The tube is removed when the urine flow stops.

Se retira el tubo cuando el flujo de orina se detiene.

Bailing out the bladder

Continuous catheterization uses a drainage tube to provide continuous drainage of urine.

El cateterismo usa un tubo que provee un drenaje continuo de orina.

The tube may produce slight discomfort, but it shouldn't be painful.

El tubo le puede causar algo de molestia, pero no es doloroso.

The urine drains into the collection bag.

La orina drena hacia dentro de la bolsa de recolección.

Position issues

(Females) Lie on your back with your knees bent. Place your feet flat on the bed.

(Mujeres) Acuéstese sobre la espalda con las rodillas flexionadas. Coloque los pies apoyados sobre la cama.

(Males) Lie on your back with your legs flat and extended.

(Los hombres) Acuéstese de espalda con las piernas planas y extendidas.

I'm going to clean the area with an antiseptic that will feel cold and wet.

Voy a limpiar el área con un antiséptico que se sentirá frío y mojado.

Procedural issues

I'm going to insert this tube into your bladder.	Voy a introducir este tubo en su vejiga.
You may feel some pressure.	Es posible que sienta presión.
The catheter will be attached to a drainage bag.	El catéter se conectará a un saco de drenaje.
The drainage bag needs to be kept below your bladder to drain properly.	La bolsa de drenaje debe permanecer debajo de su vejiga para drenar correctamente.
The catheter has a small balloon inside that's inflated to prevent it from coming out of the bladder.	El catéter tiene un pequeño globo adentro que está inflado para evitar que se salga de la vejiga.
The catheter will be taped to your leg to prevent it from being pulled out.	Se adherirá el catéter a su pierna con cinta adhesiva para evitar que se salga.

Miscellaneous procedures

Other procedures that you may need to discuss with your patient include blood transfusions, cooling treatments, electrical nerve stimulation, heat treatments, replenishing fluids with I.V. solutions, nasal irrigation, and sitz baths.

Blood transfusion

A blood transfusion adds blood to the body.	Una transfusión de sangre le añade sangre al cuerpo.
A transfusion is done to replace blood that has been lost from the body.	Se hace una transfusión para reemplazar sangre que se ha perdido.
It can also help treat anemia and other blood disorders.	También puede tratar la anemia y otros trastornos sanguíneos.
A blood sample will be drawn to determine your blood type.	Se le extraerá una muestra de sangre para determinar su tipo.

Blood bank

If you have a history of reactions to blood transfusion, you'll receive a medication before you receive the blood.	Si Ud. tiene antecedentes de reacciones a transfusión sanguínea, recibirá un medicamento antes de poder recibir la sangre.
Your vital signs are checked before and during the transfusion.	Se controlan sus señales vitales antes y después de la transfusión.
You'll have a catheter inserted into your vein.	Tendrá un catéter insertado en la vena.
The blood is delivered to your veins through special tubing.	La sangre llega a las venas por un tubo especial.
You'll be observed during and after the transfusion.	Se lo(a) observará durante y después de la transfusión.

A blood transfusion adds blood to the body.

Una transfusión de sangre le añade sangre al cuerpo.

Cooling treatments

Cooling treatments are given to lower body temperature.

Cooling treatments may be dry or moist.

If the treatment is used to reduce pain, it may not reduce the pain after the first treatment.

Los tratamientos de enfriamiento se dan para bajar la temperatura del cuerpo.

Los tratamientos de enfriamiento incluyen los secos y los húmedos.

Si el tratamiento se usa para reducir el dolor, puede no hacerlo después de la primera terapia.

Chill out

An ice pack can be used.

It works by placing it in the freezer and then applying it where needed.

Chemical ice packs need to be struck against a hard surface to turn cold.

Es posible que se use una bolsa de hielo.

Se la coloca en el congelador y luego se la aplica donde se necesite.

A las bolsas de hielo químicas hay que golpearlas contra una superficie dura para que se enfríen.

Bags and blankets

An ice bag is filled halfway with ice so it can mold to the part to be cooled.

A cooling blanket can be used to cool the entire body.

Your head won't be covered or lie on the cold blanket.

A rectal thermometer will be inserted and taped in place.

A sheet or a second cooling blanket will be placed over you.

La bolsa de hielo se llena a la mitad para que se pueda amoldar al área que se ha de enfriar.

Se puede usar una manta de frío para enfriar el cuerpo entero.

Su cabeza no estará cubierta ni se apoyará sobre la manta de frío.

Se le insertará un termómetro rectal que se fijará al lugar con cinta adhesiva.

Se lo(a) cubrirá con una sábana o una segunda manta de frío.

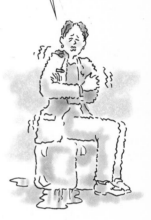

Cooling treatments are given to lower body temperature.

Los tratamientos de enfriamiento se dan para bajar la temperatura del cuerpo.

Electrical nerve stimulation

Electrical nerve stimulation relieves pain.

It uses a mild electric current to stimulate nerve fibers and blocks pain impulses to the brain.

La estimulación eléctrica al nervio mitiga el dolor.

Usa una corriente eléctrica suave para simular fibras nerviosas y bloquear los impulsos de dolor al cerebro.

Current events

The electric current is painless.

Treatments may be given three or four times per day.

La corriente eléctrica no duele.

Los tratamientos se pueden dar tres o cuatro veces al día.

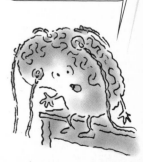

Electrical nerve stimulation relieves pain.

La estimulación eléctrica al nervio mitiga el dolor.

The treatment lasts for 30 to 45 minutes.

El tratamiento dura de 39 a 45 minutos.

The treatment may be given 6 to 8 hours apart.

El tratamiento se puede dar cada 6 u 8 horas.

Get connected

The skin is cleaned and dried.

Se limpia y seca la piel.

The area may be shaved first.

Es posible que se afeite el área primero.

An electrode is stuck to your skin in specific areas.

Se pega un electrodo a su piel en áreas específicas.

A small amount of gel is applied to the bottom of the electrode to help it work.

Se aplica una pequeña cantidad de gel a la base del electrodo para ayudarlo a funcionar.

Hotwired

You'll feel a tingling sensation when the device is turned on.

Ud. sentirá una sensación de hormigueo cuando el aparato se conecta.

The settings will be set so they relieve pain.

Se configurará de modo a aliviar el dolor.

Your pain relief will be evaluated.

Se evaluará el alivio de su dolor.

Heat treatments

Heat treatments raise body temperature.

Los tratamientos térmicos elevan la temperatura del cuerpo.

Heat causes blood vessels to expand and increases blood flow and nutrition to cells.

El calor hace que los vasos sanguíneos se dilaten y aumenta el flujo sanguíneo y la nutrición a las células.

It also helps remove waste products from cells.

También ayuda a eliminar desechos de las células.

Heat ease

Heat treatments are given to relieve pain and stiffness.

Los tratamientos térmicos se dan para aliviar el dolor y la rigidez.

Heat treatments are also given to relax muscles and increase range of motion.

Los tratamientos térmicos también se dan para relajar los músculos y aumentar la escala de movimiento.

They're also performed to promote healing.

También se dan para promover la curación.

Hot topics

You'll lie comfortably with only the area to be treated exposed.

Ud. se acostará confortablemente con sólo el área que se va a tratar expuesta.

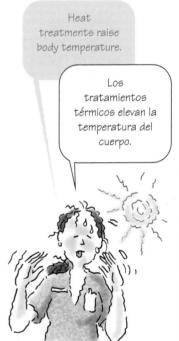

Heat treatments raise body temperature.

Los tratamientos térmicos elevan la temperatura del cuerpo.

Towels are wrapped around heat packs before they're applied.

Las compresas se envuelven con toallas antes de aplicarse.

The pack is then placed on the area to be treated.

Se envuelven las compresas calientes con toallas antes de aplicarlas.

Burning the candle at both ends

Another type of heat treatment is paraffin wax.

Otro tipo de tratamiento térmico es el de cera de parafina.

The paraffin wax is heated and maintained at room temperature.

La cera de parafina se calienta y se mantiene a temperatura ambiente.

Your hands or feet are then dipped in and out of a paraffin wax tank 8 to 10 times to form a solid coating.

Luego las manos y los pies se sumergen entrando y saliendo de la cera de parafina de 8 a 10 veces para formar una capa sólida.

A plastic bag and toweling are wrapped around the part to retain the heat.

Un saco de plástico y toallas se envuelven alrededor del área para retener el calor.

When the paraffin is cooled, it's removed.

Cuando la parafina se enfría, se le quita.

This softens the skin and increases blood flow.

Esto suaviza la piel y aumenta el flujo sanguíneo.

Hot towels

A warm pack may be a towel soaked in warm water and applied to the affected area.

Una compresa caliente puede ser una toalla empapada en agua caliente y aplicada al área afectada.

The moist towel is then covered with a hot water bottle or a chemical heat pack to maintain the temperature.

Luego la toalla remojada se cubre con una botella de agua caliente o con una almohadilla químicamente térmica para mantener la temperatura.

Sound off

Ultrasound therapy is delivered through a transducer.

La terapia de ultrasonido se administra por medio de un transductor.

Mineral oil, water, or gel is applied to the area.

Se aplica aceite mineral, agua, o gel al área.

The transducer is then applied and activated.

Luego se aplica y activa el transductor.

These treatments typically last 5 to 10 minutes.

Generalmente este tratamiento dura de 5 a 10 minutos.

Intravenous fluids

I.V. fluids are used to supply water and electrolytes to the body.

Se usan líquidos intravenosos para proveer agua y electrolitos al cuerpo.

Enter the I.V.

I'm going to insert this catheter into a vein in your hand or arm.

Voy a ponerle este catéter en una vena de la mano o del brazo.

It will be attached to tubing and a bag of I.V. fluid.

Luego el catéter se conecta a un saco con líquido intravenoso.

The I.V. may be controlled by an I.V. pump.

El tubo intravenoso puede ser controlado por una bomba intravenosa.

Medications can also be given through your I.V.

También se pueden administrar medicamentos a través de su tubo intravenoso.

The I.V. catheter can be capped and used when needed.

Se puede tapar el catéter intravenoso y usarlo cuando sea necesario.

It will need to be flushed with a solution that keeps it open.

Hay que enjuagarlo con una solución que lo mantiene abierto.

Nasal irrigation

Nasal irrigation is squirting water or saline solution into the nose.

La irrigación nasal es chorros de agua o solución salina en la nariz.

It's used to drain mucus or debris from the nose.

Se la usa para drenar mocos o residuos de la cavidad nasal.

Soothing saline

It will soothe irritated mucous membranes.

Mitigará la irritación de las membranas mucosas.

It aids breathing.

Ayuda a respirar.

You must keep your mouth open during the procedure.

Ud. debe mantener la boca abierta durante el procedimiento.

Don't speak

You shouldn't speak or swallow during the procedure.

Ud. no debe hablar ni tragar durante el procedimiento.

You'll sit upright with your head bent forward over a basin or sink.

Ud. se sentará derecho(a) con la cabeza inclinada sobre una vasija o fregadero.

Your head should be bent to your chest.

Debe doblar la cabeza en dirección al pecho.

Fluid is squirted into the nose by either a bulb syringe or an oral irrigating device.

Se echan chorros de líquido dentro de la nariz por una jeringa de bulbo o un dispositivo de irrigación oral.

Each nostril is irrigated until the return fluid is clear.

Cada narina es irrigada hasta que el líquido de retorno sea transparente.

It may be performed twice per day.

Se puede hacer dos veces al día.

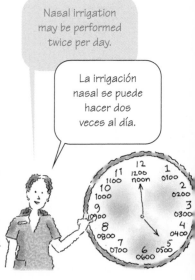

Nasal irrigation may be performed twice per day.

La irrigación nasal se puede hacer dos veces al día.

Sitz bath

In a sitz bath, the pelvic area is placed in tepid or hot water.

En el baño de asiento, se coloca el área pélvica en agua tibia o caliente.

The tube or device is usually shaped to allow the legs to remain out of the water.

El tubo o aparato normalmente tiene una forma para permitir que las piernas queden fuera del agua.

Warm relief

The sitz bath is used to relive perianal itching, swelling, or discomfort.

El baño de asiento se usa para aliviar la comezón o hinchazón perianal.

It can also be used to clean the perianal area and anus.

También se lo puede usar para lavar el área perianal y el ano.

It increases circulation and reduces inflammation.

Aumenta la circulación y reduce la inflamación.

You should urinate before the procedure.

Ud. debe orinar antes del procedimiento.

Soiled bandages should be removed.

También se le quita el vendaje sucio.

You'll sit in a tub of warm or hot water.

Ud. se sentará en una tina de agua tibia o caliente.

You'll soak for 15 to 20 minutes.

Ud. permanecerá de 15 a 20 minutos.

The water temperature will be checked periodically to ensure it hasn't cooled.

Se observará la temperatura del agua periódicamente para asegurar que no se haya enfriado.

You'll then slowly rise from the bath.

Luego Ud. se levantará de la tina despacio.

Clean dressings will be applied to the perianal area as necessary.

Se le pondrán vendajes limpios en el área según sea necesario.

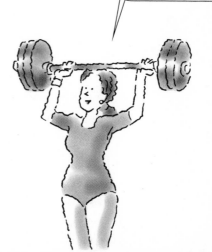

Pump up your Spanish muscles by trying the practice questions on the next page.

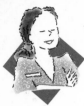

Practice makes perfecto

1. Joy is trying to tell her patient that pericardiocentesis removes fluid from the sac that surrounds the heart. Can you help her?

_____
_____
_____
_____

> La pericardiocentesis _____ del saco que rodea el corazón.

> Los tratamientos nebulizadores administran medicamentos _____.

2. Joy wants to explain that nebulizer treatments administer medication directly into the lungs. Can you supply the right phrase?

_____
_____
_____
_____

> Las enemas se dan para _____ el intestino delgado.

3. Joy needs to explain that enemas are given to clean the lower bowel. Can you add the right verb?

_____
_____
_____
_____

> Las soluciones intravenosas reponen _____.

4. Joy wants to tell her patient that I.V. solutions replenish water and electrolytes. Can you help?

_____
_____
_____
_____

Answer key

1. Pericardiocentesis removes fluid from the sac that surrounds the heart. La pericardiocentesis <u>extrae el líquido</u> del saco que rodea el corazón.

2. Nebulizer treatments administer medication directly into the lungs. Los tratamientos nebulizadores administran medicamentos <u>directamente a los pulmones</u>.

3. Enemas are given to clean the lower bowel. Las enemas se dan para <u>limpiar</u> el intestino delgado.

4. I.V. solutions replenish water and electrolytes. Las soluciones intravenosas reponen <u>agua y electrolitos</u>.

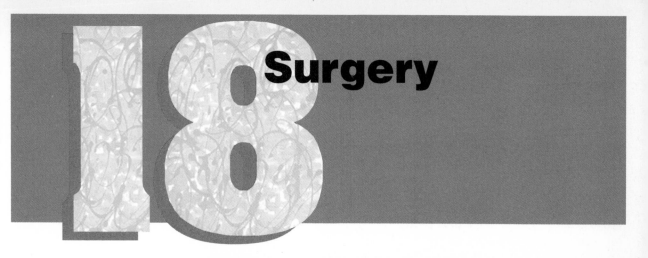

Surgery

18

General preparations

As part of general preparations for surgery, discuss the consent form with your patient and explain the different types of anesthesia.

The dotted line

Your doctor has recommended surgery to correct your problem.

Su doctor ha recomendado cirugía para corregir su problema.

The surgeon will discuss the procedure with you and your family.

El cirujano explicará el procedimiento a Ud. y a su familia.

You may receive a blood transfusion during or after surgery.

Puede dársele una transfusión de sangre durante o después de la cirugía.

You'll need to sign a consent form:
– for the surgery.
– for the blood transfusion.

Ud. tendrá que dar su autorización:
– para la cirugía.
– para la transfusión de sangre.

Feeling no pain

You'll need anesthesia during your surgery.

Ud. necesitará anestesia durante la cirugía.

Anesthesia is used to:
– keep you asleep during surgery.

La anestesia se usa para:
– que Ud. esté dormido(a) durante la cirugía.

– prevent pain.

– prevenir el dolor.

There are two kinds of anesthesia: local and general.

Hay dos tipos de anestesia: local y general.

Sometimes both are used.

A veces se usan ambos.

> Your doctor has recommended surgery to correct your problem.

> Su doctor ha recomendado cirugía para corregir su problema.

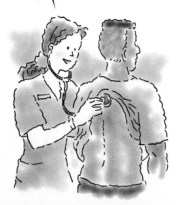

During the surgery, you'll be:
– awake.
– asleep.
(See *Part or whole?*)

Durante la cirugía Ud. estará:
– despierto(a).
– dormido(a).

Local or general

Local anesthesia will numb a certain part of your body.

General anesthesia will numb your entire body, including your breathing muscles.

A breathing tube attached to a ventilator will help you breathe if you receive general anesthesia.

The anesthesiologist inserts the tube after you're asleep; it will probably be removed before you wake up.

If you wake up with the tube still in place, it's because the anesthesia hasn't worn off or you still need assistance to breathe.

La anestesia local adormecerá cierta parte de su cuerpo.

La anestesia general le adormecerá todo el cuerpo, incluso los músculos de la respiración.

Un tubo de respiración sujeto a un respirador le ayudará a respirar si recibe anestia general.

El anestesista (doctor especialista en anestesiología) le introducirá un tubo después que se duerma, y probablemente se lo sacará antes que despierte.

Si Ud. se despertara antes que se le saque el tubo, es porque aún no se ha disipado la anestesia o porque todavía necesita ayuda para respirar.

The night before surgery

Explain to the patient about preparations the night before surgery, including establishing I.V. access, restricting eating and drinking, and cleaning the area used for surgery.

No food, no water

You'll have an I.V. catheter placed in your arm if you don't already have one.

You must not eat or drink anything:
– after midnight.
– _____ hour(s) before surgery.

Se le tendrá que poner un acceso intravenoso en el brazo si es que no lo tiene ya.

No puede Ud. tomar ni beber nada:
– después de la medianoche.
– _____ hora(s) antes de la cirugía.

Cleaning up

You may need to take a bath with a special soap before surgery.

You'll need to drink this solution to empty and clean your bowel.

Es posible que necesite bañarse con un jabón especial antes de la cirugía.

Ud. tendrá que tomarse esta solución para vaciar y limpiar su intestino.

Pump up your pronunciation

Part or whole?

Anestesia local (local anesthesia) and *anestesia general* (general anesthesia) look similar to their English equivalents, although they're pronounced slightly differently. Here are two hints to help you:

Remember that, in Spanish, the adjective typically comes after the noun—that's why it's *anestesia local*, not *local anestesia*.

Remember that the *g* in Spanish is pronounced like an English *h* whenever it's followed by an *i* or *e*.

Say it right
Here's a quick pronunciation guide:
• *anestesia local*—ah-neh-steh-see-ah loh-cahl
• *anestesia general*—ah-neh-steh-see-ah heh-neh-rahl.

You may have a catheter inserted in your bladder to drain your urine.

Es posible que se le inserte un catéter en la vejiga para drenar la orina.

The morning of the surgery

Explain to the patient about preoperative medications he'll receive the morning of the surgery.

Something to relax you

You'll receive medication before your surgery through your I.V. access.

Ud. recibirá medicación antes de su cirugía a través de su acceso intra-venoso.

You'll need to urinate before we give you the medication.

Ud. tendrá que orinar antes de que le demos la medicación.

The medication will:
– relax you.
– make you feel drowsy.
– give you a dry mouth.
– make your vision a little blurry.
– make you feel a little light-headed, disoriented, or forgetful.

El medicamento le:
– hará relajarse.
– hará sentirse soñoliento(a).
– hará que la boca se le sienta seca.
– pondrá la vista borrosa.
– lo(a) hará sentirse un poco mareado, desorientado, u olvidadizo(a).

Clear liquids only

Don't take any medications before your surgery.

No tome ningún medicamento antes de su cirugía.

Take only your _____ medication with a sip of water.

Tome sólo su medicamento _____ con un trago de agua.

We'll give you fluids through your I.V. catheter.

Se le darán líquidos por vía intravenosa.

You may have clear liquids, sips of water, or ice chips.

Ud. puede tomar líquidos claros, sorbos de agua, o pedazos de hielo.

The preoperative medicine will make you feel a little light-headed, disoriented, or forgetful.

El medicamento preoperatorio lo hará sentir un poco mareado, de desorientado, u olvidadizo.

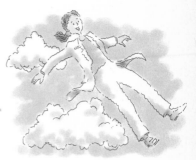

After surgery

Discuss with the patient what to expect after surgery, including the recovery room, receiving oxygen, and feeling pain, nausea, soreness, and sleepiness.

Posted to the recovery room

You'll wake up in the recovery room.

Se despertará en la sala de recuperación.

You'll remain in the recovery room for a while until your vital signs are stable, you're awake, and you're breathing on your own.

Permanecerá en la sala de recuperación un rato hasta que sus señales vitales sean estables, esté despierto(a), y esté respirando por sí solo(a).

You may be receiving oxygen through:

Es posible que esté recibiendo oxígeno a través de:

– prongs in your nose.
– a mask over your nose and mouth.

– cánulas dentro de la nariz.
– una máscara sobre la nariz y la boca.

You may have a tube, catheter, or other equipment.
(See *Postoperative tubes, catheters, and equipment.*)

Ud. puede tener un tubo, un catéter, u otro aparato.

Expected events

When you wake up, it's common to feel:

Cuando Ud. despierte, es normal que sienta:

– pain.
– nausea.
– dry mouth.
– soreness in the throat.
– groggy.
– sleepy.
– uncomfortable.

– dolor.
– náuseas.
– la boca seca.
– dolor de garganta.
– mareo.
– sueño.
– incomodidad.

Ask the nurse to give you medication for:
– nausea.
– pain.

Pídale a la enfermera que dé a Ud. medicamentos para:
– las náuseas.
– el dolor.

The nurse will closely monitor your vital signs.

La enfermera observará cuidadosamente sus signos vitales.

If the doctor wants to monitor you more closely, you may go to the intensive care unit.

Si el doctor quiere observar sus signos vitales más detalladamente, Ud. irá a la unidad de cuidado intensivo.

> When you wake up, it's common to feel sleepy.
>
> Cuando Ud. despierte, es normal que sienta sueño.

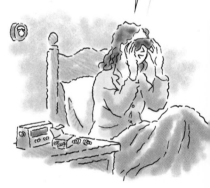

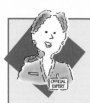

La clinica

Postoperative tubes, catheters, and equipment

Use these phrases to explain to the patient about tubes, catheters, and other equipment he may have when he returns from surgery.

Catheters and tubes

After the surgery, you may have:
- more than one I.V. catheter in your arm.
- an I.V. in your wrist, called an *arterial line*, to measure your blood pressure continuously.
- a tube in your bladder, called a *catheter*, to drain your urine.
- a tube in your nose, called a *nasogastric tube*, to drain fluids and acids from your stomach.
- an I.V. catheter in the side of your neck or in your upper chest near your shoulder or in your groin area, called a *central line*.
- a tube in the side or middle of your chest, called a *chest tube,* to reinflate your lungs or to drain fluid.
- a tube inserted near the area where surgery was performed to drain secretions.
- a very thin catheter in your back near your spine, called an *epidural catheter*, used for pain medication.
- a device with a little light taped or clipped to your finger or toe, called a *pulse oximeter*, that's used to measure oxygen levels.

Después de la cirugía, Ud. puede tener:
- un catéter intravenoso (I.V.) o más en el brazo.
- un tubo intravenoso en su muñeca, llamado *línea arterial*, para medir su presión sanguínea continuamente.
- un tubo en su vejiga, llamado *catéter*, para drenar su orina.
- un tubo en su nariz, llamado *tubo nasogátrico*, para drenar líquidos y ácidos de su estómago.
- un I.V. a un lado del cuello o en la parte superior del tórax cerca del hombro, llamada *línea central.*
- un tubo en el costado o centro de su pecho, llamado *tubo torácico,* para reinflar sus pulmones o drenar líquido.
- un tubo insertado cerca de la región donde se hizo la cirugía para el drenaje de secreciones.
- un catéter muy fino en la espalda cerca de la columna vertebral, que se llama *catéter epidural,* y que se usa para el medicamento contra el dolor.
- un aparato que se llama *pulsoxímetro,* con una pequeña luz fijada con cinta adhesiva o ganchos a un dedo de la mano o del pie, que se usa para medir el nivel de oxígeno.

Bandages, stitches, and clips

After the surgery, you may have:
- a bandage over your incision.
- no bandage over your incision, only stitches or metal clips.
- a blood pressure cuff wrapped around your upper arm attached to a machine. It will inflate and deflate to automatically measure your blood pressure and heart rate.

- a little machine called a *PCA pump* that supplies pain medication through your I.V. You can press it every _____ minutes to give yourself pain medicine.

Después de la cirugía, Ud. puede tener:
- una venda sobre su incisión.
- ninguna venda sobre su incisión, sólo puntos o grapas metálicas.
- un brazalete de medición de presión sanguínea alrededor de su brazo superior, conectado a una máquina. Se inflará y desinflará para medir automáticamente su presión sanguínea y ritmo cardiaco.
- una máquina pequeña llamada *bomba PCA* que suministra medicamentos para el dolor a través de su tubo intravenoso. Ud. puede oprimirla cada _____ minutos para administrarse medicamento para el dolor.

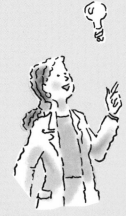

Preventing complications

Discuss with the patient potential complications after surgery, such as pneumonia, blood clots, and infections. Also discuss ways to prevent complications, such as incentive spirometry, splinting, and pain medication.

Incentive to recover

Many patients can develop pneumonia, blood clots, infections, or other complications after surgery.

A muchos(as) pacientes se les puede desarrollar una neumonía, coágulos de sangre, infecciones, u otras complicaciones después de la cirugía.

This is an incentive spirometer.

Esto es un estímulo de espirometría.

You'll use this after surgery to help you take deep breaths.

Ud. usará este aparato después de la cirugía para ayudarle a respirar profundamente.

To use the incentive spirometer, follow these steps:
– Put the mouthpiece into your mouth.
– Inhale or suck air into your mouth.
– Keep this arrow between these two lines as you inhale.
– Attempt to move this arrow up to number _____ and hold it there as long as you can.

Para usar el estímulo de espirometría siga estos pasos:
– Métase la boquilla en la boca.
– Aspire o trague aire por la boca.
– Mantenga esta flecha entre las dos rayas al aspirar.
– Trate de mover esta flecha hacia arriba hasta el número _____ y mantenerla allí todo lo que pueda.

Hug the pillow

In addition to medications, there are other ways to relieve pain.

Además de medicamentos, hay otras maneras de aliviar el dolor.

Splinting can help reduce pain with moving and coughing.

El entablillar puede aminorar el dolor al moverse o al toser.

This is how to splint:
– Take a pillow or large blanket and hold it firmly against your incision.

– Hug or squeeze it tightly and push into your incision as you move or cough.

Así se entablilla:
– Coja una almohada o manta grande y sujétela fuertemente contra la incisión.
– Apriétela o agárrela fuertemente y empújela contra la incisión al moverse o al toser.

Dealing with pain

Focus on things like reading, meditation, television, or other activities to keep your mind off of your pain.

Ask for pain medication about a half hour before you do any major activities.

If the pain prevents you from moving, breathing, or coughing, you should ask for more pain medication.

Ask for pain medication when the pain starts.

You should be comfortable soon.

Fije Ud. su atención en leer, meditar, en la televisión, u otras actividades para poder distraer su atención del dolor.

Pida Ud. medicamentos aproximadamente media hora antes de cualquier actividad de importancia.

Si a Ud. el dolor no le permite moverse, respirar, o toser, Ud. debe pedir que se le dé más analgésicos.

Pida un medicamento cuando empiece el dolor.

Pronto se sentirá cómodo(a).

Move, walk, sit up

After surgery, it will be very important to:
– move.
– walk.
– sit up.
– take deep breaths every hour.
– cough.

Take about 10 deep breaths every hour.

Después de la cirugía es importante que Ud.:
– se mueva.
– camine.
– se incorpore.
– respire profundamente cada hora.
– tosa.

Respire a fondo 10 veces cada hora.

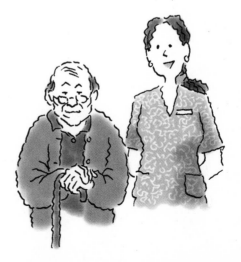

After surgery, it's important to walk.

Después de la cirugía, es importante que Ud. camine.

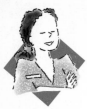

Practice makes perfecto

1. Joy is explaining to the patient that he'll be awake during his surgery. Can you fill in the right phrase?

_____

_____

_____

_____

> Ud. permanecerá _____ durante la cirugía.

> La _____ le adormecerá sólo parte del cuerpo.

2. Joy is telling this patient that local anesthesia will numb a portion of his body. Can you help Joy complete her sentence?

_____

_____

_____

_____

> Es normal que sienta _____ después de la cirugía.

3. Joy wants to explain that it's common to feel groggy after surgery. Can you supply the right phrase?

_____

_____

_____

_____

> El _____ puede aminorar el dolor al moverse.

4. Joy needs to tell this patient that splinting can reduce pain when moving after surgery. Can you help?

_____

_____

_____

_____

Answer key

1. You'll be awake during the surgery.
Ud. permanecerá <u>despierto</u> durante la cirugía.
2. Local anesthesia will numb only a portion of your body.
La <u>anestesia local</u> le adormecerá sólo parte del cuerpo.
3. It's common to feel groggy after surgery.
Es normal que sienta <u>sueño</u> después de la cirugía.
4. Splinting can help reduce pain with moving.
El <u>entablillar</u> puede aminorar el dolor al moverse.

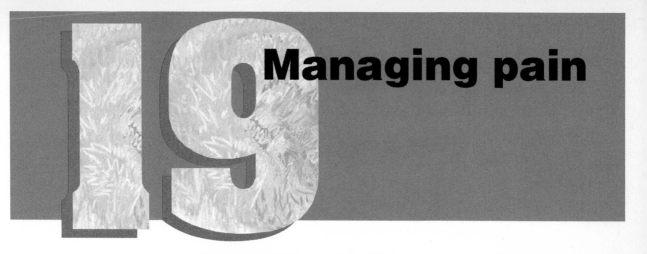

Managing pain

Fast fact

Key terms for discussing pain management include:
- *anestesia* (anesthesia)
- *dolor* (pain)
- *medicamento para el dolor* (pain medication).

Health problems

Pain alerts us to injury or illness and serves as a protective mechanism. Perceptions of pain and reactions to it vary among individuals. It's a complex process that requires a thorough assessment and a unique plan for each patient.

Feeling your pain

When did the pain start?	¿Cuándo comenzó el dolor?
Did the pain start suddenly or gradually?	¿Empezó el dolor de repente o gradualmente?
Have you seen a doctor before about this pain?	¿Vió a un doctor antes por este dolor?
Where does it hurt? – Please point to where the pain is.	¿Dónde le duele? – Por favor, señale dónde le duele.
Does it hurt anywhere else?	¿Le duele en otro lado?
On a scale of 0 to 10, with 0 being no pain and 10 being the worst pain you've ever felt, how would you rate the pain?	En una escala de 0 a 10 donde 0 no indica dolor y 10 indica un dolor intenso, ¿cómo diría usted que es el dolor?
How long does the pain last?	¿Cuánto dura el dolor?
What does the pain feel like? (See *Terms for pain*.)	¿Cómo es el dolor?

Terms for pain

Use these terms to help figure out what kind of pain the patient is feeling.
- *Repentino* (Shooting)
- *Punzante* (Stabbing)
- *Sordo* (Dull)
- *Intenso* (Aching)
- *Constante* (Constant)
- *Intermitente* (Intermittent)
- *Calambres* (Cramping)

How do you spell relief?

What do you usually do for the pain?	¿Qué hace usualmente cuando tiene dolor?
Does anything: – trigger the pain? – relieve the pain? – make the pain worse?	¿Hay algo que: – provoca el dolor? – alivia el dolor? – empeora el dolor?
Do you have other symptoms with the pain?	¿Tiene otros síntomas con el dolor?

– Nausea?   – ¿Náuseas?
– Vomiting?   – ¿Vómitos?
– Dizziness?   – ¿Mareos?

Have you had pain like this before?   ¿Ha tenido un dolor así antes?

Medical history

After the patient has described his pain, you need to establish the patient's medical history.

Past experiences

Please list all of your past medical conditions.   Por favor, enumere todas sus enfermedades médicas.

Have you had any surgeries?   ¿Fue operado?

When were these surgeries?   ¿Cuándo lo operaron?

What prescription medications do you take?   ¿Qué medicamentos bajo receta toma?

Do you take over-the counter medications?   ¿Toma medicamentos sin receta?
– Herbs?   – ¿Hierbas?
– Vitamins?   – ¿Vitaminas?
– What are they?   – ¿Cuáles son?
– Why do you take them?   – ¿Para qué los toma?
– How often do you take them?   – ¿Con qué frecuencia los toma?

Are you allergic to any medications?   ¿Es alérgico(a) a algún medicamento?

Are you allergic to anything else?   ¿Es alérgico(a) a alguna otra cosa?

The social scene

Do you: ¿Usted:
– smoke?   – fuma?
– drink alcohol?   – bebe alcohol?
– use illicit drugs?   – consume drogas?

Describe your family situation.   Describa su situación familar.

Teaching about medication

After you have established the patient's medical and social history, you may have to teach him about medications the doctor has prescribed.

What will it do?

Your doctor has prescribed: Su doctor ha recetado:
– a nonopioid pain medication.   – un medicamento no opioide para el dolor.

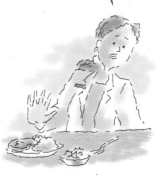

Do you have symptoms with the pain? Nausea?

¿Tiene síntomas con el dolor? ¿Náuseas?

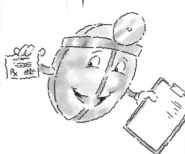

Your doctor has prescribed a nonopioid pain medication.

Su doctor ha recetado un medicamento no opioide.

This medication helps decrease joint and muscle pain, fever, and inflammation.
– an opioid pain medication.
This medication helps decrease moderate to severe pain.
– a local anesthetic.
It will cause the part of your body where it's given to become numb.
– a topical anesthetic.
This drug is applied on your skin to prevent or relieve minor pain.

You'll be receiving:
– a general anesthetic.
It will make you go to sleep.
– an epidural pain medication.

It will decrease the feeling below the level of where it's administered.

Este medicamento ayuda reducir el dolor de articulaciones y músculos, fiebre, e inflamación.
– un medicamento opioide para el dolor.
Este medicamento ayuda a aliviar el dolor moderado a intenso.
– un anestésico local.
Adormecerá la parte del cuerpo donde es aplicado.
– un anestésico tópico.
Esta medicina se aplica en su piel para prevenir o aliviar un dolor ligero.

Usted recibirá:
– un anestésico general.
Lo hará dormir.
– un medicamento epidural para el dolor.
Disminuirá las sensaciones por debajo del nivel de donde es administrado.

Taken orally

This medication should be taken by mouth. It's in:
– tablet form.
– capsule form.
– liquid form. (See *Types of oral medications.*)

Don't chew or crush this drug.

Take this medication:
– with plenty of water.
– with food.
– on an empty stomach.

You can crush this medication and mix it with applesauce or juice.

Este medicamento se debe tomar oralmente. Es:
– una tableta.
– una cápsula.
– un líquido.

No mastique ni triture este medicamento.

Tome este medicamento:
– con mucha agua.
– con comida.
– con el estómago vacío.

Usted puede triturar este medicina y mezclarlo con puré de manzana o jugo.

Sublingual meds

Place this medication under your tongue.

You may feel a tingling sensation as it dissolves.

Don't chew it.

Ponga esta medicina debajo de su lengua.

Sentirá un hormigueo cuando se disuelva.

No la mastique.

Types of oral medications

Use these terms to help describe the type of medication your patient is being prescribed.
• *Tableta* (Tablet)
• *Recubrimiento entérico* (Enteric-coated)
• *Liberación constante* (Sustained-release)
• *Masticable* (Chewable)
• *Medicamento que se desintegra* (Disintegrating)

Transdermal

This medication is an ointment. (See *Types of topical drugs*.)

Este medicamento es un ungüento.

Rub the ointment into the skin.

Pase el ungüento en la piel.

Put a dressing over the ointment.

Ponga un vendaje sobre el ungüento.

Don't put anything over the ointment.

No ponga nada sobre el ungüento.

This medication is a patch.

Este medicamento es un parche.

Apply the patch directly to the skin.

Aplique el parche directamente a la piel.

Place the patch on your:
– arm.
– chest.
– abdomen.
– leg.

Coloque el parche en su:
– brazo.
– pecho.
– abdomen.
– pierna.

Remove the patch at night.

Retire el parche a la noche.

Keep the patch on for __ hours.

Mantenga el parche por __ horas.

Remove the patch for __ hours.

Retire el parche por __ horas.

Remove the old patch before putting on the new one.

Retire el parche viejo antes de colocar uno nuevo.

> ### Types of topical drugs
> Use these terms to help describe the type of topical medication your patient is being prescribed.
> - *Parche* (Patch)
> - *Pomada* (Cream)
> - *Loción* (Lotion)
> - *Ungüento* (Ointment)
> - *Bálsamo* (Salve)

S.C. is for me

This medication is given by injection into the fat under your skin.

Esta medicina se inyecta en la grasa debajo de su piel.

Change injection sites every day.

Cambie los lugares de inyección todos los días.

Wipe the site with alcohol before giving the injection.

Limpie el lugar con alcohol antes de dar la inyección.

Rub the site after giving the injection.

Frote el sitio después de la inyección.

Don't rub the site after giving the injection.

No frote el sitio después de la inyección.

I.M., I.V., and intranasal

This medication is given by injection into the muscle.

Este medicamento se inyecta en el músculo.

You may feel pain and soreness at the injection site.

Es posible que sienta dolor y malestar en el lugar de la inyección.

This medication is injected into your vein.

Este medicamento se inyecta en su vena.

This medication is given by injection into your vein.

Este medicamento se inyecta en su vena.

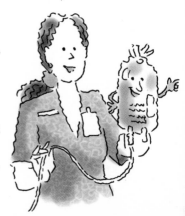

You'll inhale this medication through your nose.

Inhale este medicamento por la nariz.

You may notice some soreness or burning in your nose.

Es posible que note cierto malestar o ardor en la nariz.

Other spots...

This medication will be given through a needle in your back.

Este medicamento se le administrará a través de una aguja en la espalda.

This medication is given through your rectum.

Este medicamento se le administrará por vía rectal.

This medication will be injected directly into your joint with a needle.

Este medicamentos e inyectará directamente en su articulación con una aguja.

Patient-controlled analgesia

With this pump, you can give yourself pain medication when you feel you need it.

Con esta bomba, Ud. puede administrarse el medicamento para el dolor cuando lo necesite.

The pump is programmed so that you won't give yourself too much medication.

Esta bomba está programada para que Ud. no se administre demasiado medicamento.

Push the button when you feel pain.

Oprima el botón cuando sienta dolor.

Around-the-clock

This medication should be taken every __ hours.

Esta medicina se debe tomar cada __ horas.

Don't skip a dose.

No se saltee una dosis.

If you miss a dose:
– take the next dose as scheduled.
– take a dose when you remember, and
  then continue every __ hours.

Si se saltea una dosis:
– tome la siguiente dosis programada.
– tome una dosis cuando lo recuerde y
  luego continúe cada __ horas.

When you need it

Take this medication when you're having pain.

Tome este medicamento cuando sienta dolor.

Don't take this medication more often than every __ hours.

No tome esta medicina más seguido de cada __ horas.

Don't double the dose.

No duplique la dosis.

Becoming dependent

As you continue this medication, your body may become dependent on it.

Cuando continúe con la medicina, su cuerpo podrá volverse dependiente de ella.

Don't stop this medication suddenly without talking to your doctor.

No deje de tomar este medicamento de repente sin hablar con su médico.

If you need more medication to relieve the pain, please ask for it.

Si necesita más medicamento para aliviar el dolor, por favor pídalo.

Nonpharmacologic therapies

You may want to discuss other therapies available to the patient, including physical therapy, acupuncture, thermotherapy, cryotherapy, and transcutaneous electrical nerve stimulation (TENS).

Getting physical

Your doctor has ordered physical therapy for you.

Su médico ordenó fisioterapia para usted.

Physical therapy can help to relieve your pain.

La fisioterapia lo ayudará a aliviar su dolor.

The physical therapist will work out a plan and schedule with you.

La fisioterapeuta le preparará un plan y lo programará con usted.

In acupuncture, thin needles are inserted under the skin.

En acupuntura, se insertan agujas finitas debajo de la piel.

The needles may remain in place for 20 to 30 minutes.

Las agujas puede permanecer insertadas por 20 a 30 minutos.

Hot and cold

Hot packs can help to relieve your pain.

Las bolsas térmicas pueden ayudar a aliviar su dolor.

Make sure the hot pack doesn't directly touch your skin. You may wrap the hot pack in a towel.

Asegúrese de que la bolsa térmica no toque directamente su piel. Puede envolverla en una toalla.

Remove the hot pack if your skin becomes irritated or red.

Quite la bolsa térmica si su piel se irrita o enrojece.

Cold packs can be used to aid in pain relief.

Se puede usar bolsas de hielo para ayudar a aliviar el dolor.

Wrap cold packs so they don't directly touch your skin.

Envuelva las bolsas de hielo también para que no toquen directamente su piel.

Remove the cold pack if your skin becomes irritated or if pain worsens.

Quite la bolsa de hielo si su piel se irrita o empeora el dolor.

In acupuncture, thin needles are inserted under the skin.

En acupuntura, se insertan agujas finitas debajo de la piel.

Cold packs can be used to aid in pain relief.

Se puede usar bolsas de hielo para ayudar a aliviar el dolor.

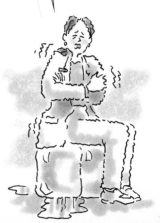

8, 9, TENS

TENS stands for *transcutaneous electrical nerve stimulation*.	TENS significa *estimulación nerviosa eléctrica transcutánea*.
A device will transmit painless impulses to your nerves or the area of pain.	Un aparato transmitirá impulsos indoloros a sus nervios o al área dolorida.
This treatment will last 3 to 5 days.	Este tratamiento durará de 3 a 5 días.
Do you have a pacemaker?	¿Tiene un marcapasos?
Have you ever had an abnormal heart rhythm?	¿Ha tenido Ud. alguna vez un ritmo cardiaco anormal?

Continuing care

Follow up with your doctor in _____ (days/weeks/months).	Haga un seguimiento con su médico en _____ (días/semanas/meses).
Please contact your doctor if your pain worsens or if you experience adverse effects.	Por favor, comuníquese con su doctor si el dolor empeora o si tiene efectos adversos.
Don't take medications for longer than prescribed.	No tome medicamentos por más tiempo que el indicado.
Don't increase or decrease your dose without talking to your doctor.	No aumente o disminuya su dosis sin hablar con su médico.
Avoid activities that increase the pain.	Evite actividades que aumenten el dolor.

Avoid activities that aggravate the pain.

Evite actividades que agravan el dolor.

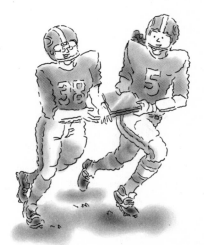

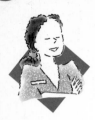

Practice makes perfecto

1. Joy wants to ask the patient if his pain started suddenly or gradually. Can you finish the question?

_____

_____

_____

> ¿Comenzó el dolor de _____ ?

2. Joy wants to know if the patient's pain is the worst he has ever felt. Can you supply the correct phrase?

_____

_____

_____

> ¿Es _____ que ha sentido alguna vez?

3. Joy wants to explain that the patient's medication should be taken orally. Can you help Joy with the correct phrase?

_____

_____

_____

_____

> Usted debe tomar esta medicina _____.

4. Joy needs to tell this patient that the doctor has ordered physical therapy for him. Can you help Joy communicate with her patient?

_____

_____

_____

_____

> Su doctor le ha ordenado _____.

Answer key

1. Did the pain begin suddenly or gradually?
¿Comenzó el dolor de <u>repente o gradualmente</u>?

2. Is the pain the worse you've ever felt?
¿Es <u>el peor dolor</u> que ha tenido?

3. You need to take this medication orally.
Usted debe tomar esta medicina <u>por vía oral</u>.

4. Your doctor has ordered physical therapy for you.
Su doctor le ha ordenado <u>fisioterapia</u>.

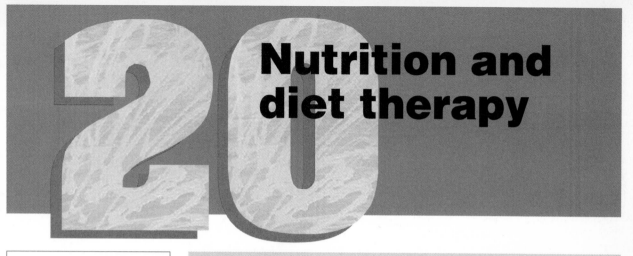

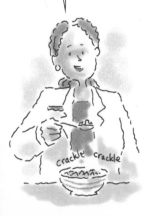

How many times a day do you eat?

¿Cuántas veces por día come?

Nutrition

Topics to discuss with your patient include eating habits, special diets the patient may follow, fluid intake, and basic nutritional knowledge.

Three squares

How many times a day do you eat?

What have you eaten during the past 3 days?

¿Cuántas veces por día come?

¿Qué ha comido Ud. en los últimos 3 días?

Under the golden arches?

Do you eat at fast-food restaurants?

– How often?
    Once per week?
    Two times per week?
    Every day?
    Less often?

¿Come Ud. en restaurantes donde se compra comida ya preparada?
– ¿Con qué frecuencia?
    ¿Una vez a la semana?
    ¿Dos veces a la semana?
    ¿Todos los días?
    ¿Menos a menudo?

Fries with that?

What items do you usually order?
– Pancakes?
– Breakfast sandwich?
– French fries?
– Hamburger?
– Cheeseburger?
– Fish?
– Tacos?
– Burritos?
– Chicken?
– Salad?

Por lo general, ¿qué platos pide?
– ¿Panqueques?
– ¿Sandwiches para el desayuno?
– ¿Patatas (papas) fritas?
– ¿Hamburguesa?
– ¿Hamburguesa con queso?
– ¿Pescado?
– ¿Tacos?
– ¿Burritos?
– ¿Pollo?
– ¿Ensalada?

Food from home

How does your ethnic or cultural background affect your diet?
– Do you eat only vegetables?
– Do you eat red meat?
– Do you eat only chicken or fish?

Does your religion restrict or otherwise affect what you eat?
– Do you fast or not eat food on any special days?

¿Cómo afectan su dieta sus antecedentes étnicos o culturales?
– ¿Come Ud. sólo Ud. verduras?
– ¿Come Ud. carne roja?
– ¿Come Ud. sólo pollo o pescado?

¿Su religión limita o de cualquier modo afecta lo que Ud. come?
– ¿Ayuna Ud. o no come nada durante días especiales?

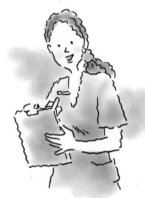

How does your ethnic or cultural background affect your diet?

¿Cómo afectan su dieta sus antecedentes étnicos o culturales?

On the scale

Have you gained weight recently?
– If so, how much?

Have you lost weight recently?
– If so, how much?

¿Ha aumentado de peso últimamente?
– Si lo ha aumentado, ¿cuánto?

¿Ha perdido Ud. peso últimamente?
– Si lo ha perdido, ¿cuánto?

Daily menu

Which foods do you eat during the day?

Are there foods that you believe you shouldn't eat?
– What are these foods?

Why do you believe you shouldn't eat these foods?

How do these foods affect you?
(See A list of foods.)

¿Qué come Ud. durante el curso de un día?

¿Hay alimentos que Ud. cree que no debiera comer?
– ¿Cuáles son éstos?

¿Por qué cree Ud. que no debiera comerlos?

¿Cómo le afectan estos alimentos si Ud. los come?

Fluid findings

How many servings do you drink each day of:
– coffee?
– tea?
– cola?
– cocoa?
– water?
– alcohol?

How much fluid do you drink during the day?

¿Cuántas porciones de las siguientes bebidas toma Ud. al día:
– café?
– té?
– cola?
– cocoa?
– agua?
– alcohol?

¿Cuánto líquido bebe Ud. al día?

A list of foods

It may be helpful to ask your patient to look at this list of foods and point to the ones he likes, ones he's allergic to, or ones he must restrict from his diet. You can also use these words to help him plan meals or adjust his diet to accommodate foods that he likes or dislikes.

The basics
- Wheat bread — Pan de trigo
- White bread — Pan blanco
- Corn bread — Pan de maíz
- Rye bread — Pan de centeno
- Rice — Arroz
- Tortillas — Tortillas
- Pasta — Pasta

Fruits of the earth
- Pear — Pera
- Cherries — Cerezas
- Apple — Manzana
- Orange — Naranja, china
- Banana — Banana, guineo
- Pineapple — Piña/ananá
- Watermelon — Sandía, mélon de agua
- Peach — Durazno, melocotón
- Strawberries — Fresas/Frutillas
- Grapes — Uvas
- Grapefruit — Toronja, pomelo
- Cantaloupe — Melón cantalupo de Castilla
- Mango — Mango
- Blueberries — Arándanos

From the garden
- Corn — Maíz
- Peas — Guisantes, arvejas

- Green beans — Ejotes, judías (habichuelas) verdes
- Refried beans — Frijoles refritos
- Pinto beans — Judías pintas
- Black beans — Frijoles negros
- Red beans — Habichuelas rojas, habichuelas coloradas
- Potatoes — Papas
- Baked potato — Papa asada
- Mashed potatoes — Puré de papas
- Squash — Zapallo
- Broccoli — Brócoli
- Carrots — Zanahorias

The cereal box
- Oatmeal — Harina de avena
- Cream of wheat — Crema de trigo
- Cold cereal — Cereal frío
- Bran — Salvado

What to drink
- Whole milk — Leche entera
- Skim milk — Leche descremada
- Low-fat milk — Leche con bajas caloriás
- Chocolate milk — Leche chocolatada
- Tea — Té
- Coffee — Café
- Orange juice — Jugo de naranja
- Grapefruit juice — Jugo de toronja

- Tomato juice — Jugo de tomate
- Cranberry juice — Jugo de arañdano
- Apple juice — Jugo de manzana
- Grape juice — Jugo de uva
- Pineapple juice — Jugo de piña
- Soda — Soda
- Water — Agua

Hearty eating
- Eggs — Huevos
- Beef — Res
- Chicken — Pollo
- Turkey — Pavo
- Pork — Cerdo
- Ribs — Costillas
- Hamburger — Hamburguesa
- Fish — Cesdo
- Shellfish — Mariscos
- Other seafood — Otros mariscos
- Tofu — Tofu
- Ham — Jamón

The good stuff
- Ice cream — Helado, mantecado
- Cake — Pastel, bizcocho
- Cookies — Galletas de dulce
- Chocolate — Chocolate
- Candy — Golosinas
- Chips — Chips
- Peanuts — Maní
- Peanut butter — Manteca de maní

Teeth and gums

Do you have all your own teeth?

¿Tiene todos sus dientes?

Do you wear dentures?
– Do they fit well?

¿Tiene dentadura postiza?
– ¿Calza bien su dentadura postiza?

How do you care for your teeth and gums?

¿Qué cuidado da Ud. a los dientes y las encías?

Do you have any problems with your teeth or gums that interfere with your ability to eat?	¿Tiene Ud. algún problema con los dientes o las encías que interfiera con su habilidad de comer?

In the kitchen

Who does the food shopping?	¿Quién hace sus compras de comestibles?
Do you have adequate storage and refrigeration?	¿Tiene Ud. un almacén y refrigerador adecuados?
Who prepares the meals?	¿Quién prepara las comidas?
Where's your food prepared?	¿Dónde se preparan los alimentos?
Do you eat alone or with others?	¿Come Ud. solo(a) o con otras personas?

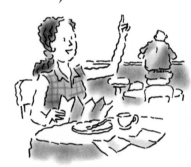

I'd like a gluten-free, high-fiber, low-calorie, low-sodium burger, please.

Quiereo una hamburguesa que no tenga gluten, de alta fibra, de pocas calorías y de poco sodio, por favor.

Special demands

Are you on a diet to lose weight? – What type of diet?	¿Está haciendo dieta para perder peso? – ¿Qué tipo de dieta?
Do you follow a special diet? – What kind of diet?	¿Tiene Ud. una dieta especial? – ¿Qué clase de dieta?
Diabetic diet?	¿Dieta para diabéticos?
Gluten-free diet?	¿Dieta sin gluten?
High-fiber diet?	¿Dieta con alto contenido de fibra?
High-protein diet?	¿Dieta con alto contenido de proteína?
Lactose-free diet?	¿Dieta sin lactosa?
Low-calorie diet?	¿Dieta con bajo contendio de calorías?
Low-carbohydrate diet?	¿Dieta con bajo contendio de carbohidratos?
Low-fat diet?	¿Dieta con bajo contendio de grasa?
Low-fiber diet?	¿Dieta con bajo contendio de fibra?
Low-protein diet?	¿Dieta con bajo contendio de proteínas?
Low-salt diet?	¿Dieta con bajo contendio de sal?
Low-cholesterol diet?	¿Dieta de colesterol bajo?
Who prescribed the diet?	¿Quién recetó a Ud. la dieta?
How long have you been on the diet?	¿Hace cuánto tiempo que tiene Ud. esta en dieta?
What's the reason for the diet?	¿Cuál es la razón por la cual sigue Ud. esta dieta?
How much salt do you use, if any?	¿Cuánta sal usa Ud., si es que la usa?
Do you limit your salt intake?	¿Limita Ud. la cantidad de sal que consume?
– Why?	– ¿Por qué?

Supplemental stuff

Do you supplement your diet with:	¿Suplementa Ud. su dieta con:
– vitamins?	– vitaminas?
– calcium?	– calcio?
– protein?	– proteína?
– other products?	– otros productos?
In what amounts?	¿En qué cantidades?

Does your current problem affect your ability to cook and eat?

¿Su habilidad de cocinar y comer es afectada por su problema actual?

Do you have difficulty opening cans or cutting meat?

¿Tiene Ud. dificultad en abrir latas o cortar carne?

How much of each of these food groups do you eat every day?	¿Cuánto de estos grupos de alimentos come todos los días?
– Grains?	– ¿Granos?
– Vegetables?	– ¿Vegetales?
– Fruits?	– ¿Frutas?
– Fats?	– ¿Grasas?
– Meats and beans?	– ¿Carnes y frijoles?
– Milk products?	– ¿Productos lácteos?

(See *Food group recommendations*, page 282.)

Diet therapy

If a patient needs a special diet, you may need to explain the diet's components, reinforce instructions, or help the patient adapt to a lifestyle change.

The diet lowdown

Your doctor has ordered a special diet for you.	Su doctor ha ordenado una dieta especial para Ud.
It's called a:	Ésta se llama:
– diabetic diet.	– dieta para diabéticos.
– gluten-free diet.	– dieta sin gluten.
– high-fiber diet.	– dieta con alto contenido de fibra.
– high-protein diet.	– dieta con alto contenido de proteínas.
– lactose-free diet.	– dieta sin lactosa.
– low-calorie diet.	– dieta con bajo contenido de calorías.
– low-carbohydrate diet.	– dieta con bajo contenido de carbohidratos.
– low-fat diet.	– dieta con bajo contenido de grasa.
– low-fiber diet.	– dieta con bajo contenido de fibra.
– low-protein diet.	– dieta con bajo contenido de proteínas.
– low-salt diet.	– dieta con bajo contenido de sal.
– low-cholesterol diet.	– dieta de colesterol bajo.

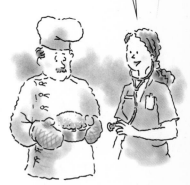

The doctor has ordered a low-protein diet.

El doctor ha ordenado una dieta con bajo contenido de proteínas.

Food group recommendations

Recomendaciones sobre grupos alimentarios

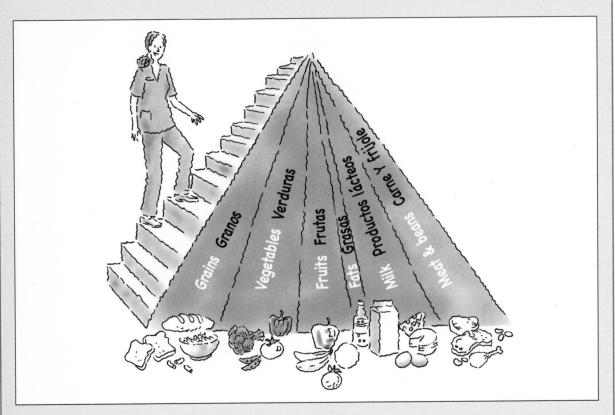

Grains
- Make half of your grains whole.
- Eat at least 3 oz of whole-grain cereals, breads, crackers, rice, or pasta every day.

- 1 oz is about 1 slice of bread, about 1 cup of breakfast cereal, or ½ cup of cooked rice, cereal, or pasta.

Vegetables
- Vary your vegetables.
- Eat more dark-green vegetables, such as broccoli, spinach, and other dark leafy greens.

- Eat more orange vegetables, such as carrots and sweet potatoes.
- Eat more dry beans and peas, such as pinto beans, kidney beans, and lentils.

Granos
- Consuma la mitad en granos integrales.
- Consuma al menos 3 onzas de cereales, panes, galletas, arroz, o pasta provenientes de granos intergrales todos los dias.
- Una onza es, aproximadamente, 1 rebanada de pan o ½ taza de arroz, cereal, o pasta cocidos.

Verduras
- Varíe las verduras.
- Consuma mayor cantidad de verduras de color verde oscuro, como el brócoli, la espinaca, y otras verduras de color verde oscuro.
- Cosuma mayor contidad de verduras de color naranja, como zanahorias y batatas.
- Cosuma mayor cantidad de frijoles y guisantes secos, como frijoles pinto, colorados, y lentejas.

Food group recommendations (continued)

Fruits
- Focus on fruits.
- Eat a variety of fruit.
- Choose fresh, frozen, canned, or dried fruit.
- Limit how much fruit juice you drink.

Milk
- Consume calcium-rich foods.
- Pick low-fat or fat-free when you choose milk, yogurt, and other milk products.
- If you don't or can't consume milk, choose lactose-free products or other calcium sources, such as fortified foods and beverages.

Meats and beans
- Go lean with protein.
- Choose low-fat or lean meats and poultry.
- Bake it, broil it, or grill it.
- Vary your protein routine; choose more fish, beans, peas, nuts, and seeds.

For a 2,000-calorie diet, you need the amounts below from each food group. To find the amounts that are right for you, go to *MyPyramid.gov.*

- Grains: Eat 6 oz every day.
- Vegetables: Eat 2½ cups every day.
- Fruits: Eat 2 cups every day.
- Milk: Get 3 cups every day; for kids ages 2 to 8, 2 cups.

- Meats and beans: Eat 5½ oz every day.

Recomendaciones sobre grupos alimentarios (continued)

Frutas
- Enfóquese en las frutas.
- Consuma una variedad de frutas.
- Elija frutas frescas, congeladas, enlatadas, o secas.
- No tome mucha cantidad de jugo de frutas.

Productos lácteos
- Coma alimentos ricos en calcio.
- Al elegir leche, opte por leche, yogur, y otros productos lácteos descremados o bajos en contenido graso.
- En caso de que no consuma o no pueda consumir leche, elija producots sin lactosa u otra fuente de calcio como alimentos y bebidas fortalecidos.

Carnes y frijoles
- Escoja proteinas bajas en grasas.
- Elija carnes y aves de bajo contenido graso o magras.
- Cocínelas al horno, a la parrilla, o a la plancha.
- Varie la rutina de proteinas que consume; consuma mayor cantidad de pescado, frijoles, guisantes, nueces, y semillas.

En una dieta de 2,000 calorías, necesita consumir las siguientes cantidades de cada grupo de alimentos. Para consultar las cantidades correctas para usted, visite *MyPyramid.gov.*

- Granos: Coma 6 onzas cada día.
- Verduras: Coma 2½ tazas cada día.
- Frutas: Coma 2 taza cada día.
- Productos lácteos: Coma 3 tazas cada día; para niños de entre 2 y 8 años, 2 tazas.
- Carnes y frijoles: Coma 5½ onzas cada día.

Adapted from U.S. Department of Agriculture. Center for Nutrition Policy and Promotion. (2005). MyPyramid Mini-Poster [Online]. Available at *http://www.mypyramid.gov/downloads/miniposter.pdf* [2006, September 5].

More of this, less of that

The doctor wants you to eat more (less) _____.

El doctor quiere que Ud. coma más (menos) _____.

Too much _____ can make your _____worse.

Demasiado(a) _____ puede empeorar su _____.

Eating more _____ can improve your _____.

El comer más _____ puede mejorar su _____.

The dietitian will speak with you about your _____ diet.

El/La dietista hablará con Ud. acerca de su dieta _____.

You need to reduce salt in your diet.	Ud. necesita reducir el contenido de sal en su dieta.
Avoid adding salt to meals.	Evite Ud. añadir sal.
Use herbs or salt substitutes to add flavor to your food.	Use Ud. hierbas de condimento o sustitutos de sal para añadirle sabor a su comida.

Bye-bye bacon

You need to reduce cholesterol in your diet.	Ud. necesita reducir el colesterol en su dieta.
Some foods that you shouldn't eat are:	Algunos de los alimentos que Ud. no debe comer son:
– butter	– mantequilla
– shortening	– grasa (manteca)
– egg yolks	– yemas de huevo
– biscuits	– panecillos
– cheese	– queso
– avocados	– aguacate
– bacon	– tocino
– sausage	– salchicha
– hot dogs	– perros calientes
– shellfish	– mariscos
– ice cream	– helado
– chocolate	– chocolate
– liver	– hígado
– most red meat.	– la mayoría de la carne roja.

Feast on fiber

You need to add fiber to your diet.	Ud. tiene que añadir fibra a su dieta.
Eating more fiber helps:	El comer más fibra le ayudará a:
– lower cholesterol.	– reducir el colesterol.
– reduce your risk of:	– aminorará su riesgo de contraer enfermedades:
heart disease.	del corazón.
colon cancer.	de cáncer del colon.
diabetes.	de diabetes.

Eat fresh fruit and vegetables.
– High-fiber fruits include apples, oranges, and peaches.
– High-fiber vegetables include carrots, string beans, broccoli, and peas.

Eat wholegrain breads such as whole wheat.

Eat wholegrain cereals, such as bran flakes, oat flakes, oatmeal, and shredded wheat.

Eat dried peas and beans, such as lentils and navy, kidney, or pinto beans.

Remember to drink at least six 8-ounce glasses of fluid per day.

Coma Ud. fruta fresca y verduras.
– Frutas con mucha fibra incluyen las manzanas, naranjas, y melocotones.
– Verduras con mucha fibra incluyen las zanahorias, ejotes, brécol, y guisantes (chícharos).

Coma pan integral como pan de trigo entero.

Como cereal es de grano integral, como hojuelas de avena, harina de avena, y trigo molido.

Coma guisantes secos y frijoles como lentejas, habichuelas rojas, frijoles negros, y judías pintas.

No se olvide Ud. de tomar por lo menos seis vasos de 8 onzas de líquido al día.

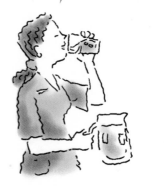

Drink at least six 8-ounce glasses of fluid per day.

Tome por lo menos seis vasos de 8 onzas de líquido al día.

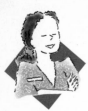

Practice makes perfecto

1. Joy wants to ask the patient what he has eaten the past 3 days. Can you finish the question?

> ¿Qué ha comido Ud. en _____?

_____

_____

_____

_____

2. Joy wants to know if the patient follows a special diet. Can you supply the correct phrase?

> ¿Tiene Ud. _____?

_____

_____

_____

_____

3. Joy wants to ask if the patient supplements her diet with vitamins. Can you add the correct phrase?

> ¿Suplementa Ud. su dieta con _____?

_____

_____

_____

_____

4. Joy needs to tell the patient to reduce salt in his diet. Can you help Joy communicate with her patient?

> Ud. tiene que _____ en su dieta.

_____

_____

_____

_____

Answer key

1. What have you eaten during the past 3 days?
¿Qué ha comido Ud. en <u>los últimos 3 días</u>?

2. Do you follow a special diet?
¿Tiene Ud. <u>una dieta especial</u>?

3. Do you supplement your diet with vitamins?
¿Suplementa Ud. su dieta con <u>vitaminas</u>?

4. You need to reduce salt in your diet.
Ud. tiene que <u>reducir la sal</u> en su dieta.

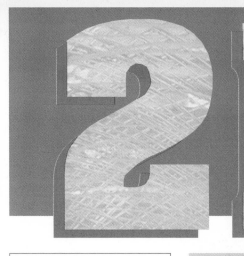

Medical equipment and supplies

Fast fact

Key terms related to medical equipment and supplies include:

- *el catéter del I.V.* (I.V. catheter)
- *una cuña* (bedpan)
- *un ventilador mecánico* (mechanical ventilator)
- *un andador* (walker)
- *un bastón* (cane).

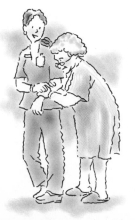

You'll need to use a walker.

Ud. necesitará un andador.

Assistive devices

Here are some common terms and phrases associated with assistive devices.

Cane

You'll need to walk with a cane.

Ud. necesitará andar con bastón.

Hold the cane on your unaffected side.

Sostenga el bastón del lado no afectado.

Hold the cane close to your body to prevent leaning.

Sostenga el bastón cerca del cuerpo para evitar inclinarse.

Move the cane and the involved leg at the same time.

Mueva Ud. el bastón y la pierna afectada simultáneamente.

Walker

You'll need to use a walker.

Ud. necesitará usar un andador.

Hold the handgrips firmly and equally.

Sostenga Ud. las manijas firme y parejamente.

Advance the walker 6″ to 8″ (15 to 20 cm).

Adelante el andador de 6 a 8 pulgadas (15 a 20 centímetros).

Step forward with the involved leg and follow with the uninvolved leg.

Dé un paso con la pierna afectada primero y después con la pierna no afectada.

Support yourself on your arms.

Apóyese Ud. en los brazos.

Take equal strides.

Dé pasos iguales.

Cardiac care equipment

Here are some common terms and phrases for equipment associated with the care of patients with cardiac disorders.

Electrocardiogram

You need an electrocardiogram so we can monitor your heart's electrical activity.	Ud. necesita un electrocardiograma para que podamos monitorear la actividad eléctrica de su corazón.
This is a heart monitor.	Esto es un monitor cardiaco.
It will help us monitor your heartbeat.	Que nos ayudará a observar continuamente el corazón.
You'll be attached to the heart monitor while you're in this unit.	Estará conectado(a) al monitor cardiaco mientras esté en esta unidad.
I need to place these electrodes on you.	Tengo que ponerle estos electrodos.
Don't be frightened if you hear the alarms.	No se asuste Ud. si oye las alarmas.
They sometimes sound with movement.	A veces suenan con el movimiento.

Pacemaker

You have an abnormal heart rhythm.	Ud. tiene un ritmo cardiaco anormal.
You need a pacemaker.	Ud. necesita un marcapasos.
I'm going to apply this external pacemaker.	Voy a ponerle este marcapasos externo.
I need to place an electrode on your chest and back.	Necesito ponerle un electrodo en el tórax y en la espalda.

Intravenous therapy equipment

Here are some terms and phrases to use when administering I.V. drugs and fluids to your patient.

I.V. catheter and pump

You need to have an I.V. line inserted.	Ud. necesita que se le ponga una intravenosa (I.V.).
This is an I.V. pump.	Ésta es una bomba I.V.
The I.V. pump will help control the flow of your I.V.	La bomba intravenosa ayudará a controlar el flujo de su tubo I.V.
I'm going to insert the I.V. catheter.	Voy a introducirle el catéter del I.V.

I need to apply a tourniquet around your arm.

Tengo que ponerle un torniquete alrededor del brazo.

You're going to feel a needle stick.

Ud. va a sentir un piquete de aguja.

I need to place a dressing over the I.V. site.

Tengo que ponerle un vendaje en el área del I.V.

Call me if you have pain at your I.V. site.

Llámeme si tiene dolor en el lugar donde tiene puesto el tubo I.V.

Try not to pull on the I.V.

Trate de no jalar la vía I.V.

I.V. drug administration

You need an I.V. catheter inserted for medication.

Necesita que se le inserte un catéter I.V. para medicación.

I need to flush your I.V. catheter to keep it open.

Necesito enjuagar su catéter I.V. para mantenerlo abierto.

Invasive devices

Here are some terms and phrases to use when caring for a patient undergoing an invasive procedure.

Arterial catheter

I need to insert an arterial catheter into your wrist to monitor your blood pressure.

Necesito insertar un catéter arterial en su muñeca para monitorizar su presión sanguínea.

I'll give you a local anesthetic before I insert the catheter.

Le pondré una anestesia local antes de insertarle el catéter.

I'm going to take a sample of blood from your arterial catheter.

Voy a tomarle una muestra de sangre de su catéter arterial.

Central venous catheter

You need a central venous catheter to get I.V. fluid.

Ud. necesita un catéter venoso central para recibir líquido I.V.

You'll receive a local anesthetic before we insert the catheter.

Le pondremos a una anestesia local antes de insertarle el catéter.

I'm going to insert the central venous catheter.

Voy a insertarle un catéter venoso central.

Pulmonary artery catheter

You need a catheter placed through a major vein into your heart.

Ud. necesita que se le ponga un catéter por la vena principal en el corazón.

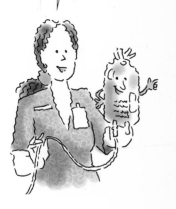

You need an I.V. catheter inserted for medication.

Necesita que le inserte un catéter I.V. para medicación.

This catheter will help us monitor your fluid status.	Este catéter nos ayudará a monitorear el estado de su líquido.
I'm going to obtain readings from your catheter.	Obtendré lecturas de su catéter.

Maternity care equipment

The following equipment is necessary for maternity care. These phrases will help you when caring for the mother and child.

Fetal monitor

This is a fetal monitor.	Esto es un monitor fetal.
I'll place it around your abdomen.	Lo pondré en su abdomen.
A small probe will be inserted into the baby's scalp.	Se le colocará una pequeña sonda en el cuero cabelludo de la criatura.
It will monitor your contractions and the baby's heartbeat.	Observaré sus contracciones y el latido cardiaco de su criatura.

Fetoscope

This is a fetoscope.	Éste es un fetoscopio.
I'll place it on your abdomen to listen to your baby's heartbeat.	Se lo pondré en el abdomen para escuchar el latido cardiaco de su criatura.
Your baby's heartbeat is _____.	El latido de su criatura es _____.

Isolette

This is an isolette.	Ésta es una incubadora.
I'll place your baby in the isolette to keep him warm.	Pondré a su criatura en la incubadora para que esté caliente.

Light therapy

Your baby is jaundiced.	Su criatura tiene ictericia.
Your baby will need to be placed under the bilirubin lights.	Su criatura se tendrá que poner bajo luces bilirrubinas.
He'll have his eyes covered while he's under the lights.	Tendrá los ojos cubiertos mientras esté debajo de las luces.

Your baby's heartbeat is _____.

El latido de su criatura es _____.

Personal care equipment

Here are some key phrases and terms that will help you communicate with your patient about personal care needs.

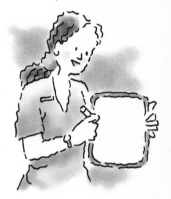

It's important to anticipate patient needs, and to be very clear...

Bedpan

Here's a bedpan if you need to move your bowels.	Aquí tiene una cuña por si Ud. tiene que evacuar.
Here's a bedpan if you need to urinate.	Aquí tiene una cuña por si Ud. tiene que orinar.
Do you need to use the bedpan?	¿Necesita Ud. usar la cuña?
Call me when you're finished with the bedpan.	Llámeme cuando acabe de usar la cuña.

Bedside commode

You can't walk to the bathroom.	Ud. no puede caminar al baño.
I can get you a bedside commode.	Le puedo traer una silla retrete.
Here's the bedside commode.	Aquí tiene una silla retrete.
Call me when you're finished using the commode.	Llámeme cuando haya acabado de usar la silla retrete.

Emesis basin

This is a basin.	Esto es una palangana.
You can use the basin if you need to vomit.	Ud. puede usar la palangana si necesita vomitar.
I'll get you a basin to wash yourself.	Le voy a traer una cubeta para que se lave Ud.
Spit into this basin.	Escupa dentro de esta palangana.
Call me when you're finished with the basin.	Llámeme cuando haya acabado de usar la cubeta.

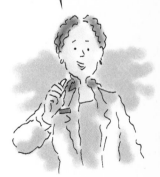

...This will make your patient more comfortable and will help alleviate embarrassment.

Enema

This is an enema.	Ésta es una enema.
You need an enema to help you move your bowels.	Ud. necesita una enema (lavativa) para ayudarle a evacuar.
Lie on your left side.	Acuéstese del lado izquierdo.
I'm going to put this tube in your rectum.	Voy a insertarle este tubo en el recto.
Take a deep breath.	Respire Ud. profundamente.

Let me know if you experience any cramping.	Dígame por favor si siente retortijones.
Try to retain the fluid.	Trate Ud. de retener el líquido.

Urinal

Here's a urinal.	Aquí está un orinal.
Do you need to use the urinal?	¿Necesita Ud. usar el orinal?
Call me when you're finished with the urinal.	Llámeme cuando acabe de usar el orinal.

Other personal items

Do you need:	¿Necesita Ud.:
– a blanket?	– una manta (frazada)?
– a comb?	– un cepillo?
– a razor?	– una rasuradora?
– soap?	– jabón?
– toilet paper?	– papel higiénico?
– a toothbrush or toothpaste?	– cepillo o pasta de dientes?
– a towel	– una toalla?
– a washcloth?	– una toallita de aseo?
– tissues?	– pañuelos de papel?
– a pillow?	– una almohada?

Respiratory care equipment

These phrases and terms will help you care for your patient with breathing problems.

Chest tube

I need to insert a tube into your chest to reexpand your lung.	Tengo que insertarle un tubo en el tórax para expandir el pulmón.
I need to insert a tube into your chest to drain fluid.	Tengo que insertarle un tubo en el tórax para extraer líquido.
This tube will help your breathing.	Este tubo le ayudará a respirar.
You'll receive a local anesthetic before I insert the tube.	Se le pondrá un poco de anestesia local antes de que yo le inserte el tubo.

Croup tent

Your child needs to be placed in a croup tent.	Es necesario poner a su hijo(a) en una cámara de crup.
It will provide warm mist and oxygen to help your child's breathing.	Le proverá vapor tibio y oxígeno para ayudarle a su criatura a respirar.

You may touch your child while he's in the croup tent.	Ud. puede tocar a su criatura mientras está en la cámara de crup.

Incentive spirometer

This is an incentive spirometer.	Éste es un estímulo de espirometría.
It will help you take deep breaths.	Le ayudará a respirar profundamente.
Breathe in deeply, hold it, and then breathe out.	Respire profundamente, contenga la respiración, y luego exhale.
You should use the incentive spirometer every hour while you're awake.	Ud. deberá usar el estimulo de espirometría cada hora mientras esté Ud. despierto.

Mechanical ventilation

We need to insert a tube through your nose or mouth into your lungs to help your breathing.	Necesitamos insertar un tubo a través de su nariz o boca y hacia los pulmones para ayudarle a respirar.
The tube will be connected to a ventilator.	El tubo estará conectado a un respirador.
A ventilator is a machine that will help you breathe.	Un respirador es una máquina que le ayudará a respirar.
You won't be able to talk while the tube is in place.	Ud. no podrá hablar mientras el tubo esté en su lugar.

Nebulizer

This is a nebulizer.	Éste es un nebulizador.
It will deliver medication into your lungs to help your breathing.	Le llevará medicamento a los pulmones para ayudarle a respirar.
Hold the mouthpiece in your mouth and breathe in the medication.	Sostenga Ud. la boquilla en su boca y aspire el medicamento.

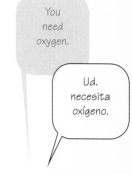

Oxygen via a mask and nasal cannula

You need oxygen.	Ud. necesita oxígeno.
This is an oxygen mask.	Ésta es una máscara de oxígeno.
The mask fits over your nose and mouth and oxygen is delivered through it.	La máscara se le pone sobre la nariz y la boca y el oxígeno se transmite por ella.
This is a nasal cannula.	Ésta es una cánula nasal.
The prongs go into your nose, and oxygen flows through them.	Las puntas se ponen dentro de la nariz, y el oxígeno pasa por ellas.

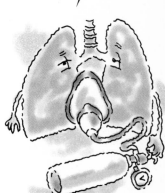

Pulse oximeter

This is a pulse oximeter.

Éste es un oxímetro.

A pulse oximeter allows us to check the oxygen level of your blood.

El oxímetro de pulso nos permite verificar el nivel de oxígeno en su sangre.

I need to put the probe on your finger.

Necesito ponerle una sonda en el dedo.

Suctioning

I need to suction your breathing tube.

Tengo que aspirar su tubo de respiración.

Suctioning will make you cough.

Esta succión le hará toser.

Tracheostomy

You need a tracheostomy.

Ud. necesita una traqueostomía.

The surgeon will make a surgical incision through your trachea and insert a tube to help you breathe.

El cirujano le hara una incisión quirúrgica por la tráquea y le insertará un tubo para ayudarle a respirar.

You'll receive an anesthetic before this procedure.

Se le pondrá un poco de anestesia local antes de este procedimiento.

I need to clean your tracheostomy.

Tengo que limpiar su traqueotomía.

I need to suction your tracheostomy.

Tengo que aspirar su traqueotomía.

Specialty beds

Debilitated patients and others at risk for pressure ulcers may require a specialty bed. These phrases will help you care for the patient who requires a specialty bed.

Air-therapy mattress

You need a special mattress called an *air-therapy mattress*.

Ud. necesita una cama especial que se llama *cama terapéutica neumática*.

It will help prevent skin breakdown and pressure ulcers.

Le evitará rupturas de la piel.

This type of mattress has air-filled compartments.

Este tipo de cama tiene partes llenas de aire.

You need to have a therapy bed temporarily.

Ud. necesita tener una cama de terapia temporalmente.

This bed will help prevent skin breakdown.

Esta cama le evitará escaras/úlceras de la piel.

Specimen collection equipment

These phrases and terms will help you communicate with your patient about specimen collection.

Arterial blood gas analysis

I need to draw blood to check your oxygen level.

Necesito extraer sangre para verificar su nivel de oxígeno.

You're going to feel a needle stick.

Ud. va a sentir un piquete de aguja.

I need to apply pressure to stop the bleeding.

Necesito aplicarle presión para detener la salida de sangre.

Glucometer

This machine is used to measure your blood sugar.

Esta máquina se usa para medir el azúcar en su sangre.

I need to prick your finger to get a drop of blood.

Necesito pincharle el dedo para obtener una muestra.

Your blood sugar is _____.

El nivel de azúcar en su sangre es _____.

I need to give you some insulin because your blood sugar is high.

Tengo que darle insulina porque el azúcar en su sangre es alto.

I need to give you some juice because your blood sugar is low.

Tengo que darle jugos porque su azúcar es baja.

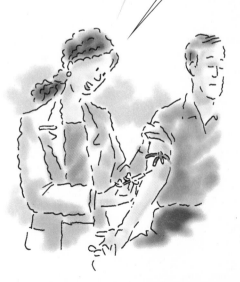

I need to draw blood to check your oxygen level.

Necesito extraer sangre para verificar su nivel de oxígeno.

Urine specimen

We need a urine specimen.

Necesitamos una muestra de su orina.

You need to urinate into this container.

Ud. debe orinar en este recipiente.

Venipuncture

I need to draw a blood sample.

Necesito sacarle una muestra de sangre.

I'm going to place a tourniquet on your arm.

Le voy a poner un torniquete en el brazo.

You're going to feel a needle stick.

Ud. va a sentir un piquete de aguja.

Wound care equipment

These phrases and terms will help you while you're providing wound care.

Drainage bag and dressing

I'm going to put a bag over your drain.

Voy a poner una bolsa sobre su drenaje.

I need to change your dressing.

Tengo que cambiarle su vendaje.

I need to irrigate your wound.

Tengo que irrigar su herida.

I'm going to clean the area around your wound.

Voy a limpiar el área alrededor de su herida.

I'm going to remove the tape.

Voy a quitarle la cinta adhesiva.

It may sting a bit.

Le puede arder un poco.

Montgomery straps

These are Montgomery straps.

Éstas son tiras de Montgomery.

I'm going to place these next to your wound so tape isn't required with each dressing change.

Voy a colocar éstas en su herida para que no sea necesario ponerle cinta adhesiva con cada cambio de vendaje.

Whirlpool bath

You need a whirlpool bath to help your wound heal.

Ud. necesita un baño de jacuzzi para sanar su herida.

Wound packing

I'm going to remove your wound packing.

Voy a quitarle el empaque de su herida.

I'm going to replace your wound packing.

Voy a cambiarle el empaque de su herida.

Wound prevention

You need to use a support surface to avoid skin breakdown.

Ud. necesita una superficie de apoyo para evitar escaras/úlceras de la piel.

These Unna boots will help keep pressure off your wound.

Estas botas "Unna" ayudarán a evitar ponerle presión a su herida.

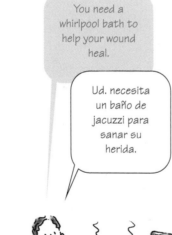

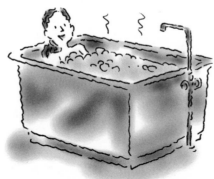

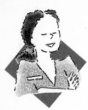

Practice makes perfecto

1. Help Joy tell the patient that he'll feel a needle stick.

_____

_____

_____

_____

> Ud. va a sentir un _____.

2. Help Joy understand what the patient is saying. What does the patient need to use?

_____

_____

_____

_____

> Quiero usar la silla retrete.

> Ésto es un _____.

3. Help Joy teach the patient about an incentive spirometer.

_____

_____

_____

_____

Appendices and index

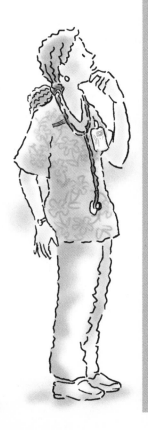

Giving eardrops to a child

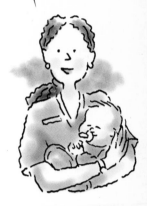

When you're giving eardrops to a baby, pull his ear down and back, not up and back.

Dear Parent or Caregiver:

To treat your child's ear infection, the doctor has ordered eardrops.

Use them exactly as directed on the label.

Checking the medicine

Wash your hands.

Then examine the medicine.

Does it look discolored or contain sediment?

If it does, notify the doctor and have the prescription refilled.

If it looks normal, you can proceed.

Inserting the drops

Warm the medicine (for the child's comfort) by holding the bottle in your hands for about 2 minutes.

Then shake the bottle (if directed), open it, and fill the dropper by squeezing and then releasing the bulb.

Place the open bottle and dropper within easy reach.

Have the child lie on his side to expose the ear you're treating.

Now gently pull the top of his ear up and back (down and back for an infant). (This will straighten his ear canal.)

Position the filled dropper above—but not touching—the opening of the child's ear canal.

Gently squeeze the dropper's bulb once to release one drop.

Watch the drop slide into the ear canal, or have the child tell you when he feels the drop enter his ear.

Then gently squeeze the dropper's bulb to release the number of drops prescribed, as shown here.

Continue holding the child's ear as the eardrops disappear down the ear canal.

Now, massage the area in front of the ear.

Ask the child to tell you when he no longer feels the drops moving in his ear.

Then release his ear.

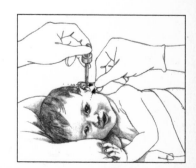

Spanish translation on opposite side

Cómo colocar gotas en los oídos de los niños

Estimado Padre o Apoderado:

Para el tratamiento de la infección de oído de su hijo, el médico recetó gotas para los oídos.

Utilícelas exactamente como indica la etiqueta.

> Al colocar gotas en el oído de un bebé, tire de su oreja hacia abajo y hacia atrás, y no hacia arriba y hacia atrás.

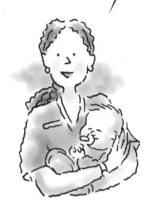

Verificación del medicamente

Lávese las manos.

Luego examine el medicamento.

¿Parece que está descolorido o que contiene sedimentos?

En caso afirmativo, informe a su médico y hágase preparar una receta nueva.

Si parece normal, puede seguir adelante.

Inserción de las gotas

Entibie el medicamento (para la comodidad del niño), sosteniendo el frasco en las manos durante unos 2 minutos.

Luego sacuda el frasco (si así lo indica la etiqueta), ábralo y llene el cuentagotas apretando y luego soltando el gotero de goma.

Coloque el frasco abierto y el cuentagotas en un lugar de fácil alcance.

Pídale al niño que se acueste de costado con el oído que tratará hacia arriba.

Ahora, tire de la parte superior de su oreja hacia arriba y hacia atrás suavemente (hacia abajo y hacia atrás si se trata de un bebé). (De esta manera, se enderezará el conducto de su oído.)

Coloque el cuentagotas sobre—pero sin tocar—la abertura del conducto del oído del niño.

Suavemente, apriete el gotero de goma del cuentagotas para que caiga una gota.

Fíjese cómo la gota se desliza hacia el canal del oído, o pídale al niño que le indique cuando sienta que la gota entró en el oído.

Luego, apriete suavemente el gotero del cuentagotas para que caiga la cantidad de gotas recetada, según se ilustra aquí.

Continúe sujetando la oreja del niño mientras las gotas bajan por el conducto auditivo.

Ahora, dele un masaje al área frente a la oreja.

Pídale al niño que le diga cuando sienta que las gotas ya no se mueven en su oído.

Luego, suéltele la oreja.

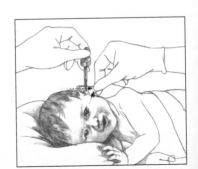

English translation on opposite side

Finishing up

Tell the child to remain on his side and to avoid touching his ear for about 10 minutes.

If the child is active, place a slightly eardrop-moistened cotton plug in his ear to help keep the medicine in his ear canal.

Don't use dry cotton because it may absorb the medicine.

If both ears require medicine, repeat the procedure in the child's other ear.

Finally, return the dropper to the medicine bottle and recap the dropper bottle.

Store the bottle away from light and extreme heat.

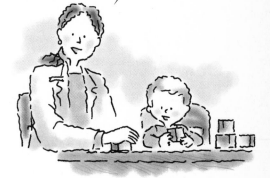

Try to keep the child still (and from touching his ear) for 10 minutes.

Spanish translation on opposite side

Pasos finales

Dígale al niño que permanezca sobre su costado y evite tocar su oído por unos 10 minutos.

Si el niño se mantiene activo, coloque en su oído un tapón de algodón ligeramente humedecido con gotas para los oídos, para ayudar a mantener el medicamento en su canal auditivo.

No use algodón seco pues puede absorber el medicamento.

Si ambos oídos requieren medicamento, repita el procedimiento con el otro oído del niño.

Finalmente, vuelva a colocar el cuentagotas en el frasco de medicamento y tape el frasco.

Guarde el frasco lejos de la luz y de calor extremo.

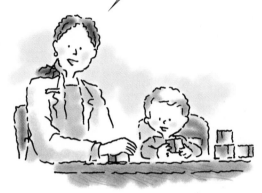

Trate de mantener al niño quieto, (y que no se toque la oreja) por 10 minutos.

English translation on opposite side

Giving yourself eyedrops

Dear Patient:

Your doctor has ordered eyedrops for you. Here's how to place the drops in your eye.

Getting ready

Wash your hands.

Hold the medication bottle up to the light and examine it. (If the medication is discolored or contains sediment, don't use it. Instead, take it back to the pharmacy and have it examined.)

If the medication looks okay, warm it to room temperature by holding the bottle between your hand for 2 minutes.

A quick clean

Moisten a cotton ball or a tissue with water, and clean any secretions from around your eyes.

Wipe outward in one motion, starting from the side near your nose.

Use a fresh cotton ball or tissue for each eye.

Dropping in

Squeeze the bulb of the eyedropper and slowly release it to fill the dropper with medication.

Some eyedrops may be given directly from the bottle, if it's attached to the dropper.

Then stand or sit before a mirror or lie on your back, whichever is most comfortable for you.

Tilt your head slightly backward and toward the eye you're treating.

Pull down your lower eyelid and position the dropper between your lower lid and the white of your eye.

Steady your hand by resting two fingers against your cheek or nose.

Look up at the ceiling.

Then squeeze the ordered number of drops into the eye. (Be careful not to touch the dropper to your eye, eyelashes, or finger.)

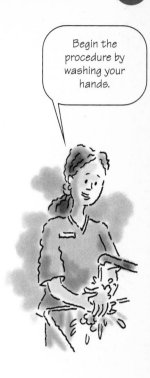

Begin the procedure by washing your hands.

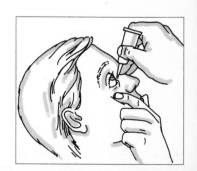

Spanish translation on opposite side

Cómo colocarse gotas en los ojos

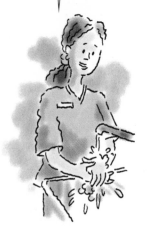

Comience Ud. el procedimiento lavándose las manos.

Estimado(a) Paciente:

Su médico ha ordenado que se aplique gotas en los ojos. Así es como se puede colocar las gotas en el ojo.

La preparación

Lávese las manos.

Ponga Ud. la botella de medicamento contra la luz y examínela. (Si el medicamento está descolorido o contiene sedimento, no lo use. Devuélvalo a la farmacia y haga que lo examinen.)

Si el medicamento parece estar en buen estado, llévelo a temperatura ambiente sosteniendo el frasco entre las manos durante 2 minutos.

Una limpieza rápida

Moje en agua un pedazo de algodón o un pañuelo de papel, y limpie toda secreción alrededor de los ojos.

Limpie hacia afuera con un movimiento, comenzando del lado cerca de la nariz.

Use un algodón o pañuelo limpio para cada ojo.

Cómo poner las gotas

Apriete el gotero y suéltelo despacio para llenar el gotero de medicamento.

Algunas gotas para ojos se pueden administrar directamente desde el frasco, si tiene el gotero incorporado.

Luego pá cese o siéntese frente a un espejo o acuéstese de espaldas, lo que sea más cómodo para Ud.

Mueva la cabeza un poco para atrás hacia el ojo que Ud. va a tratar.

Tire hacia abajo su párpado inferior y coloque el gotero entre su párpado inferior y la parte blanca del ojo.

Mantenga la mano firme descansando dos dedos contra la mejilla o la nariz.

Mire hacia el techo.

Luego vierta la cantidad indicada de gotas en el ojo. (Tenga cuidado de no tocar el ojo, las pestañas o el dedo con el gotero.)

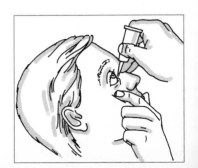

English translation on opposite side

Making it work

Close your eye briefly, but don't squeeze it shut.

Release the lower lid.

Wipe away excess medication with a clean tissue.

Try to keep your eye open and not blink for at least 30 seconds.

Apply gentle pressure to the corner of your eye at the bridge of your nose for 1 minute. This will stop the drops from draining into the tear duct.

If both eyes need drops, repeat the procedure in the other eye.

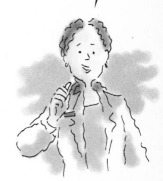

Final steps

Recap the bottle and store it away from light and heat.

If you're using more than one kind of drop, wait 5 minutes before you use the next one. (*Remember:* Never put medication in your eyes unless the label reads "For Ophthalmic Use" or "For Use in Eyes.")

Spanish translation on opposite side

Hacerlo funcionar

Apenas cierre el ojo, pero no lo cierre fuertemente.

Suelte el párpado inferior.

Limpie el exceso de medicamento con un pañuelo de papel limpio.

Trate de mantener el ojo abierto y sin parpadear por lo menos 30 segundos.

Aplique una ligera presión en el ángulo de su ojo que está en el caballete de la nariz durante 1 minuto. Esto evitará que las gotas se vayan por el lagrimal.

Si ambos ojos necesitan gotas, repita el procedimiento en el otro ojo.

Últimos pasos

Vuelva a tapar el medicamento y guárdelo lejos de la luz y el calor.

Si está usando más de un tipo de gotas, espera 5 minutos antes de usar el próximo tipo. (Recuerde: Nunca coloque medicamento en los ojos, a no ser que la etiqueta diga "Para Uso Oftalmológico" o "Para Uso en Los Ojos").

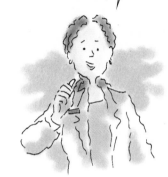

Trate de mantener el ojo abierto y sin parpadear por lo menos 30 segundos.

English translation on opposite side

How to breast-feed properly

Dear Patient,

Breast milk contains the best nutrition for your baby.

To breast-feed properly, follow these guidelines.

Getting ready

Wash your hands.

Relax and make yourself comfortable.

Sit with your back straight or bent slightly forward.

You may wish to support your back with a pillow or use a pillow on your lap to raise your baby to breast level.

Feeding your baby

Rest your baby's head in the bend of your elbow and support his back with your hand.

Turn his body toward you and cup your breast with your other hand. (See the breast-feeding positions shown at right.)

Cradle position

For the cradle position, cradle the baby's head in the crook of your arm.

Place a pillow on your lap for the baby to lie on.

Place a pillow behind your back; this provides comfort and also puts your breasts in the correct position for feeding.

Side-lying position

Lie on your side with your stomach facing the baby's.

As the baby's mouth opens, pull him toward the nipple.

Place a pillow or rolled blanket behind the baby's back to prevent him from moving or rolling away from your breast.

Football position

Sitting with a pillow in front of you, place your hand under the baby's head.

As the baby's mouth opens, pull the baby's head near your breast.

This position may be more comfortable if you've have had a C-section.

Spanish translation on opposite side

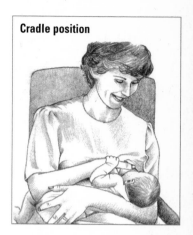
Cradle position

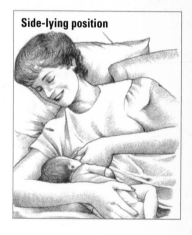
Side-lying position

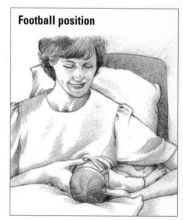
Football position

Cómo amamantar correctamente

Estimada paciente,

La leche materna contiene los mejores nutrientes para su bebé.

Para amamantar correctamente, siga estas instrucciones.

Cómo prepararse

Lávese las manos.

Relájese y póngase cómoda.

Siéntese con la espalda derecha o inclinese ligeramente hacia adelante.

Usted puede apoyar su espalda contra una almohada o usar una en su regazo para levantar al bebé a la altura del seno.

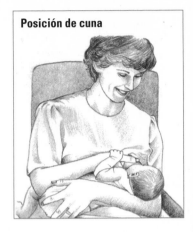

Posición de cuna

Cómo alimentar a su bebé

Coloque la cabeza de su bebé en la parte interna de su codo y apóyele la mano en la espalda para brindarle soporte.

Gire el cuerpo del bebé hacia usted y sostenga su seno con la oltra mano. (Véase las posiciones de amamantamiento, ilustradas a la derecha.)

Posición de cuna

Para esta posición, apoye la cabeza del bebé en la parte interior de su brazo.

Coloque una almohada en su regazo para que el bebé se acueste sobre ella.

Coloque una almohada detrá de su espalda; esto la hará sentir cómoda y también permite que sus senos estén en la posición correcta para amamantar.

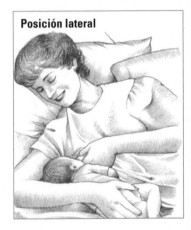

Posición lateral

Posición lateral

Acuéstese sobre un costado con su estomago ubicado hacia el bebé.

Cuando se abre la boca del bebé, llévelo hacia el pezón.

Coloque una almohada o manta enrollada detrás de la espalda del bebé para impedirle que se mueva o se aleje de su seno.

Posición de "fútbol americano"

Siéntese con una almohada enfrente de usted y coloque su mano debajo de la cabeza del bebé.

Cuando se abre la boca del bebé, empuje la cabeza del mismo hacia su seno.

Esta posición puede ses más cómoda si se le hizo una cesácea.

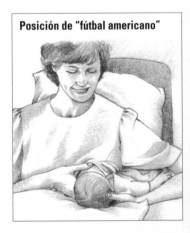

Posición de "fútbal americano"

English translation on opposite side

Basic nursing tips

Touch your baby's cheek with your nipple to make him turn his head and then touch your nipple to his mouth.

When your baby opens his mouth, insert your nipple into his mouth.

The tip of his nose should touch the top of your breast.

When your baby is done nursing, gently pull his chin downward or insert a finger into the side of his mouth to break the suction.

Allow your baby to feed from both breasts at each feeding.

Burp your baby after he finishes feeding from each breast.

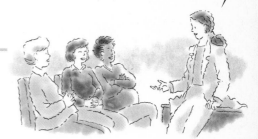

Allow your baby to feed from both breasts at each feeding.

Storing breast milk

Refrigerated breast milk must be used within 24 hours.

Frozen breast milk should be used within a few weeks.

Thaw frozen breast milk under lukewarm tap water and use it within 3 hours.

Never thaw breast milk in a microwave oven and don't refreeze it after thawing. Instead, discard any leftover thawed breast milk.

Keep your breasts healthy

Allow your breasts to air dry after each feeding.

Wear a comfortable, supportive bra.

Wear nursing pads or a soft cloth in your bra if your breasts leak milk.

Keep yourself healthy

Try to get adequate sleep. Rest while your baby is sleeping and enlist the help of others with cooking and other household chores.

Increase your fluid intake and eat well-balanced meals.

Avoid alcohol, caffeine, and over-the-counter medications.

Tell your doctor that you're breast-feeding if he plans to order any medications.

You may not get your menstrual period while you're breast-feeding. However, you can still get pregnant, so an effective birth control method is necessary.

Spanish translation on opposite side

Sugerencias básicas para el amamantamiento

Toque la mejilla del bebé con su pezón para hacer que gire la cabeza, y luego lleve su pezón a la boca del bebé.

Cuando su bebé abra la boca, insértele su pezón en la boca.

La punta de la nariz del bebé debe tocar la parte superior de su pecho.

Cuando su bebé termine de amamantar, tire suavemente su mentón hacia abajo o inserte un dedo en el costado de su boca para cortar la succión.

Permita que su bebé se alimente de ambos pechos en cada amamantamiento.

Haga que el bebé eructe después de terminar de amamantar en cada pecho.

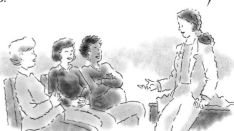

> Permita que su bebé se alimente de ambos senos en cada amamantamiento.

Cómo guardar la leche materna

La leche materna refrigerada se debe usar dentro de las 24 horas.

La leche materna congelada se debe usar dentro de unas semanas.

Desconegele la leche materna debajo del agua tibia del grifo y úsela dentro de las 3 horas.

Nunca descongele leche materna en un horno de microondas, ni vuelva a congelaria después. En cambio, elimine cualquier resto de leche materna descongelada.

Mantenga sus senos sanos

Permita que sus pechos se sequen al aire después de cada amamantamiento.

Use un sostén cómodo que sostenga bien los pechos.

Si tiene pérdidas de leche en sus pechos, límpiese con una almohadilla o una toallita suave.

Mantégase sana

Trate de dormir lo suficiente. Descanse mientras su bebé está durmiendo y pida la ayuda de otras personas cuando cocine y haga los quehaceres domésticos.

Beba más liquidos y coma alimentos bien equilibrados.

Evite el alcohol, la cafeína y los remedios de venta libre.

Informe a su médico que usted está amamantando si él prevé prescribirle medicamentos.

Es posible que no tenga su menstruación mientras esté amamantando. Sin embargo, aún podrá quedar encinta; por ello, es necesario contar con un método anitconceptivo eficaz.

English translation on opposite side

Giving yourself an insulin injection

Dear Patient:

To give yourself an insulin injection, follow these guidelines.

Assembling equipment

Wash your hands.

Place this equipment in a clean area:
–a sterile insulin syringe and needle
–a sharps container or a metal or plastic container (a coffee can with a tight-fitting lid or a laundry detergent bottle) to dispose of the needle safely
–insulin
–alcohol pads or wipes (or rubbing alcohol and cotton balls).

Check the labels on the syringe and bottle of insulin to make sure they match. (If you're using U-100 insulin, you must use a U-100 insulin syringe.)

Also check that you have the correct type of insulin, such as NPH or Lente.

If your insulin is the cloudy-looking type, roll the bottle gently between your hands to mix it. Never shake the insulin vial.

Wipe the top of the insulin bottle with an alcohol pad or a cotton ball and rubbing alcohol.

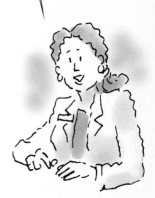

Remember to make sure you have the correct type of insulin.

Cleaning the skin, preparing the syringe

Select an appropriate injection site. (Remember to alternate injection sites.)

Then, using a circular motion, clean the skin with an alcohol pad or wipe with a cotton ball dampened with rubbing alcohol.

Remove the needle cover. (To prevent possible infection, don't touch the needle.)

Touch only the barrel and plunger of the syringe.

Pull back the plunger to the prescribed number of insulin units. (This draws air into the syringe.)

Spanish translation on opposite side

Cómo aplicarse una inyección de insulina

Estimado(a) Paciente:

Para transferir el medicamento del frasco a la jeringa, y luego darse a sí mismo una inyección de insulina, siga Ud. estas instrucciones.

Reunir el material

Lávese las manos.

Coloque estos equipos en un área limpia:
–una jeringa para insulina y una aguja estériles
–un recipiente cerrado (como una lata de café con tapa bien ajustada o un frasco de jabón para la ropa) para objetos con filo
–insulina
–almohadillas de algodón y paños limpiadores (o alcohol fino y bolitas de algodón).

Controle las etiquetas de la jeringa y el frasco de insulina para asegurarse de que concuerden. (Si usa insulina U-100, debe usar una jeringa U-100.)

También asegúrese de tener el tipo correcto de insulina, como NPH o Lente.

Si usa la insulina turbia, mueva suavemente el frasco entre las manos para mezclarla. No sacuda nunca el vial de insulina.

Limpie la parte superior del frasco de insulina con una toallita o pompa de algodón humedecida con alcohol.

> Verifique que Ud. tiene el tipo correcto de insulina.

Limpiar la piel, preparar la jeringa

Escoja Ud. el lugar apropiado para la inyección. (Recuerde alternar los lugares de inyección.)

Luego, con un movimiento circular, limpie Ud. la piel con la gasa o con la bolita de algodón mojada en alcohol.

Quítele la cubierta a la aguja. (Para evitar una posible infección, no toque Ud. la aguja.)

Toque sólo el barril y el émbolo de la jeringa.

Retire el émbolo hacia atrás hasta el número de unidades de insulina recetadas. (Esto aspira aire dentro de la jeringa.)

English translation on opposite side

If you're mixing two types of insulin (clear and cloudy), withdraw the clear insulin first and then the cloudy.

Insert the needle into the rubber stopper on the insulin bottle, and push in the plunger. (This pushes air into the bottle and prevents a vacuum.)

Hold the bottle and syringe together in one hand; then turn them upside down so the bottle is on top.

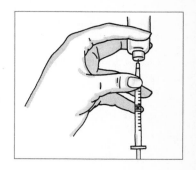

Using one hand, you can hold the bottle between your first and middle finger and hold the syringe between your thumb and fourth and fifth fingers.

Injecting insulin

Using the other hand, pull back on the plunger until the top, black portion of the barrel corresponds to the line that indicates you have withdrawn your correct insulin dose.

Remove the needle from the bottle. (If air bubbles appear in the syringe after you fill it with insulin, tap the syringe and push lightly on the plunger to remove them.)

Draw up more insulin, if necessary.

Using your thumb and forefinger, pinch the skin at the injection site.

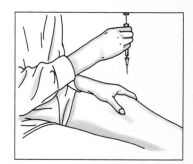

Then quickly plunge the needle (up to its hub) into the site at a 90-degree angle.

Cleaning up

Place an alcohol pad or cotton ball over the injection site.

Press down on the pad or cotton ball lightly as you withdraw the needle. (Don't rub the injection site when withdrawing the needle.)

Dispose of the needle and syringe in the sharps container, metal can, or plastic bottle.

Important info

If you travel, keep a bottle of insulin and a syringe with you at all times.

Don't place insulin near heat (above 90° F [32° C]).

Insulin may be left at room temperature for up to 1 month.

Keep extra bottles of insulin refrigerated.

Refrigerated bottles may be used for up to 3 months.

Spanish translation on opposite side

Si está mezclando dos tipos de insulina (clara y turbia), saque la insulina clara primero, y luego la turbia.

Inserte la aguja dentro del tapón de hule del frasco de insulina, y empuje el émbolo hacia dentro. (Esto empuja el aire dentro del frasco y evita un vacío.)

Sostenga Ud. el frasco y la jeringa con una mano; luego inviértalas para que el frasco quede arriba.

Ud. puede sostener el frasco entre el pulgar y el índice y la jeringa entre el anular y el dedo meñique.

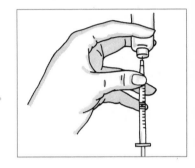

Inyectar insulina

Retire Ud. el émbolo hasta que la porción negra del barril que está arriba corresponda a la línea que indica que ha sacado su dosis correcta de insulina.

Saque Ud. la aguja del frasco. (Si aparecen burbujas de aire en la jeringa después de haberla llenado de insulina, déle un golpecito a la jeringa y empuje el émbolo ligeramente para eliminarlas.)

Saque Ud. más insulina si es necesario.

Con el pulgar y el índice, pellizque la piel en el lugar donde se va a poner la inyección.

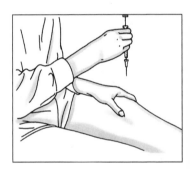

Luego presione la aguja (hasta el tope) en el sitio en un ángulo de 90 grados.

Limpiar

Ponga Ud. un pedazo de gasa o una bolita de algodón con alcohol en el lugar donde se puso la inyección.

Comprima la gasa o bolita de algodón ligeramente al sacar la aguja. (No frote el lugar de la inyección al sacar la aguja.)

Tire Ud. la aguja y la jeringa en un recipiente cerrado para esa clase de objetos.

Información importante

Si Ud. viaja, siempre tenga consigo un frasco de insulina y una jeringa.

No la ponga cerca del calor (más alto de 90° F [32° C]).

La insulina puede quedar a temperatura ambiente por hasta 1 mes.

Mantenga refrigerados los frascos adicionales de insulina.

Los frascos refrigerados pueden usarse por hasta 3 meses.

English translation on opposite side

Using an oral inhaler

Dear Patient:

Inhaling your medication through this metered-dose nebulizer will help you breathe more easily.

Use it exactly as your doctor has directed.

Here's how.

Preparing the inhaler

Shake the inhaler well immediately before each use.

Remove the cap from the mouthpiece.

The strap on the cap will stay attached to the plastic case. If the strap is lost, the inhaler's mouthpiece should be inspected for the presence of foreign objects.

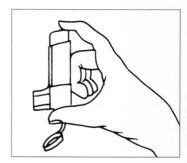

Taking a breath

Make sure the canister is fully and firmly inserted into the plastic case.

Breathe out fully through pursed lips.

Holding the nebulizer upright, as shown, close your lips around the mouthpiece.

Tilt your head back slightly.

Take a slow, deep breath at the same time that you slowly depress the top of the canister with your index finger.

Continue inhaling until your lungs feel full.

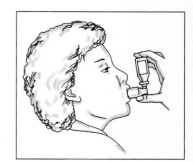

Holding the breath

Take the mouthpiece away from your mouth, and hold your breath for several seconds.

Purse your lips and breathe out slowly.

If your doctor wants you to take more than one dose, wait a few minutes and then repeat.

When finished, rinse your mouth, gargle, and drink a few sips of fluid.

Spanish translation on opposite side

Uso del inhalador oral

Estimado(a) Paciente:

El inhalar su medicamento por este nebulizador (atomizador) medidor de dosis le ayudará a respirar con más facilidad.

Úselo exactamente como se lo ha indicado su médico.

Hágalo de esta manera.

Preparar el inhalador

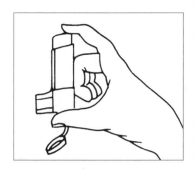

Agite el inhalador bien inmediatamente antes de cada uso.

Quítele la tapa a la boquilla.

La correa de la tapa se quedará conectada al accionador. Si la correa se pierde, la boquilla del inhalador se debe examinar para ver si tiene objetos extraños.

Inhalar

Asegúrese de que el bote esté metido total y firmemente dentro del accionador.

Expire completamente con los labios fruncidos.

Ponga el nebulizador verticalmente, como se muestra, y sujete los labios alrededor de la boquilla.

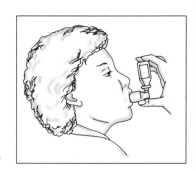

Incline la cabeza hacia atrás un poco.

Haga una inspiración lenta y profunda mientras baja lentamente la parte superior de la lata con el dedo índice.

Siga Ud. inhalando hasta que sus pulmones se sientan llenos.

Contener la respiración

Sáquese la boquilla de la boca, y contenga la respiración por algunos segundos.

Frunza los labios y expire lentamente.

Si su médico quiere que Ud. tenga más de una dosis, espérese unos minutos y luego repita.

Cuando haya terminado, enjuáguese la boca, haga gárgaras y tómese unos sorbos de líquido.

English translation on opposite side

Cleaning up

Remember to clean the inhaler once a day by removing the canister and rinsing the plastic case and cap under warm running water for 1 minute.

Shake off the excess water and allow the parts to dry.

Then gently replace the canister with a twisting motion and put the cap back over the mouthpiece.

Precautions

Discard the canister after you have used the labeled number of inhalations.

Important: Never overuse your oral inhaler.

Follow your doctor's instructions exactly.

Notify your doctor if your inhaler isn't working.

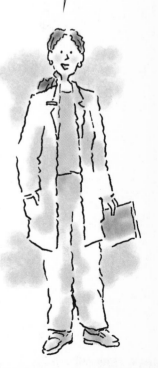

Remember to clean your inhaler once a day.

Spanish translation on opposite side

Limpiar

Recuerde limpiar el inhalador una vez al día quitando la lata y enjuagando el envase de plástico y la tapa bajo agua tibia durante 1 minuto.

Sacúdales el exceso de líquido y deje que las partes se sequen.

Luego ponga la caja en su lugar dándole unas vueltas, y vuelva a poner la tapa sobre la boquilla.

Precauciones

Tire la caja después de haber hecho el número indicado de inhalaciones.

Importante: Nunca use el inhalador oral demasiado.

Siga Ud. exactamente las instrucciones de su médico.

Notifique a su médico si su inhalador no funciona.

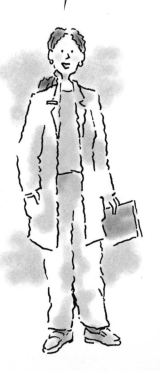

Acuérdese Ud. de limpiar el inhalador una vez al día.

English translation on opposite side

Taking your pulse

Dear Patient:

The doctor wants you to take your pulse (the number of times your heart beats per minute).

Take your pulse at rest and during exercise, or before taking medicine, if ordered by the doctor.

By comparing these two pulse rates, the doctor can evaluate how well your heart is pumping.

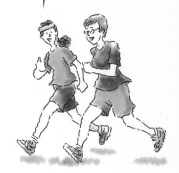

Taking your pulse after exercise can help you develop a good fitness program.

Taking your pulse at rest

Don't check your pulse right after eating a big meal. When you're ready to take your resting pulse rate, be sure you have a watch or a clock with a second hand.

Sit quietly and relax for 2 minutes.

Then place your index and middle fingers on your wrist, as shown here. Don't use your thumb.

Count the beats for 30 seconds and multiply by 2 or count for 60 seconds. If you have an irregular heart rhythm, your doctor may instruct you to count for 60 seconds.

Write down this number and the date.

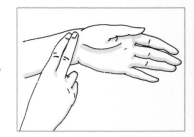

Taking your pulse during exercise

As soon as you stop exercising, find your neck (carotid) pulse.

To do this, place two or three fingers on your windpipe and move them 2″ to 3″ (5 to 8 cm) to the left or right.

Feel for the pulse point low on your neck and don't press too hard. (You can stop blood supply to the brain or cause an irregular heartbeat.)

Count the beats for 6 seconds; then add a zero to that number. Don't count your pulse for a whole minute because your heart rate slows quickly when you rest.

Write down this number and the date.

If your heart rate during exercise is 10 or more beats above your target rate, don't exercise so hard the next time.

If your working heart rate is lower than your target rate, exercise a little harder next time.

Always consult your doctor before beginning a new exercise program.

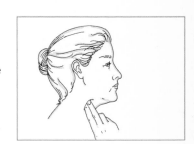

Spanish translation on opposite side

Cómo tomarse el pulso

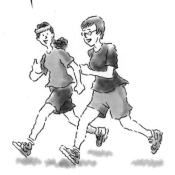

El tomarse el pulso después de ejercitarse le puede ayudar a desarrollar un buen programa de ejercicios.

Estimado(a) Paciente:

El médico quiere que Ud. se tome el pulso (el número de veces que su corazón late por minuto).

Tómese el pulso en reposo y durante el ejercicio, o antes de tomar medicamentos, si así lo indica el médico.

Al comparar estas dos frecuencias del pulso, el médico puede evaluar si el corazón está bombeando la sangre correctamente.

Cómo tomarse el pulso en reposo

No se controle el pulso justo después de una gran comida. Cuando esté listo para tomarse el pulso en reposo, asegúrese de tener un reloj con segundero.

Siéntese quieto(a) y relajado(a) por dos minutos.

Luego ponga los dedos índice y del corazón en la muñeca, como se ve aquí. No use el dedo pulgar.

Cuente los latidos durante 30 segundos y multiplíquelos por 2 o cuente durante 60 segundos. Si usted tiene un ritmo cardiaco irregular, es posible que su médico le indique que cuente durante 60 segundos.

Escriba el número y la fecha.

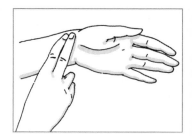

Cómo tomarse el pulso al hacer ejercicio

En cuanto pare de hacer ejercicio, busque el pulso (en la carótida) del cuello.

Para hacer esto, ponga dos o tres dedos en la tráquea y muévalos de 2 a 3 pulgadas (5 a 8 centímetros) a la izquierda o a la derecha.

Búsquese el pulso en el cuello y no presione demasiado fuerte. (Puede detener el suministro de sangre al cerebro o provocar un ritmo cardiaco irregular.)

Cuente los latidos durante 6 segundos; después agregue un cero a ese número. No se cuente el pulso por un minuto porque el ritmo cardiaco baja rápidamente en reposo.

Escriba el número y la fecha.

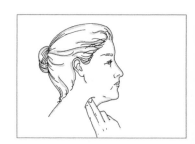

Si la frecuencia de su corazón mientras hace ejercicio es 10 o más latidos por eneima de la frecuencia de interés, no haga ejercicios tan vigorosos la siguiente vez.

Si la frecuencia de su corazón mientras hace ejercicio es menos que esa, haga ejercicios algo más vigorosos la próxima vez.

Siempre consulte el médico antes de comenzar un programa de ejercicios nuevo.

English translation on opposite side

Using a condom correctly

Dear Patient:

Sexual abstinence is the only sure way to prevent sexual transmission of HIV and AIDS.

However, if you use a new condom every time you have sex—and use it correctly—this will help protect you from infection.

The suggestions below will help you choose, store, and use condoms.

Buying condoms

Buy American-made, latex condoms. However, if you are allergic to latex, please talk to your doctor about alternatives.

Avoid condoms made of lambskin.

Be sure the condom has a reservoir tip (or receptacle end).

Check that the package has a manufacturer's date—and an expiration date if the product contains a spermicide.

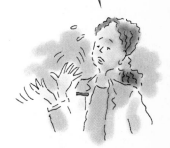

Heat can damage condoms, so store them in a cool place.

Storing condoms

Store unused condoms in a cool, dry place.

Don't keep them in a warm place, such as your hip pocket or the glove compartment of your car, because heat can damage the latex.

Using condoms

Follow these steps to apply and remove a condom.

Open the wrapper carefully to avoid tearing the condom.

Hold the rolled condom by the reservoir tip to squeeze out the air and make room for the semen when you ejaculate.

If the condom isn't lubricated inside, apply a water-based lubricant or plain water to your penis to increase sensation.

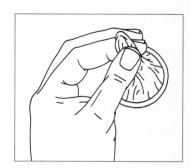

Once you have an erection, pull back the foreskin if you're uncircumcised. Next, place the rolled condom on the end of your penis.

Hold the reservoir tip with one hand, and unroll the condom onto your erect penis with the other hand.

Spanish translation on opposite side

Cómo usar un condón correctamente

Estimado(a) Paciente:

La abstinencia sexual es el único modo seguro de prevenir la transmisión sexual de VIH y SIDA.

Sin embargo, si usa un preservativo nuevo cada vez que tiene sexo—y lo usa correctamente—estará protegido frente a infecciones.

Las sugerencias que siguen le pueden ayudar a escoger, guardar, y usar condones.

Comprar condones

Compre sólo los condones hechos en EE.UU. de látex. Sin embargo, si Ud. es alérgico(a) al látex, por favor converse con su médico sobre alternativas.

Evite Ud. los que están hechos de piel de cordero.

Asegúrese de que el condón tenga un recipiente extremo.

Observe Ud. si el empaque tiene una fecha del fabricante—y una fecha de vencimiento si el producto contiene un espermicida.

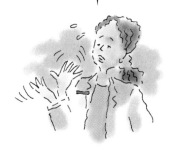

El calor puede dañar los condones, de manera que guárdelos en un lugar fresco.

Guardar los condones

Guarde los condones que no ha usado en un lugar fresco y seco.

No los guarde en un lugar caliente, tal como el bolsillo de su pantalón o en la guantera de su auto, porque el calor puede dañar el látex.

Uso de los condones

Siga estos pasos para ponerse y quitarse un condón.

Abra el envoltorio con cuidado para evitar rasgar el preservativo.

Detenga la parte enrollada del condón por el extremo para sacarle el aire y tener lugar para el semen cuando Ud. eyacule.

Si el condón no está lubricado por dentro, aplíquele al pene un lubricante a base de agua o agua sola para aumentar la sensación.

Una vez que tenga una erección, empuje el prepucio hacia atrás si Ud. no está circuncidado. Luego ponga el condón enrollado en la punta del pene.

Detenga el extremo del condón con una mano, y desenróllelo sobre el pene en erección con la otra mano.

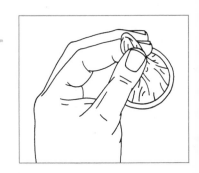

English translation on opposite side

Unroll the condom until it touches your pubic hair. If the condom doesn't have a reservoir tip, keep ½″ (0.5 cm) free at the end to collect semen.

If you need extra lubrication, rub it on the outside of the condom after applying the condom.

Use a water-based lubricant such as K-Y Jelly, not petroleum jelly or oil; these materials can weaken the latex.

If the condom breaks, tears, or slips off during intercourse, stop intercourse immediately.

If you have already ejaculated, your partner may be protected if she or he inserts spermicide immediately.

After you ejaculate, hold the condom firmly while withdrawing your penis.

To reduce the risk of spilling semen, withdraw your penis while it's still erect.

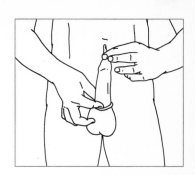

Removing the condom

To remove the condom, pinch the tip with one hand to keep the semen from spilling, and roll the condom off your penis with the other hand.

Flush the condom down the toilet immediately or discard it in a closed, rigid plastic or metal container such as a coffee can.

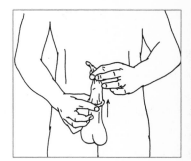

Additional info

Never use a condom twice.

Wash your penis with soap and water.

Then wash and dry your hands.

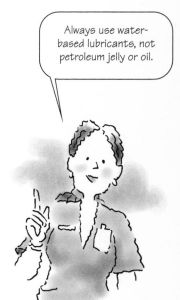

Always use water-based lubricants, not petroleum jelly or oil.

Spanish translation on opposite side

Desenrolle el condón hasta que toque el vello púbico. Si el condón no tiene un recipiente extremo, deje libre ½″ (0.5 cm) para retener el semen.

Si Ud. necesita lubricación extra, aplíquela afuera del condón después de habérselo puesto.

Use un lubricante acuoso como K-Y Jelly, no uno con vaselina o aceite, ya que estos materiales pueden debilitar el látex.

Si el condón se rompe, se rasga o se resbala durante el contacto sexual, suspenda las relaciones sexuales inmediatamente.

Si Ud. ya ha eyaculado, su compañero(a) puede obtener protección si él o ella usa espermicida inmediatamente.

Después de eyacular, sostenga firmemente el condón al sacar el pene.

Para reducir el riesgo de que el semen se derrame, saque Ud. el pene mientras aún tiene una erección.

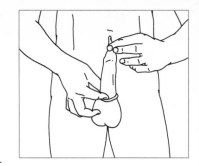

Quitarse el condón

Para quitarse el condón, pellizque la punta con una mano para evitar que el semen se derrame, y con la otra mano quítese el condón enrollándolo.

Póngalo en el retrete y tire de la cadena inmediatamente o tírelo en un bote de plástico o de metal, tal como un bote de café.

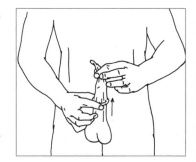

Información adicional

Nunca use un condón más de una vez.

Lávese el pene con agua y jabón.

Luego lávese y séquese las manos.

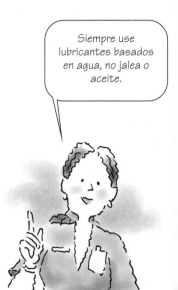

Siempre use lubricantes basados en agua, no jalea o aceite.

English translation on opposite side

Testing your blood sugar level

Dear Patient:

Testing blood sugar levels will tell you whether your diabetes is under control.

Follow these steps to learn how to obtain blood for testing and how to perform the test.

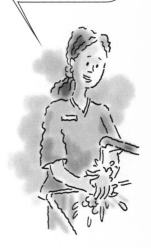

Holding your finger under warm water for a couple of minutes will enhance blood flow.

Getting ready

Begin by assembling the equipment:
–your glucose meter
–a lancet
–test strip.

Remove a test strip from the vial.

Then replace the cap, making sure it's tight.

Turn on the glucose meter and insert the test strip according to the manufacturer's instructions.

Then wait for the display window to show that the meter is ready for the blood sample.

Obtaining blood

Choose a site on the end or side of any fingertip.

Wash your hands thoroughly and dry them.

To increase blood flow, hold your finger under warm water for a minute or two.

Hold your hand below your heart, and press the fingertip you plan to pierce with the thumb of the same hand.

Place your fingertip (with your thumb still pressed against it) on a firm surface such as a table.

Twist off the lancet's protective cap.

Then grasp the lancet and quickly pierce your fingertip just to the side of the fingertip.

Remove your thumb from your fingertip to permit blood flow.

Then press your finger gently until you get a large, hanging drop of blood.

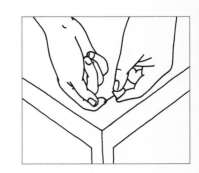

Spanish translation on opposite side

Cómo analizar el nivel de azúcar en la sangre

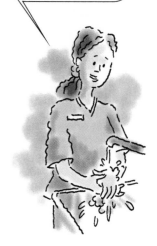

Si pone el dedo de bajo del agua tibia por unos dos minutos, el flujo de sangre aumentará.

Estimado(a) Paciente:

Un análisis de los niveles de azúcar en sangre le dirán si su diabetes está bajo control.

Siga Ud. estos pasos para saber cómo obtener sangre para examinarla y cómo hacer el análisis.

La preparación

Primero arme el equipo:
–su medidor de glucosa (azúcar)
–una lanceta
–tira de prueba.

Quite una tira de prueba del vial.

Luego vuelva a tapar el frasco para que quede bien cerrado.

Encienda el medidor de glucosa e inserte la tira de prueba según las instrucciones del fabricante.

Luego espere hasta que la abertura le indique que el medidor está listo para la muestra de sangre.

Cómo obtener la sangre

Escoja un lugar en la punta o a un lado de la yema de cualquier dedo.

Lávese las manos muy bien y séqueselas.

Para incrementar el flujo sanguíneo, coloque su dedo debajo de un chorro de agua tibia durante uno o dos minutos.

Sostenga la mano debajo del corazón y presione la punta del dedo que va a pinchar con el pulgar de la misma mano.

Ponga la yema (mientras la aprieta con el pulgar) sobre una superficie firme, tal como una mesa.

Quite la tapa protectora a la lanceta.

Agarre la lanceta y pinche rápidamente la punta de su dedo, apenas hacia el costado.

Quite el pulgar de la yema del dedo para permitir el flujo de sangre.

Luego presione ligeramente el dedo hasta obtener una gran gota de sangre colgando.

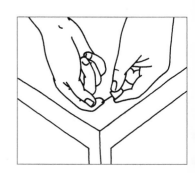

English translation on opposite side

Testing blood

When the display window indicates that the meter is ready, touch the drop of blood to the test strip at the indicated spot.

The drop of blood will start the meter's timer.

After the meter has finished the test, you can read the results on the display window.

The meter will store the date, time, and results of the test and will also keep a diary of the test results.

Call your doctor if the test results are low or extremely high.

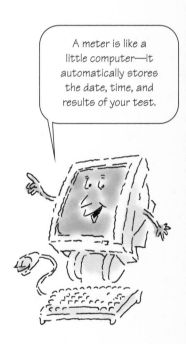

A meter is like a little computer—it automatically stores the date, time, and results of your test.

Spanish translation on opposite side

Análisis de la sangre

Cuando la pantalla indique que el medidor está listo, toque la tira de prueba con la gota de sangre en el punto indicado.

La gota de sangre activará el temporizador del medidor.

Después de que el medidor haya terminado la prueba, usted puede leer los resultados en la pantalla.

El medidor almacenará la fecha, la hora y los resultados de la prueba y también llevará un diario de los resultados de la prueba.

El medidor automáticamente conservará la fecha, la hora y los resultados.

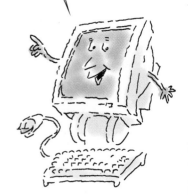

Un medidor es como una pequeña computadora — automáticamente conserva la fecha, la hora y los resultados del análisas.

English-Spanish quick-reference guide

abortion	el aborto	emphysema	el enfisema
abscess	el absceso	encephalitis	la encefalitis
acquired immunodeficiency syndrome	el síndrome de inmunodeficiencia adquirida	epilepsy	la epilepsia
		fainting spell	el desmayo
addiction	la adicción	fatigue	la fatiga
adenoids	los adenoides	fever	la fiebre
adenoma	el adenoma	fistula	la fístula
allergy	la alergia	flu	la influenza, la gripe
anemia	la anemia	fluid	el fluido, líquido
angina	la angina	food poisoning	el envenenamiento por comestibles
appendicitis	la apendicitis		
arteriosclerosis	la arteriosclerosis	fracture	la fractura
arthritis	la artritis	frostbite	la congelación
asthma	el asma	gallbladder attack	el ataque de la vesícula biliar
backache	el dolor de espalda		
blindness	la ceguera	gallstone	el cálculo biliar
bronchitis	la bronquitis	gangrene	la gangrena
burn (first-, second-, or third-degree)	la quemadura (de primer, segundo o tercer grado)	gastric ulcer	la úlcera gástrica
		glaucoma	el glaucoma
bursitis	la bursitis	gonorrhea	la gonorrea
cancer	el cáncer	hallucination	la alucinación
chest pain	el dolor de pecho	harelip	el labio leporino
chickenpox	la varicela, las viruelas locas	hay fever	la fiebre de heno
chills	los escalofríos	headache	el dolor de cabeza
cholesterol	el colesterol	heart attack	el ataque al corazón
chorea	la corea	heartbeat	el latido
cold	el catarro, el resfriado	fast (tachycardia)	taquicardia
cold sores	las úlceras de la boca	irregular	irregular
confusion	la confusión	rhythmical	rítmico
constipation	el estreñimiento	slow	lento
convulsion	la convulsión	heartburn	las agruras (el ardor), acedía
cough	la tos		
cramps	los calambres	heart disease	la enfermedad cardiaca
deafness	la sordera	heart failure	el fallo cardiaco
diabetes	la diabetes	heart murmur	el soplo al corazón
diarrhea	la diarrea	hemorrhage	la hemorragia
diphtheria	la difteria	hemorrhoids	las almorranas, las hemorroides
disability	la discapacidad		
discharge	el flujo	hepatitis	la hepatitis
diverticulitis	diverticulitis	hernia	la hernia
dizziness	el vértigo, el mareo	herpes	el herpes
eczema	el eccema	high blood pressure	la presión alta
embolism	el embolismo	hit (on face)	la bofetada
		hives	la urticaria

hoarseness	la ronquera
human immunodeficiency virus	el virus de inmunodeficiencia humano
ill	enfermo(a)
illness	la enfermedad
immunization	la inmunización
infantile paralysis	la parálisis infantil
infarction	el infarto
infection	la infección
inflammation	la inflamación
injury	el daño la lastimadura, la herida
itch	la picazón, la comezón
jaundice	la piel amarilla, la ictericia
kidney stone	el cálculo en el riñón, la piedra en el riñón
kidneys	riñones
laceration	la laceración
laryngitis	la laringitis
lesion	la lesión, el daño
leukemia	la leucemia
lice	los piojos
liver	el hígado
lump	el bulto
lungs	los pulmones
malaria	la malaria
malignancy	el tumor, maligno
malignant	maligno(a)
malnutrition	la malnutrición
manic-depressive	maníaco-depresivo(a)
measles	el sarampión
medication	la medecinal, el medicamento
meningitis	la meningitis
menopause	la menopausia
menstruation	la menstruación
metastasis	la metástasis
migraine	la migraña, la jaqueca
mite	el ácaro
mononucleosis	la mononucleosis infecciosa
multiple sclerosis	la esclerosis múltiple
mumps	las paperas
muscular dystrophy	la distrofia muscular
mute	mudo(a)
myocardial infarction	el infarto cardiaco
myopia	la miopía

nausea	la náusea
nephritis	la nefritis
neuralgia	la neuralgia
obese	obeso(a)
obstruction	la obstrucción
ophthalmia	la oftalmia
osteomyelitis	la osteomielitis
overdose	la sobredosis
overweight	el sobrepeso
pain	el dolor
burning pain	el dolor que arde
growing pain	el dolor de crecimiento
intense pain	el dolor intenso
intermittent pain	el dolor intermitente
labor pain	el dolor de parto
phantom limb pain	el dolor de miembro fantasma
referred pain	el dolor referido
severe pain	el dolor severo
sharp pain	el dolor agudo
shooting pain	el dolor punzante
throbbing pain	el dolor palpitante
painful	doloroso
palpitation	la palpitación
palsy	la parálisis
palsy, Bell's	la parálisis facial
palsy, cerebral	la parálisis cerebral
paralysis	la parálisis
Parkinson's disease	la enfermedad de Parkinson
pellagra	la pelagra
pernicious anemia	la anemia perniciosa
pertussis	la tos convulsiva
pill	la píldora
pimple	el grano de la cara, el barrito
pneumonia	la pulmonía
poison ivy	la hiedra venenosa
poison oak	zumaque venenoso
polio	a poliomielitis
polyp	el pólipo
postmenopausal	postmenopaúsico
premenopausal	premenopáusico(a)
premenstrual syndrome	síndrome premenstrual
psoriasis	la psoriasis
pus	el pus
pyorrhea	la piorrea
rabies	la rabia

rash	la roncha, el salpullido, la erupción
relapse	la recaída
renal	renal
rheumatic fever	la fiebre reumática
roseola	la roséola
rubella	la rubéola
rupture	la ruptura
scab	la costra
scabies	la sarna
scar	la cicatriz
scarlet fever	la escarlatina
scratch	el rasguño
senile	senil
sexually transmitted disease	enfermedad de transmisión sexual
canker sore	la postemilla
chancre	el chancro
chlamydia	la clamidia
cold sore	los fuegos en la boca
condyloma	el condiloma
cytomegalovirus	el citomegalovirus
genital herpes	el herpes genital
genital wart	la verruga genital
gonorrhea	la gonorrea
moniliasis	la moniliasis
syphilis	la sífilis
trichomonas	el tricomonas
shaking	la tembla
shock	el choque
sinus congestion	la congestión nasal
sinuses	la sinusitis
slipped disc	el disco desplazado
smallpox	la viruela
snakebite	la mordedura de culebra
sore	la llaga
spasm	el espasmo
spider bite	la picadura de araña
spotted fever	la fiebre púrpura
sprain	la torcedura
stomach ache	el dolor del estómago
stomach ulcer	la úlcera del estómago
suicide	el suicidio
sunburn	la quemadura del sol
sunstroke	la insolación
surgery	la cirugía
swelling	la hinchazón
syphilis	la sífilis
tachycardia	la taquicardia
tapeworm	la lombriz solitaria
tetanus	el tétano
thrombosis	la trombosis
thrush	el afta
tonsillitis	la tonsilitis, la amigdalitis
toothache	el dolor de muela
toxemia	la toxemia
trauma	el trauma
tuberculosis	la tuberculosis
tumor	el tumor
typhoid fever	la fiebre tifoidea
typhus	el tifus, el tifo
ulcer	la úlcera
unconsciousness	la pérdida del conocimiento
undulant fever	la fiebre ondulante
uremia	la uremia
uterus, prolapsed	el prolapso de la matriz
varicose veins	las venas varicosas, várices
virus	el virus
vomit	el vómito, los vómitos
wart	la verruga
weakness	la debilidad
weal	el verdugón, el moretón
wheeze	el jadeo, la silba
whiplash	la concusión de la espina-cervical, lesión de latigazo
whooping cough	la tos ferina
worm(s)	la lombriz (las lombrices)
wound	la herida
yellow fever	la fiebre amarilla

Incredibly Easy picture dictionary

crutches
muletas

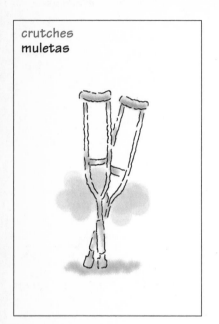

cane
bastón

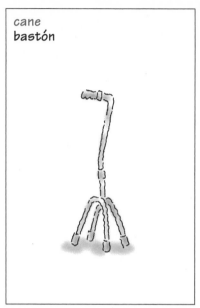

walker
andador

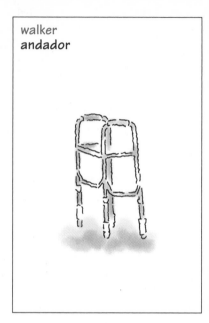

TV off
TV apagada

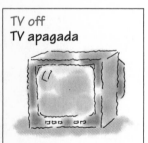

TV on
TV prendida

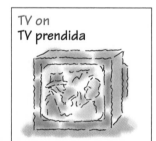

hot water bottle
bolsa de agua caliente

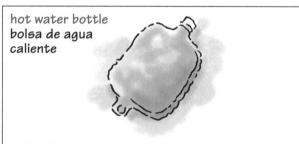

I want to get back in bed.
Quiero volver a la cama.

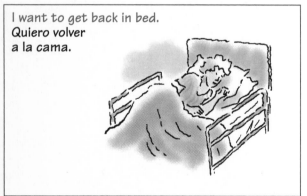

jugo
juice

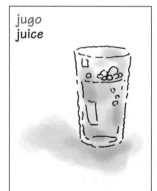

pillow
almohada

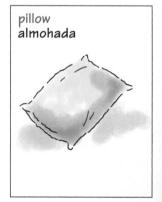

334

bed higher
cama más alta

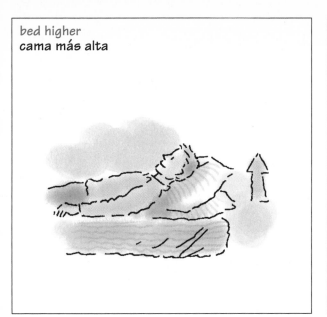

bed lower
cama más baja

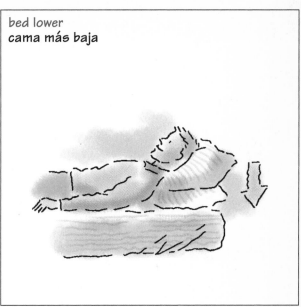

I want to see my doctor.
Quiero ver a mi médico.

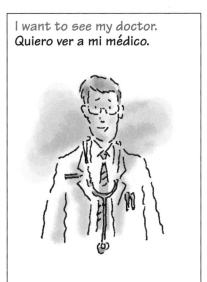

I want to see my nurse.
Quiero ver a mi enfermero(a).

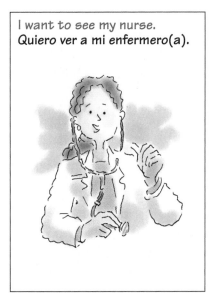

I need my inhaler.
Necesito mi inhalador.

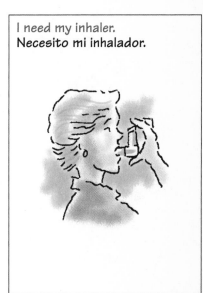

urinal
orinal

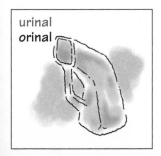

blanket
manta

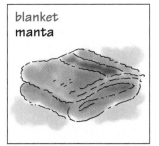

pencil and paper
lápiz y papel

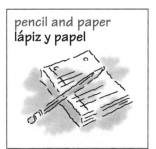

bedpan
chata

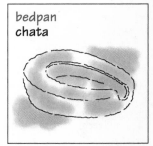

sitz bath
baño de asiento

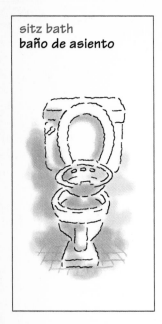

I want to go for a walk.
Quiero caminar.

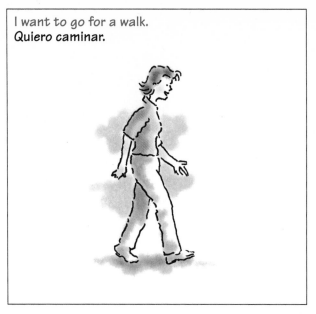

wheelchair
silla de ruedas

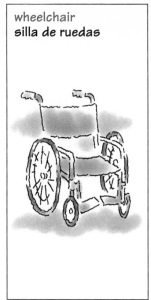

pain
dolor

mild
leve

bothersome
molesto

throbbing
pulsante

intense
intenso

commode
silla retrete

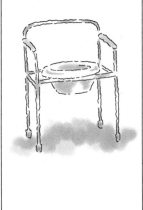

ice chips
cubitos de hielo

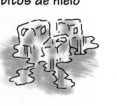

ice pack
bolsa de hielo

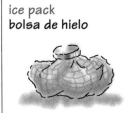

telephone
teléfono

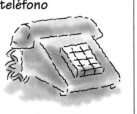

cold
frío(a)

hot
caliente

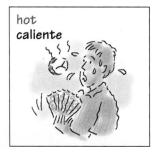

slippers
pantuflas, chanclas

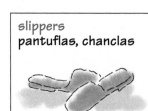

water
agua

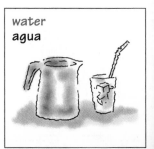

call light
luz de llamada

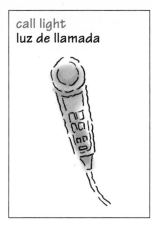

light on
luz prendida

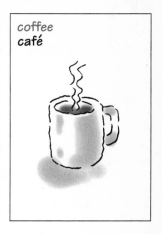

light off
luz apagada

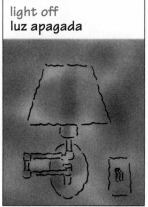

coffee
café

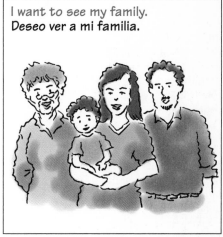

I would like to eat.
Me gustaria comer.

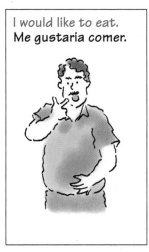

I want to sit in the chair
Quiero sentarme en la silla.

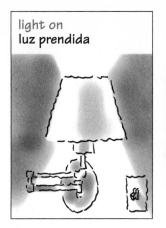

I want to see my family.
Deseo ver a mi familia.

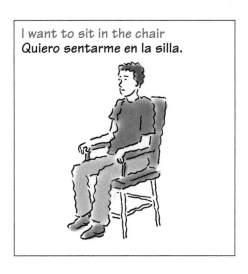

I need pain medicine.
Necesito analgésicos.

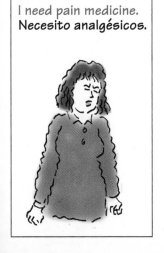

I feel nauseous.
Me siento con nausea.

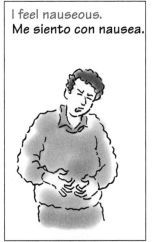

bath
baño

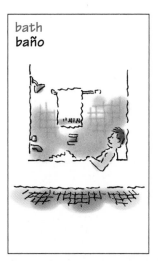

shower
ducha

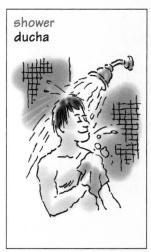

Index

i refers to an illustration.

i refers to an illustration.

i refers to an illustration.

Indice

i refers to an illustration.

i refers to an illustration.